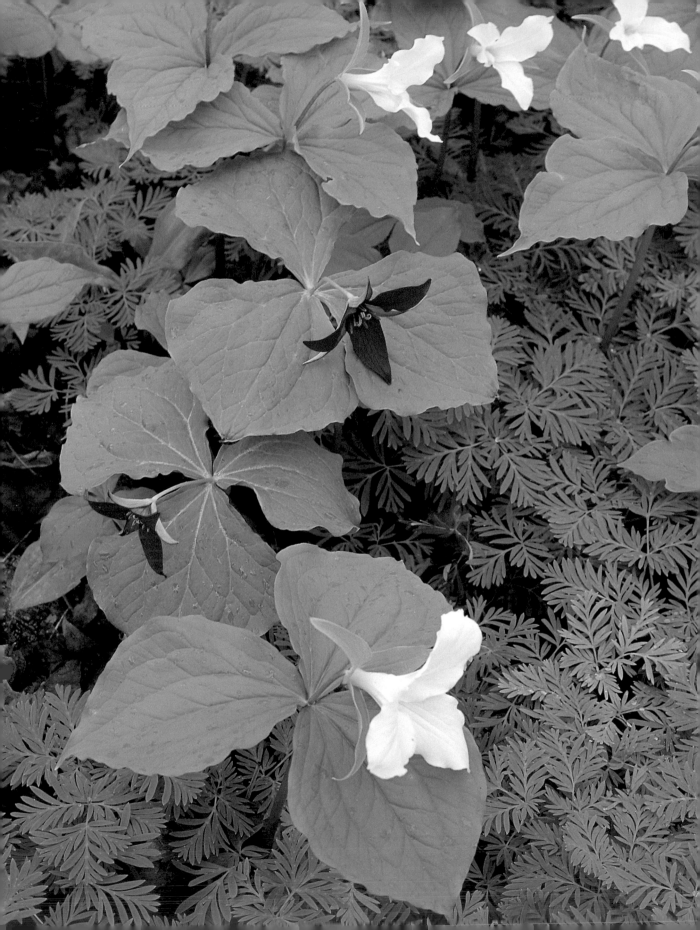

The Complete

WOMAN'S HERBAL

A Manual of Healing Herbs and Nutrition for Personal Well-being and Family Care

ANNE McINTYRE

A Henry Holt Reference Book
Henry Holt Company
New York

Henry Holt and Company, Inc.
Publishers since 1866
115 West 18th Street
New York, New York 10011

Henry Holt ® is a registered
trademark of Henry Holt and Company, Inc.

First published in the United States in 1995 by
Henry Holt and Company, Inc.
Published in Canada by Fitzhenry & Whiteside Ltd.,
195 Allstate Parkway, Markham, Ontario L3R 4T8.
Originally published in the United Kingdom in 1994 by
Gaia Books Ltd.

Library of Congress Cataloging-in-Publication Data
McIntyre, Anne.
The complete woman's herbal : a manual of healing herbs
and nutrition for personal well-being and family care /
Anne McIntyre – 1st American ed.
p.cm. – (Henry Holt reference book)
Includes bibliographical references and index.
1. Herbs–Therapeutic use. 2. Women–health and hygiene.
I. Title. II. Series.
RM666.H33M39 1995   94-29291
615'.321 '082–dc20   CIP

ISBN 0-8050-3537-0

Henry Holt books are available for special promotions and premiums.
For details contact: Director, Special Markets.

First American Edition–1995

Printed in Hong Kong
All first editions are printed on acid-free paper. ∞

10 9 8 7 6 5 4 3 2 1

Frontispiece: A bed of white (*T. grandiflorum*)
and red (*T. erectum*) trilliums.

Foreword

What a pleasure it is to read this wonderful book! Anne McIntyre brings to her writing the deep compassion and professional excellence that her many patients have benefitted from during her years of clinical practice. The reader can be confident that the insights and information contained in this herbal for women is based on a wealth of experience, clinical competence, and phytotherapeutic understanding.

Anne has that rare and enviable ability of making the most obtuse medical and herbal concepts readily understandable, leading the reader to their practical application. Unlike many modern herbals, The Complete Woman's Herbal empowers the reader on a number of levels by not only making therapeutic suggestions but clearly explaining the rationale that underpins them.

The more we turn our attention towards our relationship with the environment, the more profound become the insights into the close embrace we share. Of the numerous ways in which our inter-relatedness shows itself, the art and science of herbal medicine is for many people the most unexpected.

Herbalism is the medicine of belonging, the direct experience of the whole healing the part. Our world blesses us with herbs, with leaves of life. The medieval herbalist and Christian mystic, Hildegard Von Bingen, talks of Viriditas, the "greening power". By greening power, I interpret her to mean a vital energy that is life, the spirit of the planet, the divine in form, and one that heals humanity. From this perspective it comes as no surprise that Nature is rich in plants that nurture women and especially the process of conception and birth. After all, this creative process is the very keynote of life.

Herbalism abounds with opportunities to experience the reality of the healing presence of Nature, whether in treating disease or in hugging a tree.

It is a field of human endeavour that is a weaving of the miraculous and the mundane, a therapy that encompasses anthraquinone laxatives, the spiritual ecstasy of the Amazonian shaman, and the beauty of the flower. The limits to what might be called the path of the herbalist are only those imposed by parochial vision and constipated imagination!

A new understanding of health – often referred to as holistic medicine – is developing. The World Health Organization, for example, has defined health as being more than simply the absence of illness. It is the active state of physical, emotional, mental, and social wellbeing. This is a wonderfully precise encapsulation of the perspectives of holistic medicine. This approach to medicine starts from the assumption that health is a positive state, that it is an inherent characteristic of whole and integrated human beings.

From a holistic standpoint, a person is not merely a patient with a disease syndrome but a whole being; and therapists need to appreciate not only the physical but also the mental, emotional, spiritual, social, and environmental aspects of their patients' lives.

Herbal medicine fits perfectly into this emerging holistic paradigm. A healing technique that is inherently in tune with Nature, it has been described as "ecological healing" because it shares an ecological and evolutionary heritage with the plant kingdom. The book you hold in your hand is a practical, grounded expression of the holistic vision.

The author is to be commended on a job well done, and the reader congratulated on finding such a competent and reliable guide to the uses of herbs for women.

Thank you Anne!

David Hoffmann B.Sc., MNIMH
Santa Rosa, California

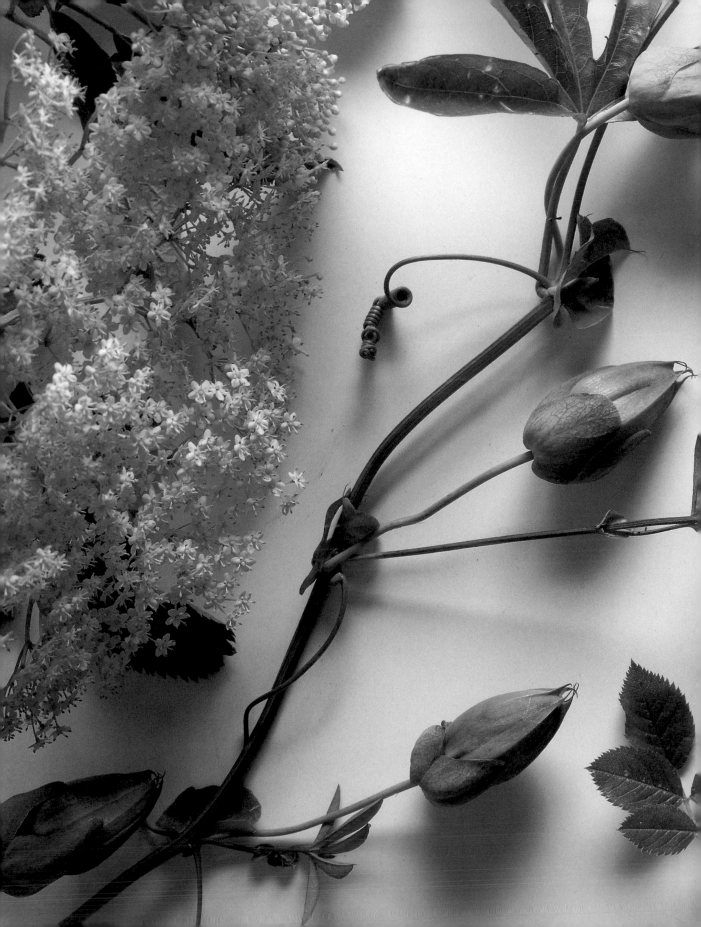

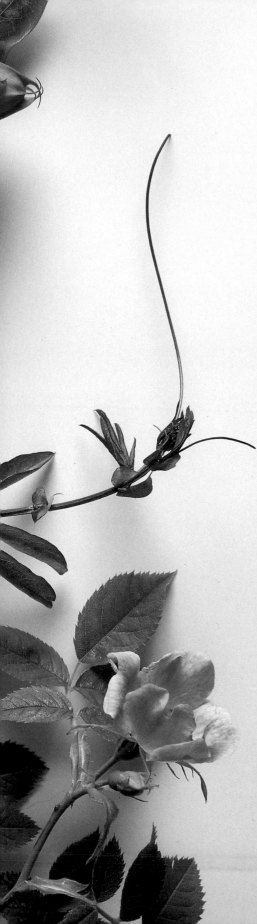

Contents

Introduction

Most women have a variety of roles to play in life. A woman is a female, may be a lover, wife, mother, creator of others, medicine woman, healthcare provider, wise woman, and counsellor. She is the heart of every family unit. Part of her very femininity is a wisdom about how to care for herself and others, and strength to do it. The ancient herbalists or healers who gathered roots and herbs for medicinal use were generally women.

The pressures of modern everyday life often make it difficult for women to maintain the level of health and vitality necessary for playing such crucial roles. The innate wisdom and strength of a woman needs to be complemented by a lifestyle that enhances these qualities rather than draining her vital resources.

Increasingly, women are seeking knowledge and information to deepen their understanding about how their bodies work, and how they change from one phase of life to another. They want to know how best to care for themselves, so that they can also care for those around them.

This book is intended as a manual for women to give them knowledge of what constitutes a healthy diet and lifestyle, coupled with information on the use of medicinal herbs. It aims to provide a sound basis for the role of healer and carer, and to enhance women's health and wellbeing.

Knowledge about diet, lifestyle, and herbs can be used both to prevent health problems, and also to treat imbalances and illnesses if they occur. Those who adopt the practices advised should be able to become less reliant on orthodox drugs. Quite simple dietary measures and herbal remedies can relieve a variety of ills.

Women and herbs – the art of Artemis

In myth and legend all over the world, the moon has always been the woman's symbol. The moon is the essential feminine principle, while the sun is seen as masculine. This is probably because women swell in pregnancy like a waxing moon and both have a monthly cycle. In many languages the words for menstruation and for moon have the same root. In English, "menstruation" signifies "moon change"; in rural Germany a menstrual period is simply "the moon", while in France it is called "le moment de la lune".

In Greek mythology, Artemis is the moon goddess, the twin sister of Apollo, the sun god. In Roman mythology she is Diana. Since ancient times the moon goddess has been regarded as the protector of women. The moon was held to influence fertility, and to be the source of women's power to bear children.

In many ancient civilizations women had (and in some still have) charge of all matters concerned with food supply. They searched for wild roots and fruits to eat and medicinal plants to remedy ills. It was believed that only women could make things grow as they are under the direct guardianship of the moon. Plants and seeds, it was thought, could not grow without the influence of the moon, whilst animals and women could not bear young without its energizing power.

Artemis is also the goddess of chastity, the protector of young maidens, who punishes those who offend against her, and against the morality of all she represents. She is a healing, purifying divinity, a nature goddess of fertilizing moisture, who influences lakes, rivers and springs. As the goddess of agriculture she promotes increase in fruits of the field, protects the grain and is friend to the reaper. She is the goddess of trees and all vegetation. She is also goddess of childbirth, watching over the birth of every child. Women in childbirth over thousands of years have evoked her aid and given prayers and offerings to secure a safe delivery and have given thanks to her afterwards.

Herbs named after Artemis, used for centuries, are still in use today to aid childbirth and for the treatment of a variety of women's ailments. *Artemisia abrotanum* (southernwood), *Artemisia vulgaris* (mugwort), and *Artemisia absinthium* (wormwood) all facilitate childbirth. They regulate and strengthen contractions, and help to bring away the afterbirth. The first English gynecological handbook, *A Medieval Woman's Guide to Health*, recommended the following for a difficult birth:

"Make her a bath of mallows, fenugreek, linseed, wormwood, southernwood, pellitory and mugwort, boiled in water, and let her bathe in it for a good time".

The qualities of Artemis reflect much of our feminine nature, our connection with healing and the world of plants. Femininity tends to be more subjective than objective, more inner than outer, more concerned with the inner mysteries of creation and nurture than the laws and principles of the outer world. In the West today greater emphasis is laid on the value of the outer, more objective, masculine approach to life. Almost as a prerequisite for holding their heads up, Western women have tended to develop the more masculine side of their nature, so that they can earn a living, practise a profession or follow a trade. This has meant that women have moved away from their ancient feminine spirits causing much inner conflict between the urge to express themselves through their work as men do, and the inner necessity to live in accordance with their feminine nature. Women who are consciously trying to get in touch with their lost feminine side are finding that the use of herbs can enhance this process. By using herbs to benefit our health, to heal us when sick, to regulate our menstrual cycles, enhance fertility, prepare for and support us during pregnancy and childbirth, we can go some way to reclaiming our knowledge of the mysteries of women and plants. We can enhance the "wise woman" in all of us with a new-found ability to heal ourselves, our families and one another. Although we may have temporarily lost much of the knowledge of therapeutic plants and healing skills, the instinct and wisdom to use plants to redress our imbalances is still there.

Up until only a hundred years ago it was customary for the woman of the house to prepare medicines from the natural resources around her for the majority of the healthcare needs of her family, selecting herbs from her garden and wild plants from the fields and hedgerows. Although many may have dismissed the value of such "grandmother's secrets" (believing only in those remedies whose benefits can be scientifically proved), herbalists can now look the world of science squarely in the face. Pharmacological research has, in the majority of cases, proved rather than ridiculed the ancient use of herbs, bringing traditional herbal lore smartly into the twentieth century.

Feeling reassured by such scientific evaluation and at the same time looking to retune themselves to their feminine natures, women are increasingly turning to the world of herbs for their healing benefits. They are looking towards playing a larger part in their own health care and understanding their imbalances and illnesses from a holistic viewpoint.

The philosophy of herbal healing

Central to the philosophy of holistic and herbal medicine is the recognition of an inherent healing wisdom within all of us, that imbues our every cell, and permeates our energy reserves. It manifests itself in the amazing feats that our bodies perform daily, as they continually protect, heal and regulate themselves. We maintain a steady state within ourselves, known as "homeostasis", in, for example, our blood sugar levels, temperature, fluid balance, blood chemistry, heart rate, and respiration rate, despite the constant variables that could otherwise severely upset our equilibrium. Junk food, pollution in the atmosphere, contaminants in our water, overwork, stress, and tension can all contribute to imbalance us, but despite these factors we perennially demonstrate our powers of adaptation and self-healing.

Within all the different traditions of medicine these powers are recognized and are variously known as the vital force, the life force, Qi, or Prana. When a surfeit of pathogenic factors is sufficient to overcome our homeostatic mechanisms, imbalances occur, and if these are ignored, illness can result. When a specific symptom manifests itself, it is often an expression of disharmony within our whole being, not simply of the part involved. To be able to assist our self-healing and restore harmony, we need to examine how our physical dysfunction relates to the different aspects of ourselves and our lives – physical, mental, emotional and spiritual. Only then will we understand how to enhance and not hinder our healing energies.

By observation of ourselves, life within and without us, we may begin to see how we are subject to natural laws and forces. By understanding these, we will be able to live our lives in accordance with them, rather than in isolation from them, not only when we fall ill, but also in our daily lives.

Such observation will necessarily involve expanding our awareness to observe our interconnection with the world around us, our families, our community, our place in the world, the natural world around us and ultimately the entire planet itself. We know that all life depends for its existence on the sun, the masculine life force. Plants have the unique ability to store this solar energy. Through the process of photosynthesis they use sunlight, carbon dioxide and water, to make sugars, proteins, enzymes, hormone-like substances, oils, and a whole range of other constituents. Plants provide us with our food and with invaluable medicines. In addition, from the soil plants take up elements which are vital for our diet. In the process of manufacturing their food plants give out the other essential ingredient for life – oxygen. By trapping the sun's energy, plants make it accessible to every inhabitant of the earth.

It is not difficult therefore to understand the central role that medicinal plants have held in our lives throughout history. The use of herbs reflects our dependence on the plant world, and their role in healing reflects holism in its wider aspects. By using the healing power of plants to redress the imbalances which contribute to our ill-health, we can restore harmony within ourselves and with the world around us.

How to use this book

Many commonly used herbs have several popular names. Each herb recommended in the book has a one-page profile, which can be located through the index, and which gives alternative names some of which may be more familiar. The twenty most popular herbs are featured together in Part One. Although herbs are recommended for use only where appropriate, you should always refer to the herb profile page before use, as any cautions or contraindications are listed there.

Throughout the book, readers are given recommendations for dietary measures and herbal treatments for ailments. These are summarized in The Herbs and Ailments on p.274-277.

In order to make a more readable text, the author has avoided the now customary use of "s/he" when referring to a baby boy or girl, and has used the male pronoun throughout.

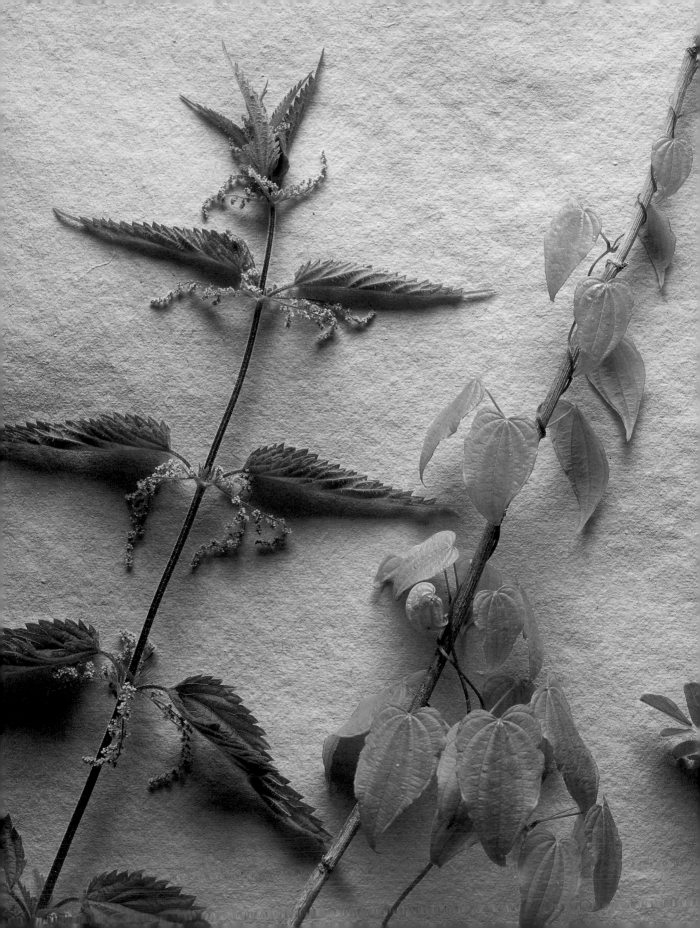

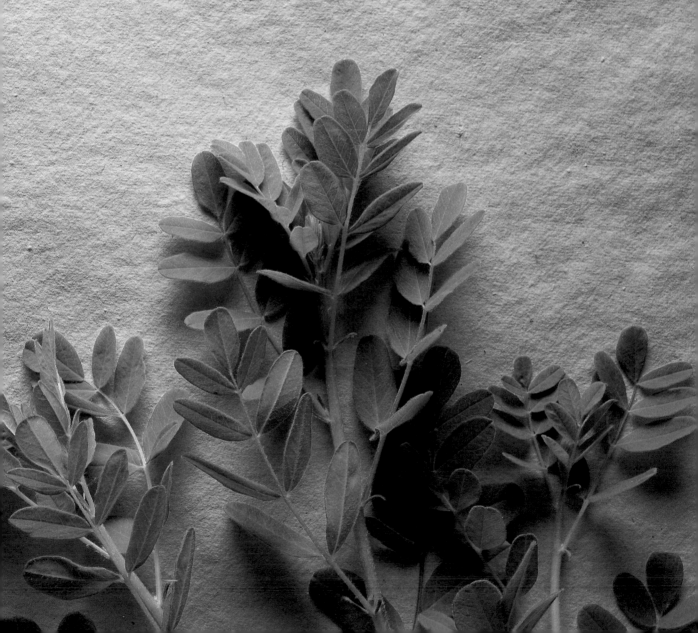

PART ONE

Herbal Wellbeing

About Herbs
The Well Woman

1 *About Herbs*

Herbal medicine is among the most respected of the ancient natural therapies, and has stood the test of time, despite the introduction of modern medical science. Herbs are compatible with the chemistry of the human body which has adapted over thousands of years to assimilate them. Today there is an enormous resurgence of interest in all things herbal, and a rediscovery of the traditional use of medicinal herbs. Treatment with herbs can often provide a gentle and safe alternative, or complement, to modern drugs and other orthodox medical treatments.

Women in particular are concerned to find natural, safe remedies for the various problems that arise during the gestation period, such as morning sickness, heartburn, varicose veins, and constipation. Many want to find effective remedies when their babies and children fall sick with the minor ailments of childhood, which often do not warrant the use of harsh, powerful drugs.

Over the centuries we have developed an enormous wealth of information on the uses and efficacy of herbal medicines. Passed down from generation to generation, it has survived until the present day, when (the World Health Organization informs us) 85 per cent of the world's population still use herbs as their main form of medical treatment. And this is very fortunate, for in the late 1970s, after worldwide surveys by international health agencies, the Director General of the WHO stated that to achieve and maintain adequate healthcare for the world by the year 2000, we need to encourage and develop the use of traditional systems of medicine, for western orthodox medicine alone will not meet our medical needs. Even industrialized countries, such as the USA and Japan, are looking to herbs and their potential for primary health care.

Here in the West we can combine the best of both worlds, with a blend of old and new – the folklore of ancient herbalism vindicated by the results of modern scientific research. The modern herbal practitioner has replaced the old wise woman, and is well versed not only in the tradition of herbal medicine, but also in its biochemistry and pharmacology. In addition, such practitioners are well trained in conventional medical science which they use as part of a holistic approach to healing.

Many traditional and attractive garden plants are useful medicinal herbs.

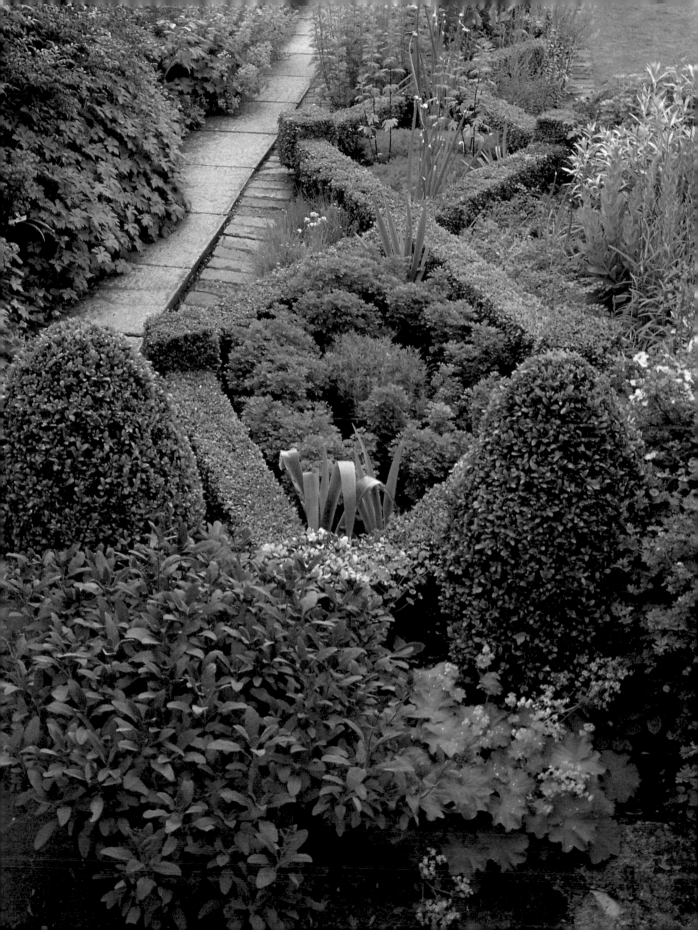

The chemistry of herbs

Herbs are very much like foods, and in many cases are indistinguishable from them. They contain a variety of different nutritious and therapeutic constituents – vitamins, minerals, trace elements – as well as active ingredients with a variety of medicinal actions. These include volatile oils, tannins, mucilage, alkaloids, bitters, and flavonoids. It may be helpful to know a little about the function of these ingredients.

Volatile oils

Volatile oils lend their wonderful aroma and taste to the herbs we all know from their use in food – rosemary, marjoram, parsley, dill, basil, thyme, mint, and sage. While we are enjoying our pasta with fresh basil, fish with parsley sauce, potato soup with fresh coriander leaves, and tomatoes with oregano, we are unwittingly taking in substances with a wide variety of medicinal actions.

Volatile or essential oils are made up of numerous different chemical compounds, the many combinations of which account for the variation in their fragrance, taste and actions. All volatile oils have antiseptic and antimicrobial properties, enhancing the body's ability to fight off a range of infections. Many oils, such as in chamomile and yarrow, have anti-inflammatory and antispasmodic effects, others are expectorant, such as those in thyme and hyssop; some are diuretic, as in chamomile and parsley. Some volatile oils, such as in rosemary, fennel, and marjoram, are tonics, enhancing the appetite, and the digestion and absorption of food by their beneficial action throughout the digestive system. Some – as in ginger, rosemary, and thyme – stimulate the heart and circulation.

You can take volatile oils into the body through a variety of different pathways. They may enter the bloodstream through the gut when taken in food, drinks, or in herbal medicines, or directly into the bloodstream when placed under the tongue. They can enter via the pores of the skin in a massage, or inhaled. They are rapidly dispersed, particularly in the digestive, respiratory, circulatory, and urinary systems. During pregnancy and lactation, the oils are passed to the baby through the placenta and breastmilk.

When we inhale the wonderful scents of volatile oils, nerve endings in the upper part of the nose are stimulated to carry messages to the brain, particularly an area known as the limbic system which relates to our thoughts and emotions. When we take oils in via the skin in baths and massage, they stimulate nerve endings in the skin which send messages to underlying tissues – muscles, blood, lymphatic vessels and nerves. Their actions are relayed to the pituitary gland, which governs the function of all other endocrine glands in the body. It is not difficult to see the enormous value of the therapeutic use of oils in relieving stress and enhancing general health.

Treatment with aromatic oils is called aromatherapy, and is usually a massage with oils. Rose oil is particularly beneficial to women, relieving tension and anxiety, problems related to femininity and sexuality, and symptoms in the reproductive system including menstrual problems, anxiety around childbirth, postnatal depression and low libido. Scents are some of the most delightfully evocative sensations we can enjoy from nature. The aromatic flowers that scent our gardens and country lanes and the tasty, often pungent, herbs and spices which enliven our food, are not hard to appreciate. By inhaling the wonderful aromas around us we can lift our spirits and enhance our wellbeing immeasurably.

Tannins

The main therapeutic action of tannins is astringent, as a result of their ability to bind albumen, a protein present in the skin and mucous membranes of the body, to form an insoluble, protective layer that is resistant to disease. This protective layer can separate micro-organisms, such as bacteria which threaten to invade the body, from the source of their nutrition, either on the skin, or in the linings of the mouth, digestive, respiratory, urinary, and reproductive systems.

Tannins also have a healing action, protecting areas treated from irritation, while at the same time reducing inflammation. They are the main therapeutic ingredients in astringents such as oak bark, witch hazel, and beth root.

Such herbs can be used in compresses for cuts and wounds, hemorrhoids, varicose veins, and in medicines for diarrhea, catarrh, heavy periods, and inflammatory conditions of the digestive tract.

Bitters

There are many herbal remedies containing bitter ingredients. These mainly exert their beneficial effect in the digestive tract, stimulating the secretion of digestive juices and enzymes in the stomach and intestines, and the flow of bile from the liver. They enhance the appetite, improve digestion and absorption. They are prescribed for poor appetite, sluggish bowels, indigestion, gallbladder and liver problems, gastritis, nervous exhaustion, and to aid convalescence after flu or other debilitating illness.

Many bitter herbs have other therapeutic actions; some benefit the immune system, acting as natural antimicrobials and antineoplastic (anti-tumour) remedies, some have a relaxing effect on the nervous system, some have an anti-inflammatory action. Well-known bitter tonics include dandelion, dock root, rosemary, burdock and wood betony. Their beneficial action on the digestive system begins with their effect on the bitter receptors in the mouth, so for good effect they are best tasted, despite our squeamish palates.

Mucilage

Mucilage is a sweet, gel-like substance which has hydroscopic properties, that is, it draws water to it, so that on the addition of water it swells up to form a viscous fluid. Mucilage has wonderful demulcent and emollient properties, forming a protective layer over the mucous membranes and skin, effectively soothing irritation and relieving inflammation.

Plants with a high mucilage content such as flax or psyllium seeds draw water into the bowel and thereby bulk out the stool and make effective laxative remedies which soothe the gut.

Saponins

Saponins are glycosides found widely among medicinal plants which, like soap, form a lather when mixed with water. Soapwort (*Saponaria officinalis*) has a high saponin content and can be used to make a natural soap. Saponins have a wide variety of different therapeutic actions in the body. Some, such as in cowslips and mullein, have an expectorant effect; others, such as in horsetail and asparagus, act as diuretics. Some, as in horse chestnut, benefit the circulatory system, reducing fragility of blood vessel walls.

The most interesting and most appropriate for treating a wide variety of women's problems are the steroidal saponins. These are similar in structure and function to human sex hormones, produced by the ovaries, adrenal glands, and in men by the testes. There are steroidal saponins which resemble estrogen, cortisone, cholesterol, and progesterone and there are some known as tri-terpenoid saponins which act to regulate the steroidal hormone activity in the body and to counter stress.

Remedies which contain hormone-regulating properties are known as "adaptogens", the most famous of which is ginseng. Other adaptogenic herbs include false unicorn root, partridge berry, blue and black cohosh, wild yam, and licorice.

Anthraquinones

These are glycosides which are yellow, and were often used in the past to produce dyes. They act to stimulate muscular contraction of the large intestine and so have a laxative effect. Herbs such as dock, cascara, senna, and aloes contain anthraquinones, which taken alone can cause griping in the bowel. For this reason they are best combined with carminative (flatulence-treating) herbs such as ginger or fennel which prevent this from happening. Such laxative herbs are best used for short term treatment of constipation while the underlying causes are dealt with, for longer use can reduce normal bowel reflexes and cause habituation.

Flavonoids

Flavonoids or flavonoid glycosides are responsible for the yellow or orange in herbs such as cowslips, fruits such as oranges and lemons, and vegetables such as carrots. Many flavonoids, as in parsley, have a diuretic action; some, as in licorice, are antispasmodic and anti-inflammatory; others are antiseptic.

Bioflavonoids are well-known constituents of some plants rich in vitamin C, such as citrus fruits, rose hips, blackcurrants, and cherries. In such plants, bioflavonoids act with ascorbic acid (vitamin C) to enhance its absorption and metabolism by the body.

Bioflavonoids have a strengthening and healing effect on the walls of blood vessels and are used to treat problems such as capillary fragility, tendency to bruising and nosebleeds, and high blood pressure.

Alkaloids

Alkaloids vary widely from one plant to another in their components and their actions, but are all compounds that contain nitrogen. They tend to have potent effects and in some cases are toxic in large amounts – they are frequently found in herbs whose use is restricted to qualified medical herbalists and doctors in specified doses, and are often unsuitable for home use. They include morphine from the opium poppy, nicotine in tobacco, atropine in deadly nightshade, caffeine and theobromide in coffee, black tea, and cocoa.

Alkaloids also occur in small non-toxic amounts in some medicinal herbs where they act as catalysts to other healing agents without being involved themselves – pyrrolizidine alkaloids in comfrey and coltsfoot are good examples.

How to prepare herbal remedies

There is a wide variety of ways we can use herbs in order for them to exert their beneficial influence – just being amongst them in a fragrant herb garden, or picking wild herbs in a country lane in summer, is enough for us to feel their wonderful effects. The easiest way to take herbs is of course to eat them, which most of us do daily – parsley in salads, dill with fish, marjoram with pizza, mint with lamb, horseradish with beef, basil with pasta, garlic with everything. They are absorbed from the digestive tract into the bloodstream and circulate round the body.

Preparations for internal use

Apart from culinary use, herbs can be taken internally as teas, tinctures, or in tablet form.

Infusions

These are made in the same way as a cup of tea using the soft parts of plants – the leaves, stems and flowers. The standard dose is 1 oz (25 g) of dried herb, or 2 oz (50 g) of fresh herb to 1 pint (600 ml) boiling water. You can vary this according to taste – it is important to make your herb teas palatable so that you drink them regularly when you need to. Put the herbs in a warmed teapot, pour on boiling water, leave covered to infuse for ten minutes and then strain. A cupful is generally taken three times daily for chronic conditions, and six times daily or more in acute illness. An infusion will keep for up to two days in a refrigerator.

Some herbs, particularly those with a high mucilage content, such as comfrey, need to be prepared in the same way but with cold water. Most infusions are taken hot, except when treating the urinary system, when they need to be drunk lukewarm to cold.

When making infusions you can blend several herbs together to make a tasty brew; the addition of aromatic herbs such as mints, lemon balm, lemon verbena, fennel, lavender, and licorice to more bitter medicinal herbs is recommended to make them more palatable, especially for children.

Decoctions

These are similar to infusions but prepared from the hard woody parts of plants, such as the bark, seeds, roots, rhizomes, and nuts, which require greater heat to impart their constituents to water. Break or hammer them first with pestle and mortar, or chop them if fresh, then place in a pan with the water, bring to the boil, cover and simmer for ten minutes and strain. Use a little over a pint of water per ounce of herb to make up for any lost in the simmering. The dosage is the same as for infusions.

Using infusions and decoctions

You can use infusions and decoctions in eyebaths, gargles, mouthwashes, and lotions generally. Such treatments are given about two to three times daily for chronic problems and every two hours in acute cases.

Syrups

These are often preferred by children. Give two teaspoons (double for adults) three or four times daily in chronic problems and twice as much in acute illness.

You can use an infusion or decoction to make a syrup by mixing 12 oz (325 g) sugar into a pint (600 ml) of the liquid and heat until the sugar dissolves. Store the syrup in a refrigerator. Alternatively, you can weigh your infusion or decoction and add a quarter of its weight of honey to it. Heat this slowly and stir as it starts to thicken, skimming off scum that forms on the surface.

Another way to make syrup is to pour a pint (600 ml) of boiling water over 2½ lb (1.25 kg) of soft brown sugar and stir over a low heat until the sugar is dissolved and the solution starts to boil. Remove from the heat. Add one part herbal tincture (see below) to three parts syrup and this will keep indefinitely.

Tinctures

These are concentrated extracts of herbs, usually using a mixture of water and alcohol to extract the constituents of the remedy and act as a preservative. The ratio of alcohol to water varies from one remedy to another; 25 per cent alcohol is used for simple glycosides and tannins, while 90 per cent alcohol is needed for resins and gums.

To make a tincture, use dried herbs at a ratio of one part herb to five parts of liquid, or fresh herbs at a ratio of one part herb to two of liquid. Place the herb in a large jar and pour the alcohol and water mixture over it. Leave to macerate, shaking daily for two weeks. Then, using a wine press, press out the liquid and discard the herb – which makes very good compost. Store in labelled, dark bottles or glass jars, away from heat and light.

When making tinctures at home you can use undiluted alcohol such as brandy, gin or vodka. Alternatively you can use glycerol (glycerine) which gives a sweet taste to the extracts and makes them more palatable. Use equal parts of water and glycerol for dried herbs, and 80 per cent glycerol for watery, fresh herbs such as borage to ensure they do not deteriorate or become contaminated by infection.

A standard dose is one teaspoon of tincture diluted with a little water with or after food three times daily in chronic conditions, and every two hours in acute illness. Children should be given half dosages, and babies a quarter of the adult dose.

Tinctures generally keep well for about two years, and although more time-consuming to prepare than teas, they have the advantages of being easy to store, and of needing to be taken only in small amounts.

Tinctures can also be used to make gargles and mouthwashes, lotions and douches. Use half to one teaspoon in a cupful of water two or three times daily in chronic problems and every two hours for acute conditions.

Suppositories

Both local and systemic problems can be treated quickly and simply by this method. Suppositories bypass the alimentary canal and are absorbed quickly into the system. The herbal remedy is absorbed directly into the bloodstream through the mucosa of the rectum.

You can prepare suppositories easily at home by adding finely powdered dried herbs to a base of melted cocoa butter. Pour this into moulds, made in the required shape from aluminium foil, and allow to cool. Store in a refrigerator. It is a good idea to make a row of suppositories in the foil at one time.

Tablets and capsules

Herbs in tablet or capsule form can often be bought from herb suppliers or health food shops. You can also make capsules at home using gelatin capsules filled with powdered mixtures of the herbs you require. The process is made easier by using a capsule maker which enables you to make up a large quantity at a time. The two standard capsule sizes are 0 and 00. Size 0 holds about 0.35 g of powder, so that three capsules should be taken three times daily to achieve the standard dose. Size 00 holds about 0.5 g of powder, requiring two capsules to be taken three times daily.

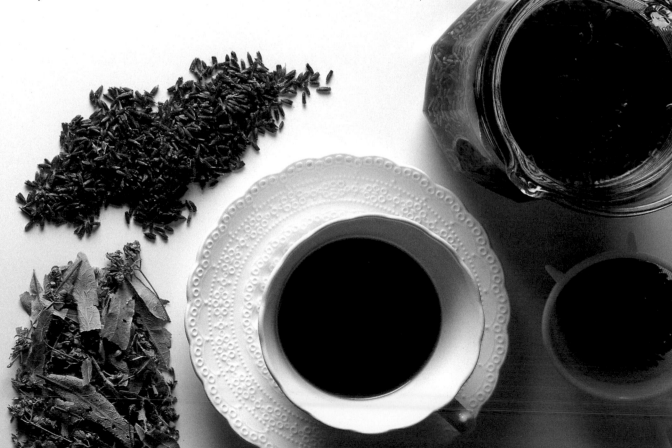

Preparations for external use

The skin is highly absorbent; constituents of any herbal preparation applied to it will be carried by tiny capillaries under the skin surface into the bloodstream and then round the body. There are various ways in which you can employ this pathway into the body.

Herbal baths

A fragrant warm bath is a wonderfully luxurious and relaxing way to take herbal medicines and a very easy way to treat babies and children. You can hang a muslin bag filled with fresh or dried herbs under the hot tap. Alternatively you can add strong herb infusions to the bathwater. Soak in the water for 15-30 minutes. You can also add a few drops of your chosen essential oil to the bathwater – always dilute the oils first for babies and children, or if you have a sensitive skin.

In a herbal bath the plant constituents are absorbed through the skin's pores which are opened by the warmth of the water. Volatile oils are carried on the steam to be inhaled through the nose and mouth into the lungs and from there into the bloodstream. From the nose, the oils send messages via nerve receptors to the brain and have a rapidly relaxing and soothing effect, easing mental and emotional strain. Lavender, chamomile, and ylang ylang are wonderfully relaxing and smell lovely, while rosemary is also relaxing but has a stimulating edge sending blood to the brain and enhancing alertness.

Hand and foot baths

Our hands and feet are very sensitive areas, with plenty of nerve endings. Despite some thickening of the skin from use, herbal constituents pass easily from these areas into the bloodstream.

Mustard foot baths are an old English remedy for all afflictions of cold and damp, from colds and flu to poor circulation and arthritis. The famous French herbalist Maurice Messegue advocates this therapeutic pathway for the use of herbs in his several books on herbal medicine and recommends foot baths for eight minutes in the evening and hand baths for eight minutes in the morning.

Hand and foot baths are excellent ways to treat babies and children who only need to remain in the water for half the time recommended for adults – four minutes in the morning and again in the evening.

Salves and creams

To make a simple salve, herbs are macerated in oil. Put 16 oz (450 ml) of olive oil and 2 oz (50 g) of beeswax into a heatproof dish, add as much of the herb as the mixture will cover, and let it heat gently for a few hours in a bain-marie. This allows time for the constituents of the remedy to be absorbed into the oil. Press out through a muslin bag, discard the herb, and pour the warm oil into jars where it will quickly solidify.

You can also make up creams very easily by stirring tinctures, infusions, decoctions or a few drops of essential oil into a base of aqueous (water-based) cream from the pharmacist.

Poultices

A poultice is a soft, damp mixture applied to part of the body. You can use fresh or dried herbs as a poultice, placed between two pieces of gauze. When using fresh leaves, stems or roots, make sure to bruise or crush them first. When using dried herbs, add a little hot water to the powdered or finely chopped herbs to make a paste to spread over the gauze.

Then bind the gauze poultice to the affected part using a light cotton bandage and keep it warm with a hot-water bottle. You can use cabbage leaves in this way for painful, arthritic joints or tender, engorged breasts, while a bran poultice will ease mastitis.

Compresses

Take a clean cloth or towel, and soak it either in a hot or cold herbal infusion or decoction, or in water to which a few drops of essential oil have been added. Then wring it out and apply to the affected area, such as the site of a headache, period pain, backache, inflamed joints, or varicose veins. Repeat several times for good effect.

Liniments

Liniments, also called embrocations, are rubbing oils used in massage to relax or stimulate muscles and ligaments or soothe away pain from inflammation or injury. They consist of extracts of herbs in an oil or alcohol base, or a mixture of herbal oils and alcohol tinctures of your chosen herbs. They are intended to be absorbed quickly through the skin to the affected part and for this reason often contain stimulating oils or cayenne to increase local circulation.

Oils

Essential oils are extracted from aromatic plants by a process of steam distillation and so cannot be prepared at home. You can buy them from many different sources including health food shops and mail order companies (see p.281 for sources).

You can easily make herbal oils, however, by infusing finely chopped herbs in a pure vegetable oil such as almond, sunflower or olive oil, for about two weeks. Place the herbs in a glass jar with a tight-fitting lid and cover them with oil. Place

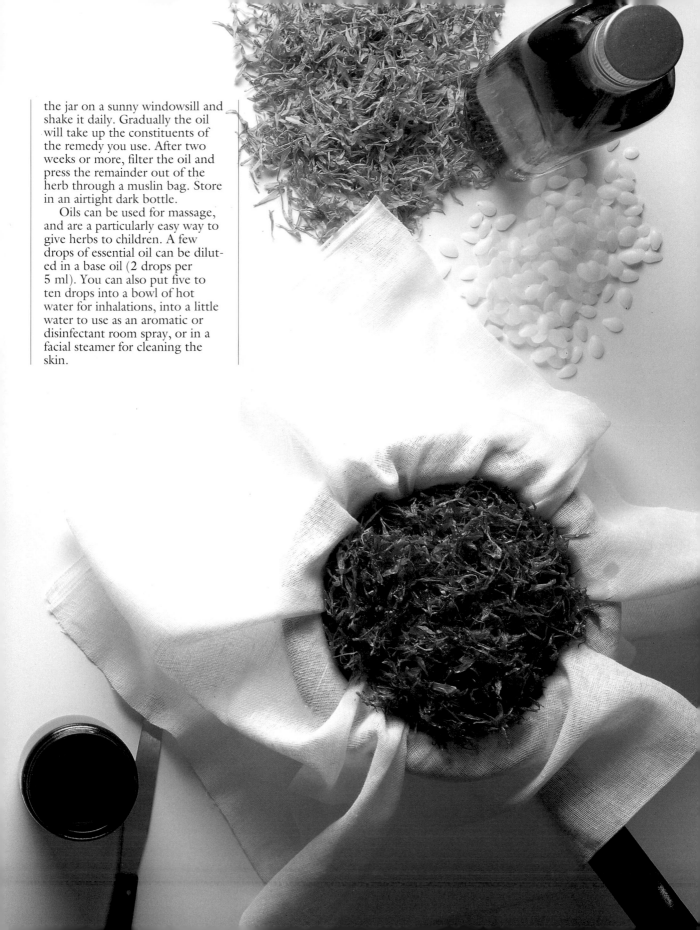

the jar on a sunny windowsill and shake it daily. Gradually the oil will take up the constituents of the remedy you use. After two weeks or more, filter the oil and press the remainder out of the herb through a muslin bag. Store in an airtight dark bottle.

Oils can be used for massage, and are a particularly easy way to give herbs to children. A few drops of essential oil can be diluted in a base oil (2 drops per 5 ml). You can also put five to ten drops into a bowl of hot water for inhalations, into a little water to use as an aromatic or disinfectant room spray, or in a facial steamer for cleaning the skin.

Chaste tree

Vitex agnus-castus

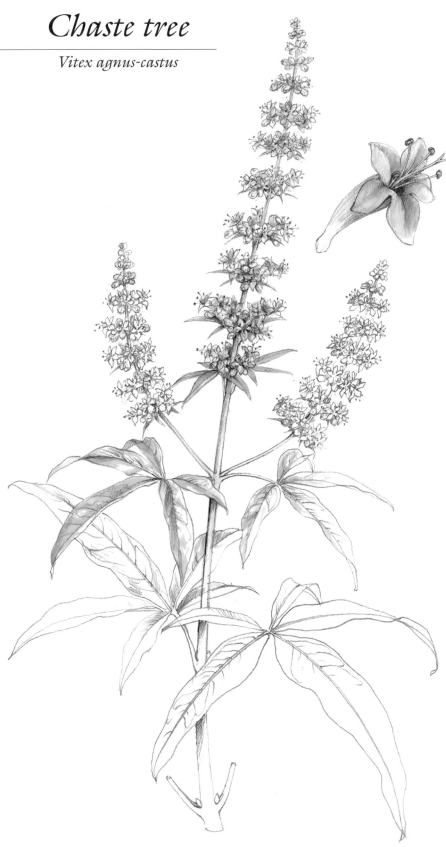

ALSO KNOWN AS: Chasteberry, monk's pepper

PART USED: Seeds

CONTAINS: Volatile oil, bitter principle (castine), alkaloids, iridoid glycosides (including aucbin and agnoside), flavonoids (including casticin, isovitexin and orientin)

KEY USES: Hormone regulator, galactagogue, reproductive tonic

Chaste tree is a beautiful Mediterranean shrub with the wonderful ability of stimulating and balancing the function of the pituitary gland, particularly in relation to female sex hormones. It has a normalizing (often known as amphoteric) effect on the female hormone balance by its effect on follicle stimulating hormone (FSH) and luteinizing hormone (LH) produced by the anterior pituitary gland. It acts to support the corpus luteum of the ovaries in its work of producing hormones in the second half of the menstrual cycle. In practice, it appears to have a more progesteronic than estrogenic action and makes a fine remedy for PMS and a range of menstrual and gynecological problems that are related to hormone imbalance.

It can be used effectively for irregular and painful periods, heavy bleeding, fibroids, and to re-establish hormone balance after stopping use of the contraceptive pill. It is a good remedy for menopausal problems and stimulates milk production in nursing mothers, and because it has a calming and relaxing effect it can be used for any emotional distress associated with the reproductive system, such as PMS and menopausal depression.

False unicorn root

Chamaelirium luteum

ALSO KNOWN AS: Helonias root, devil's bit, blazing star, *Veraticum luteum, Helonias dioica, Helonias lutea*

PARTS USED: Root and rhizome

CONTAINS: Yellow bitter principle, steroidal saponins, including chamelirin, fatty acids

KEY USES: Ovarian and uterine tonic, digestive, diuretic, anthelmintic, emetic

False unicorn root is another herb inherited from the Native American tradition. It contains hormone-like saponins which partly account for its long tradition as an excellent ovarian and uterine tonic. It was used specifically for uterine weakness and over-relaxation, characterized by a dragging sensation, a feeling of downward pressure in the pelvis, often associated with irritability and depression. It has also been used to encourage fertility in women and treat impotence in men. It has an adaptogenic or balancing effect on sex hormones, helping to relieve many disorders of the reproductive tract, menstrual irregularities and premenstrual syndrome, which are related to hormonal imbalance. It improves the secretory responses and cyclical functions of the ovary and has been used in infertility caused by dysfunction in follicular formation in the ovary.

The bitter principle has a tonic effect on the liver and digestive tract, which benefits appetite and digestion and helps to relieve nausea and vomiting in pregnancy.

False unicorn root has also been used to prevent threatened miscarriage and to stop hemorrhage.

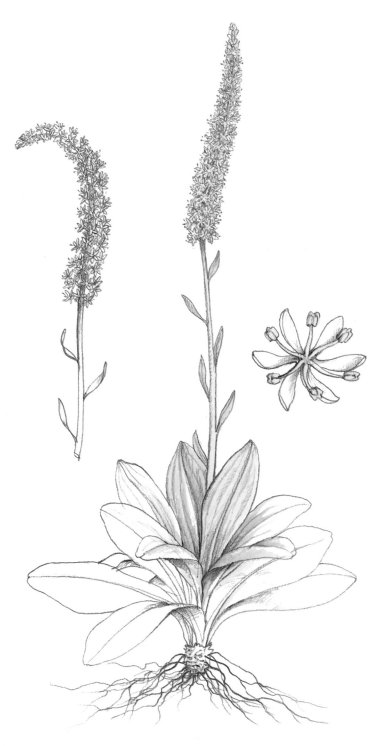

Partridge berry

Mitchella repens

ALSO KNOWN AS: Squaw vine, squawberry

PARTS USED: Whole plant

CONTAINS: Saponins, mucilage, resin, wax, dextrine, tannins, bitter principles

KEY USES: Astringent, tonic, diuretic, digestive, emmenagogue, nervine

Partridge berry tones and strengthens the uterine and pelvic muscles, and primes them for contraction. It also relaxes the uterus, and stops uterine cramping during pregnancy, while acting as a tonic generally to the nervous system.

Partridge berry helps to maintain the right balance between relaxation and contraction of the uterine muscles and tissues. It helps to relieve back pain during pregnancy, and is recommended particularly for anxiety and tension during pregnancy, or related to birth, and possible consequences such as false labour pains. It is also a good urinary tonic, it regulates the bowels, and improves appetite and digestion.

Partridge berry can be drunk as a tea, a cupful two to three times daily in the last six weeks of pregnancy, to ease and speed childbirth. Alternatively, half a teaspoon of the tincture can be taken two to three times daily.

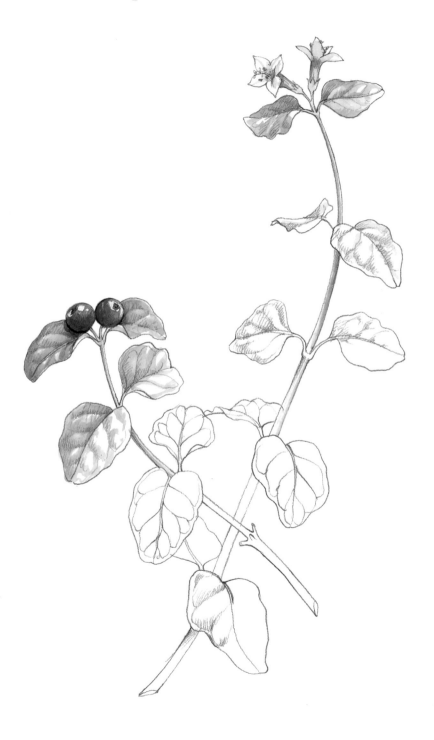

Raspberry leaves

Rubus idaeus

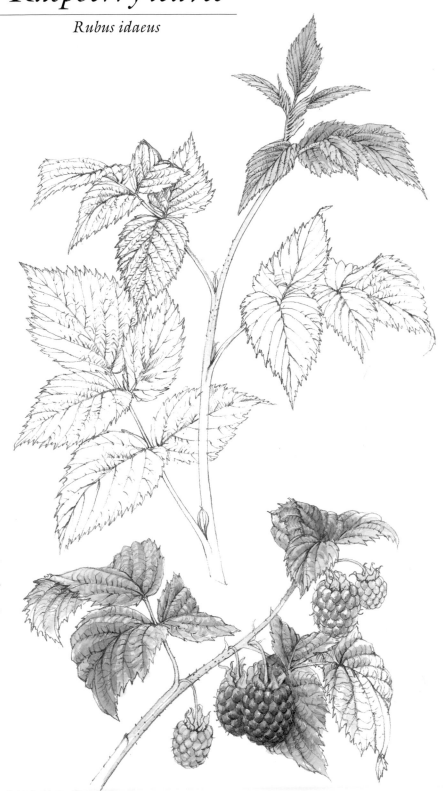

PARTS USED: Leaves and fruit

CONTAINS: Fragarine, volatile oils, tannin, fruit acids, minerals (including potassium, calcium, magnesium, zinc)

KEY USES: Astringent, toning, pelvic and uterine relaxant

Raspberry leaves are the most famous of all herbs used during pregnancy. They have both relaxing and toning or astringent actions, with a particular affinity for the uterus. Their astringent and stimulating properties help to strengthen and tone up the uterine and pelvic muscles, while the relaxing and more soothing properties relax the uterus at the same time. Raspberry leaves also tone the mucous membranes throughout the body, soothe the kidneys and urinary tract and are useful for allaying diarrhea and stopping hemorrhage. They have digestive properties which are effective in quelling nausea in pregnancy and are also sedative and relaxant.

Throughout history, raspberry leaves have been used principally to encourage a safe, easy and speedy childbirth, as well as afterwards to stimulate milk production and to speed recovery from the birth. Their tonic and relaxant actions on the smooth muscle of the uterus act to reduce the pain of uterine contractions during childbirth and also make the contractions more effective and productive, thereby easing and shortening the duration of the birth.

Raspberry leaves are best taken as a warm infusion. From the third month onwards you can take a cupful once a day, and from the sixth month, three times daily. When the birth is imminent, one teaspoon of composition essence can be added to each cup of tea, and, once contractions begin, it should be taken one cupful an hour while you can. Once the digestive system shuts down, sips of the tea, or a few drops on the tongue taken as often as possible will be helpful. Continue with this mixture after the birth, once to three times daily, to tone and strengthen the pelvic tissues.

Blue cohosh

Caulophyllum thalictroides

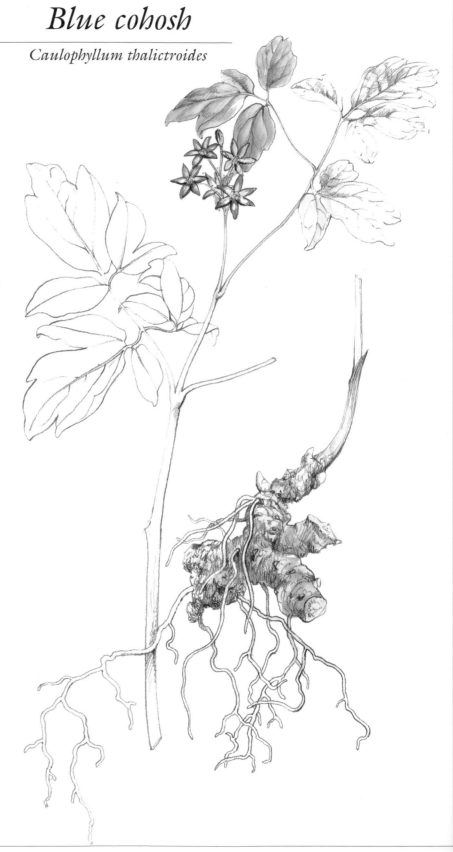

ALSO KNOWN AS: Squaw root, woman's best friend, papoose root, blue ginseng, yellow ginseng

PARTS USED: Root and rhizome

CONTAINS: Methylcytisine (caulophylline), baptifoline, anagyrine, magnoflorine, tannin, steroidal saponins, resins and gums, laburnine

KEY USES: Antispasmodic, laxative, anti-rheumatic, emmenagogue, uterine tonic, partus preparator

Like raspberry leaves and black cohosh, blue cohosh has both stimulating and relaxing properties which facilitate childbirth. It produces contractions which are regular and effective, interspersed with a good relaxation period.

Its tonic properties improve sluggish labour pains and are most helpful when delay in childbirth is due to weakness, fatigue or lack of uterine power. Similarly, the relaxant effects of this plant prove useful when tension produces uterine irritability, with spasmodic pains, false labour pains and over-strong Braxton-Hicks contractions. It was a favourite remedy amongst Native American women for false pains and after-pains. They drank the tea regularly a few weeks before the birth was due, as a partus preparator, to ease and speed labour. It is used particularly to relax women in childbirth and ease the pain, but also to soothe restlessness, tension and pain during pregnancy. The antispasmodic action helps ensure that the uterus holds the growing baby, and so it prevents premature delivery. Its antispasmodic properties are also used for stomach and menstrual cramps. Blue cohosh has a good reputation for helping to prevent miscarriage, particularly when used with black haw or cramp bark. The plant acts as a relaxant and tonic to the nervous system.

Blue cohosh may be taken alone or in conjunction with other partus preparators, for a few weeks prior to the birth, three times daily.

Note Never use in early pregnancy.

Black cohosh

Cimicifuga racemosa

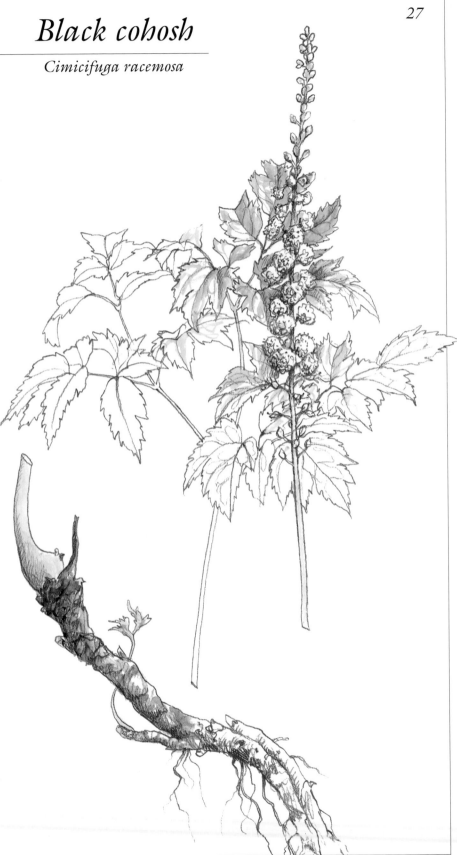

ALSO KNOWN AS: Squaw root, black snakeroot, bugbane

PARTS USED: Dried root and rhizome

CONTAINS: Triterpene glycosides, including actein and cimigoside, resins, volatile oil, tannin, salicylates, ranunculin (which yields anemonin)

KEY USES: Anodyne, antispasmodic, anti-inflammatory, hypoglycemic, hypotensive, sedative (cardiac), uterine tonic, parturient

Black cohosh is a powerful painkiller which can be put to good use in childbirth. It is specific for nerve and muscle pain, and was widely used very successfully by the Native Americans for treating neuralgia. Its anodyne (painkilling) and sedative properties can also help relieve headaches and tinnitus. It is also one of the best remedies for reflex mammary pains during pregnancy, mastitis, and for ovarian and uterine pain.

The antispasmodic action eases cramping and muscle tension and is usefully employed in asthma, whooping cough, menstrual cramps and childbirth. Black cohosh is an ideal regulator of uterine contractions during childbirth. It produces natural intermittent uterine contractions, and for best results should be used as a partus preparator for several weeks prior to the birth. The antispasmodic action is matched by the tonic properties of the plant. It is famous for its power of increasing and normalizing weak and erratic uterine contractions, and to tone the reproductive tract. It has been used for painful periods, sore and inflammatory conditions of the reproductive tract, infections, and lack of functional power in the uterus leading to infertility.

The resinous compound in the plant has been found to dilate the peripheral blood vessels and to lower blood pressure. The salicylates have shown in research to have an anti-inflammatory effect.

Note Never use in early pregnancy.

Beth root

Trillium erectum

ALSO KNOWN AS: Birth root, wake-robin

PARTS USED: Rhizome and root

CONTAINS: Steroidal saponins (including diosgenin), fixed oil, gum, volatile oil, tannins

KEY USES: Astringent, antiseptic, uterine tonic, alterative, expectorant

Beth root is a well-known Native American remedy used to lessen the pain during childbirth. It contains natural precursors or building blocks of female sex hormones, explaining its use for a variety of menstrual disorders. It acts as an excellent tonic for the uterus, and its astringent properties are particularly useful for heavy bleeding, and post-partum hemorrhage. It is excellent for excessive menstruation around the menopause. It can also be used for bleeding elsewhere in the body - such as the digestive tract, bladder, nose and mouth, and to stem diarrhea and dysentery. During childbirth it is excellent to stimulate contractions and get the birth going properly, but for this reason should not be used during pregnancy.

Externally, its antiseptic properties make beth root useful for treating vaginal discharges and infections such as thrush and trichomonas. It will speed healing of skin problems, ulcers, bleeding, hemorrhoids and varicose veins, and soothe irritation of insect bites and stings.

Note Beth root should not be used during pregnancy.

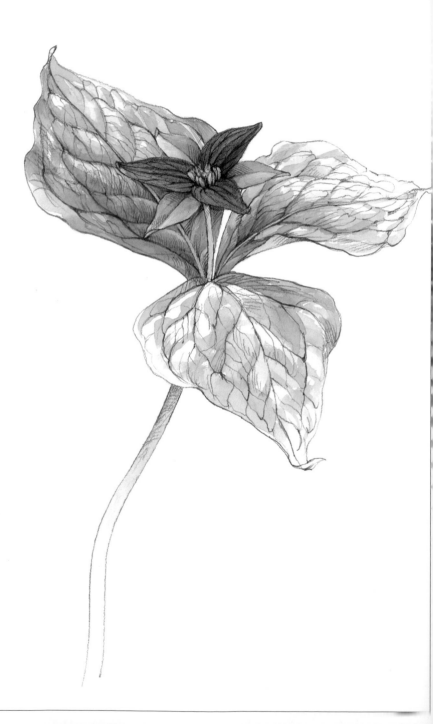

Wild yam

Dioscorea villosa

ALSO KNOWN AS: Colic root, rheumatism root

PARTS USED: Root and rhizome

CONTAINS: Steroidal saponins, including dioscin and trillin, which yields diosgenin, alkaloids, tannins, starch

KEY USES: Antispasmodic, diuretic, anti-inflammatory, cholagogue, relaxant, peripheral vasodilator

Wild yam was until 1970 the sole source of the hormone material diosgenin, used in the contraceptive pill and other steroid hormones. This would suggest that wild yam has a significant effect on the balance of the female hormones. It was traditionally used for easing menstrual cramps and, because of its antispasmodic action, can be used for any kind of muscular spasm and colic, such as intestinal and bilious colic, flatulence, ovarian and uterine pain. The steroidal saponins are also anti-inflammatory, making it a useful herb when treating rheumatoid arthritis and inflammatory conditions of the bowel. Its diuretic effect, combined with the antispasmodic action, soothes painful conditions of the urinary tract.

In all areas of the body, it seems best adapted to irritable and excitable conditions, and less efficient when due to lack of tone. This applies particularly to pregnancy and childbirth. It has been used for any kind of cramping in pregnancy, particularly when it is related to stress and tension. It has also been used traditionally in threatened miscarriage. It has also been used with effect in nausea in pregnancy.

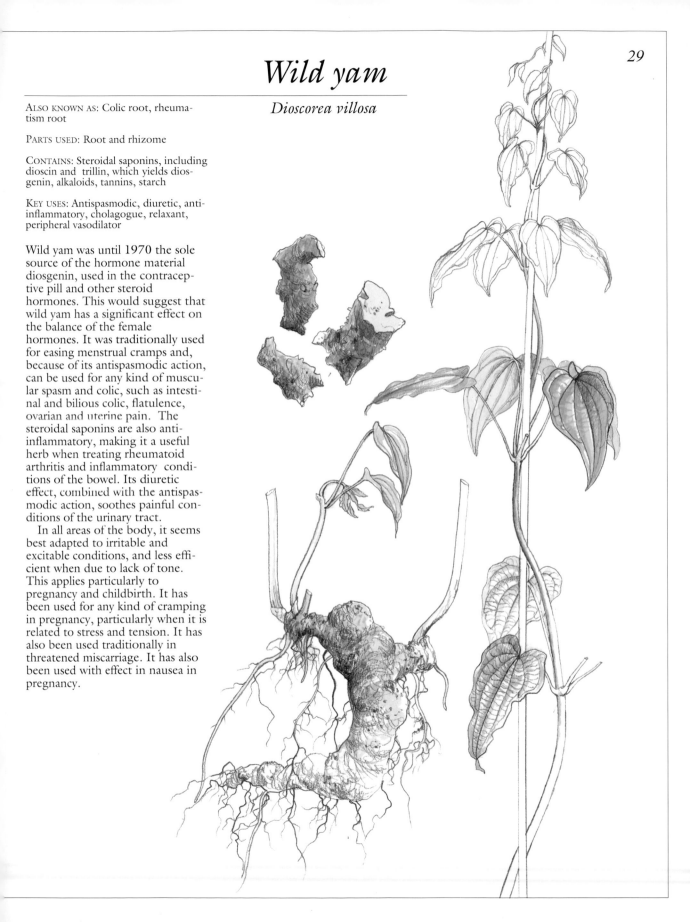

Ginseng

Panax ginseng

ALSO KNOWN AS: Oriental ginseng, Chinese ginseng, Korean ginseng, Japanese ginseng

PART USED: Root

CONTAINS: Hormone-like saponins (called ginsenosides or panaxosides), volatile oil, sterols, starch, pectin, vitamins B1, B2, B12, D choline, fats, minerals (iron, calcium, manganese, vanadium, magnesium, copper, zinc), antioxidant

KEY USES: Nervine, antidepressant, tonic, adaptogen, aphrodisiac

This famous tonic is used in traditional Chinese medicine for debility, insomnia, weakness and breathlessness which may result from stress, a debilitating illness or advanced years. In the West extensive research has found that ginseng has the amazing ability to increase resistance to stress. It acts on the pituitary gland and stimulates the adrenal glands, and by enhancing the function of the nervous system it increases mental performance, concentration and memory and decreases fatigue. It is excellent for short term use while studying for exams, or during a stressful time. It has an adaptogenic effect, being simultaneously stimulating and sedative, depending on what is required.

Ginseng has a reputation as a rejuvenating tonic, a longevity herb, delaying the aging process. The presence of the antioxidant substance will contribute to this action. Certainly the best results from ginseng are seen in the elderly and those in depleted states from stress or illness. It has a stimulating action on sexual energy, particularly if low libido is associated with stress or general debility. It can be used to reduce nervous tension and anxiety, and for nervous exhaustion and depression. It is useful during the menopause where stress is contributing to symptoms such as hot flashes. It can be used during childbirth to help pushing at second stage particularly if you are feeling exhausted and at the end of your tether.

Note Ginseng should be avoided in acute inflammatory conditions and bronchitis as it may drive the disease further into the body and aggravate the symptoms. Avoid caffeine and other stimulants while taking it, and only take for short periods, no more than 2-3 months if young, robust and active.

Cramp bark

Viburnum opulus

ALSO KNOWN AS: Guelder rose

PART USED: Bark

CONTAINS: A bitter (viburnin), valeric acid, salicylates, tannin, resin

KEY USES: Antispasmodic, partus preparator

Like black haw, cramp bark acts as a uterine sedative and a tonic at the same time. It is used traditionally where there is a tendency to miscarriage and as a partus preparator (to prepare the uterus for childbirth). However, cramp bark is a stronger antispasmodic, recommended for relieving cramps and spasmodic uterine pain, uterine irritability, over-strong contractions, false labour pains and afterpains.

Cramp bark is a specific remedy for pains in the thighs and back and a bearing-down, expulsive pain in the uterus, whether during pregnancy and childbirth or during menstruation. In menstruation, it can be used to relieve painful periods. It allays cramping pain in the legs and bladder.

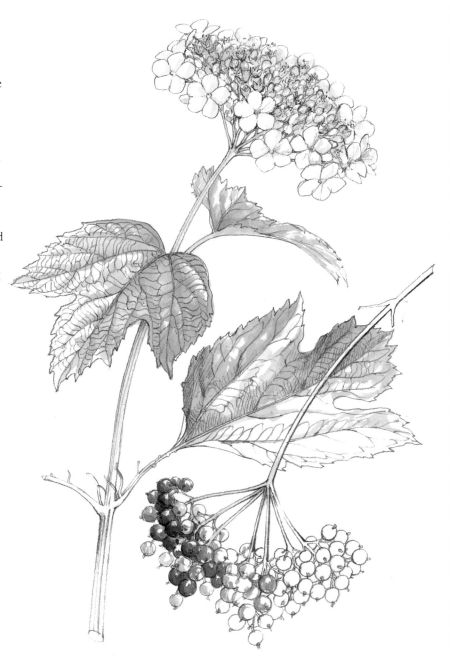

Dang gui

Angelica sinensis

ALSO KNOWN AS: Chinese angelica, women's ginseng, Tong kuei, Dong quai

PART USED: Root

CONTAINS: Beta-carotene, vitamins B and E, volatile oils, ferulic acid, succinic acid, beta-sitosterol, angelic acid, myristic acid, angeol

KEY USES: Sedative, antispasmodic, hormone balancing, detoxifying, nourishing, blood tonic, emmenagogue, analgesic

This is the best Chinese tonic herb for women, although it can also be used for men, and is the most highly valued blood tonic in the East. It is used to tonify the reproductive system and maintain normal function of the sex organs. It regulates hormones, menstruation, brings on delayed or suppressed periods, relieves menstrual cramps, and can be used during the menopause. Eaten raw or taken as a tincture, it relaxes the uterus, used with water it tones the uterus and stimulates uterine contractions, increasing circulation and relieving congestion in the pelvic area. It is best not to take it during pregnancy.

When cooked, dang gui is stimulating, antispasmodic and warming. It improves the circulation, speeds tissue repair, lowers blood pressure, slows the pulse, helps prevent atherosclerosis and blood clots and relaxes the muscles of the heart. It also acts as a sedative. It is nourishing, containing vitamins, and aids the absorption and utilization of vitamin E. It is used for anemia and angina.

Dang gui stabilizes blood sugar levels and enhances the function of the immune system. It has bactericidal, antiviral and antifungal properties and is a wonderful remedy for a whole range of infections, including colds and flu. It is a valuable blood purifier and a moistening remedy to relieve constipation. It has rejuvenative properties and helps to relieve arthritis and rheumatic pain. As a tonic it is recommended in convalescence, and to speed recovery and increase energy after childbirth.

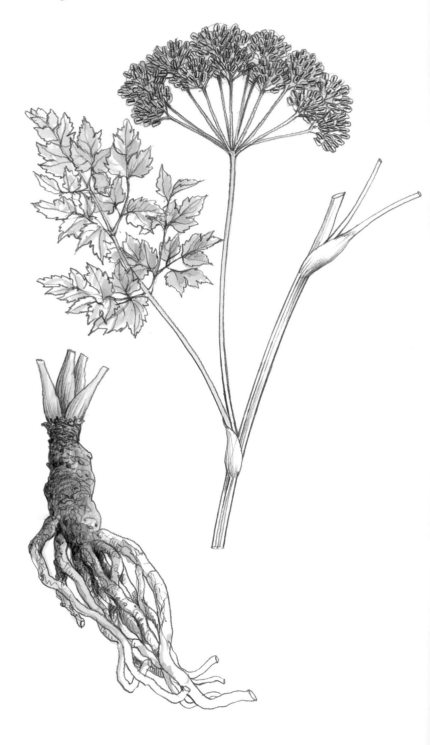

Black haw

Viburnum prunifolium

ALSO KNOWN AS: Stag bush, sweet
viburnum

PARTS USED: Bark of root

CONTAINS: Scopoletin, fruit acids, tannin, bitter resins, arbutin

KEY USES: Uterine antispasmodic,
diuretic, astringent, sedative, tonic, partus preparator

Black haw is another tonic to the
reproductive tract, toning over-
relaxed muscles while being sedative for spasmodic pain of the
uterus. It improves circulation to
the uterus and ovaries, and thereby
promotes nutrition to the pelvic
area.

Several of the plant's constituents
have been shown to have uterine
relaxant effects, notably scopoletin.
It is specific for uterine colic,
threatened abortion, lumbar and
bearing-down pelvic pain, false
pains and afterpains. During menstruation, black haw relieves
dysmenorrhea with cramping pelvic
pains and scanty flow. It is also recommended for uterine cramping
during pregnancy as well as noctur-
nal cramping of the leg muscles.

It has had a good reputation for
strengthening the reproductive system in women who have had previous miscarriages. As a uterine sedative, it was used to avert threatened
miscarriage – it has been claimed
that, once hemorrhage has started,
cure is still possible if bedrest is
insisted on, providing there are no
fetal abnormalities. Black haw has a
generally beneficial effect upon the
nervous system, and helps to calm
anxieties related to miscarriage.

If taken in the latter part of
pregnancy, it helps promote normal uterine contractions and antag-
onizes irregular ones. It prevents
afterpains, post partum hemorrhage
and helps ensure normal involution
of the uterus. Other benefits
include relief of morning sickness,
and lowering of arterial blood pressure.

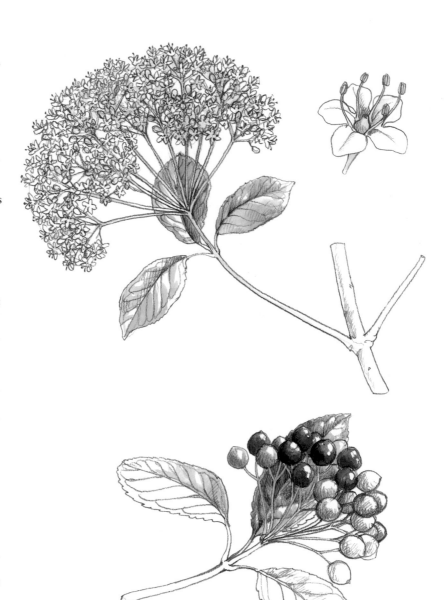

Licorice

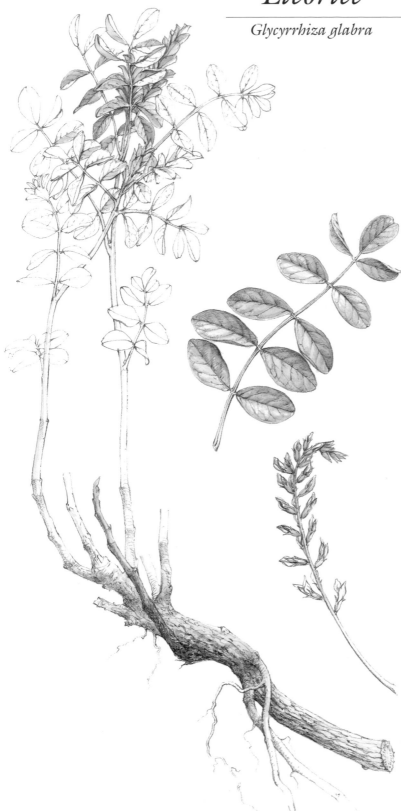

Glycyrrhiza glabra

PARTS USED: Roots and runners

CONTAINS: Glycyrrhizin (calcium and potassium salts of glycyrrhizic acid), triterpenoid saponins, flavonoids, bitter principle (glycymarin), estrogenic substances, asparagin, volatile oil, coumarins, tannins

KEY USES: anti-inflammatory, antipyretic, diuretic, expectorant

Licorice is the most remarkable herb with an affinity for the endocrine system. Glycyrrhizin has a similar structure to hormones produced by our adrenal glands, giving licorice an anti-inflammatory, anti-allergic and anti-arthritic effect similar (but without the side effects) of cortisone. The steroid-like compounds in licorice can change to estradiol and estrone which are estrogen precursors, giving licorice mild estrogenic properties – very helpful during the menopause. It is useful for people coming off orthodox steroid drugs.

Licorice has a well-documented reputation for healing ulcers. It lowers stomach acid levels and relieves heartburn and indigestion. It also acts as a mild laxative. It can be used for irritation, inflammation and spasm in the digestive tract. Through its beneficial action on the liver, it increases bile flow and lowers cholesterol levels.

In the respiratory system it has a similarly soothing and healing action, reducing irritation and inflammation and has an expectorant effect, useful in irritating coughs, asthma and chest infections. It has an aspirin-like action and is helpful in relieving fevers and soothing pain such as headaches. Its anti-allergenic effect is very useful for hay fever, allergic rhinitis, conjunctivitis and bronchial asthma.

Possibly by its action on the adrenal glands, licorice has the ability to improve resistance to stress. It should be thought of during times of both physical and emotional stress, after surgery or during convalescence, or when feeling tired and run down.

Note Avoid during pregnancy.

Echinacea

Echinacea angustifolia
Echinacea purpurea
Echinacea pallida

ALSO KNOWN AS: Purple coneflower, coneflower, black samson, rudbeckia, Missouri snakeroot

PARTS USED: Root and rhizome

CONTAINS: Essential oil, polyacetylenes, polysaccharide, glycoside, isobutylalk-lamines, resin, betain, inulin, sesquiter-pene, vitamin C

KEY USES: Immune enhancer, alterative, antimicrobial, diaphoretic, anti-allergenic

Echinacea's ability to enhance the immune system is well document-ed. It has an antibiotic and interfer-on-like antiviral action, an antifun-gal effect and an anti-allergenic action. It has also been shown to have antitumour activity.

Echinacea was used by the Native Americans for healing wounds and treating snake bites, infected conditions, sore throats and burns. Today it can be used as a blood cleansing remedy for skin problems such as boils and abscess-es, allergies such as eczema and urticaria, infections such as tonsili-tis, colds, flu, chest infections, and viral diseases such as glandular fever, as well as candidiasis and post-viral fatigue syndrome. Its beneficial effect in treatment of HIV and AIDS is currently being researched.

Echinacea has a stimulating effect on the circulation, particularly when taken in hot infusion, and by stimulating sweating it helps bring down fevers while enhancing our defenses to shake off whichever infection has caused fever in the first place.

The anti-inflammatory effect of echinacea can be put to good effect in treatment of arthritis and gout and for any inflammatory condition of the reproductive system, such as pelvic inflammatory disease.

Because of its immune-enhanc-ing properties, echinacea should be thought of at the first signs of infection to clear it quickly, and also for those whose immune sys-tems are run down and deficient and who are prone to one infection after another.

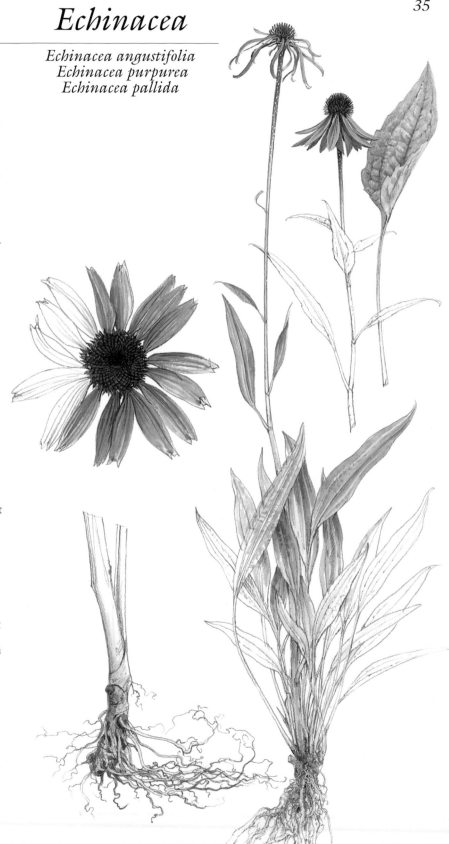

Ginger

Zingiber officinale

PART USED: Root

CONTAINS: Volatile oil (including borneol, cineole, phellandrene, zingiberole, zingiberene), starch, resin, mucilage

KEY USES: Antiseptic, diaphoretic, expectorant, digestive, antioxidant, circulatory stimulant, hypotensive, decongestant, carminative, rubefacient

Ginger has pungent and warming properties that make it a valuable medicine. It has a stimulating effect on the heart and circulation, creating a feeling of warmth and wellbeing and restoring vitality, especially for those feeling the cold in winter. Hot ginger tea promotes perspiration, brings down a fever and helps to clear catarrh. It has a stimulating and expectorant action in the lungs, expelling phlegm and relieving catarrhal coughs and chest infections.

Ginger is a wonderful warming aid to the digestion. It invigorates the stomach and intestines, stimulating the appetite and enhancing digestion by encouraging secretion of digestive enzymes. It moves stagnation of food and subsequent accumulation of toxins, which has a far-reaching effect throughout the body, increasing general health and vitality and enhancing immunity.

Ginger is famous for relieving nausea and vomiting, from whatever cause. It settles the stomach, soothes indigestion and calms wind. Its pain-relieving and relaxing effects in the gut relieve colic and spasm, abdominal pain, distension and flatulent indigestion and help to relieve griping caused by diarrhea. In the uterus it promotes menstruation, useful for delayed and scanty periods as well as clots. It relaxes spasm and relieves painful ovulation and periods, and is recommended to invigorate the reproductive system. Ginger also inhibits clotting and thins the blood; it lowers blood pressure and cholesterol.

Note Because of its heating properties ginger is not recommended for those who do not tolerate heat well or those with gastritis or peptic ulcers.

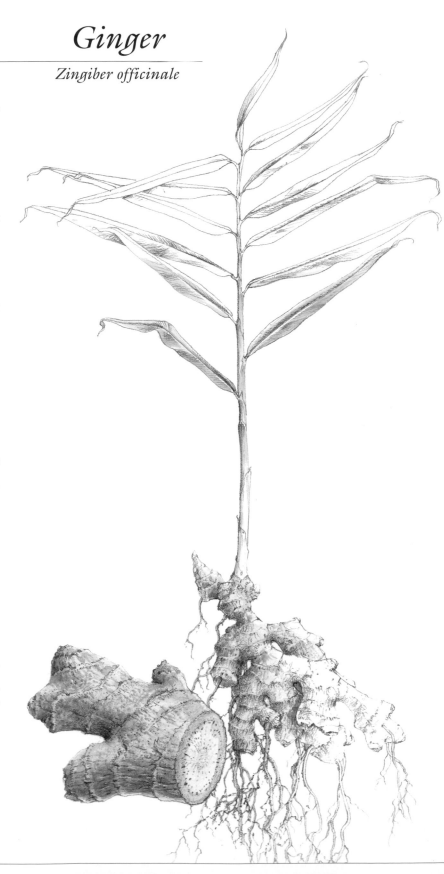

Golden seal

Hydrastis canadensis

ALSO KNOWN AS: Yellow root, orange root, Indian turmeric, eye root

PARTS USED: Root and rhizome

CONTAINS: Alkaloids (hydrastine, berberine, canadine), resin, volatile oil

KEY USES: Tonic, alterative, laxative, stomachic, astringent

Golden seal is a famous North American Indian remedy, first used for treating arrow wounds and ulcers. It acts as a tonic to the mucous membranes throughout the body, resolving inflammation and clearing phlegm. In the respiratory system it can be used for catarrh, sinusitis, colds and flu, tonsilitis, pharyngitis, laryngitis, and catarrhal coughs. In the digestive tract it reduces catarrh, gastritis, ulceration, and inflammation.

The bitters enhance liver function, and stimulate the appetite and improve digestion. In the reproductive tract its tonic and astringent action is useful for treating heavy periods, and hemorrhage, and since it stimulates the uterine muscles, it is useful during childbirth. Locally it can be used as a lotion or douche for vaginal infections such as thrush and trichomonas. In the bladder it soothes inflammation and resolves infection, and in the nervous system it acts as a tonic and sedative.

Research has shown its ability to lower blood pressure and that it possesses powerful antibacterial and antiviral properties, making it applicable to a wide range of infections. It is useful in any congested condition, including sluggish venous conditions, varicose veins and hemorrhoids, as it enhances the circulation.

Externally, use for infected gums, mouth ulcers, and sore throats, as a mouthwash or gargle. It can be used in eye lotions with rosewater or chamomile for inflammatory eye problems, and in eardrops for earache. Used as a lotion or decoction it soothes irritated and infected skin conditions.

Note Avoid during pregnancy.

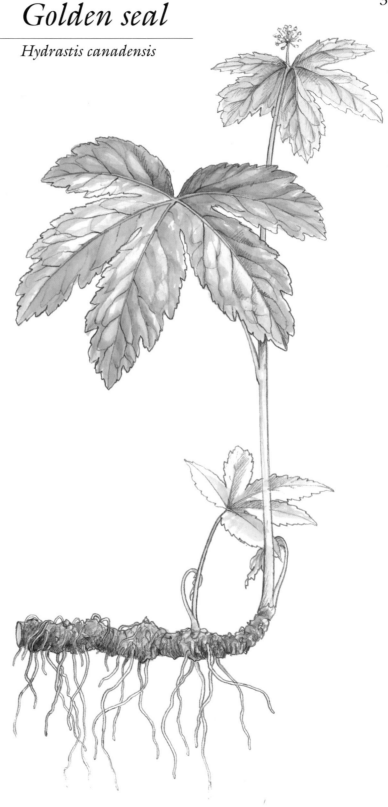

Skullcap

Scutellaria laterifolia

ALSO KNOWN AS: Helmet flower, mad-dogweed, Virginian skullcap

PARTS USED: Aerial parts

CONTAINS: Flavonoid glycosides (including scutellonin and scutellanein), volatile oil, bitter principles, tannin, iron, silica, calcium, potassium, magnesium

KEY USES: Mild astringent, tonic, nervine, antispasmodic, diuretic

Skullcap is one of the best nourishing tonics for the nervous system. It is rich in minerals necessary for a healthy nervous system, and is greatly strengthening and supportive during stressful times. It is a wonderful remedy for all states of nervous tension, for headaches, agitation, anxiety, insomnia, hysteria, neurasthenia, exhaustion and depression. Its antispasmodic action is useful for twitching or jerking muscles, trembling, epilepsy – both petit and grand mal – as well as heart palpitations. It is well worth using to aid withdrawal from orthodox tranquilizers and antidepressants, and is excellent when combined with hormone balancing herbs such as chaste tree or false unicorn root for PMS.

Skullcap also acts as an anti-inflammatory herb, and can be used for arthritis, particularly where it is aggravated by stress. It is also said to reduce fevers, to enhance the digestion and to stimulate liver function, due to the presence of bitters. It was used traditionally in North America to treat bites of poisonous insects and snakes, and for rabies, as well as to quieten sexual over-excitement and relieve menstrual cramps.

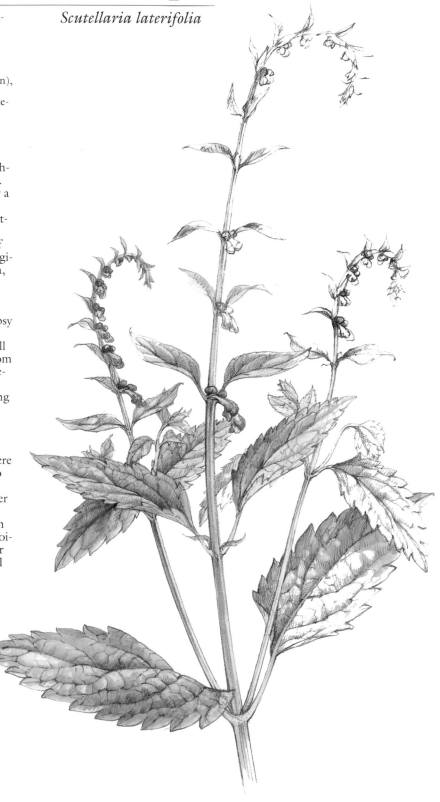

Nettle

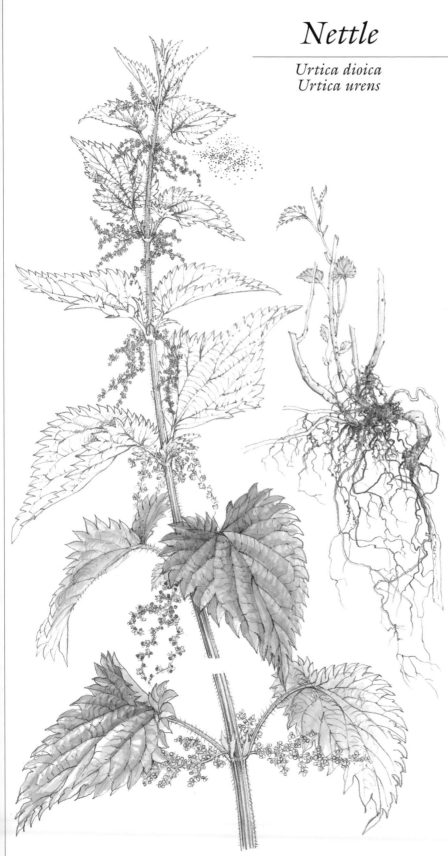

Urtica dioica
Urtica urens

PART USED: Aerial parts of young plants

CONTAINS: Formic acid, histamine, acetylcholine, vitamins A and C, 5-hydroxytryptamine, glucoquinones, chlorophyll, minerals

KEY USES: Nutrient, diuretic, detoxifying, astringent, galactagogue, decongestant, hypoglycemic

Nettles are highly nutritious, high in vitamins and minerals, particularly iron, silica and potassium, and have been used for centuries as a nourishing tonic for weakness and debility, convalescence and anemia.

Through their stimulating action on the bladder and kidneys, nettles help to cleanse the body of toxins and wastes. Nettles relieve fluid retention, bladder infections, stones and gravel. By aiding excretion of uric acid they make an excellent remedy for gout and arthritis as well as skin problems.

Their astringent action helps check bleeding. An infusion, tincture or fresh juice can be applied externally to cuts and wounds, hemorrhoids, to nostrils for nosebleeds, and to soothe and heal burns and scalds. They have been used to stem heavy periods, and interestingly to bring on delayed or absent periods. As a galactagogue they stimulate milk production; they can also make a good restorative remedy during the menopause.

In the respiratory system nettles help clear catarrhal congestion and relieve allergies such as hayfever and asthma. In the digestive tract they help remedy diarrhea, wind, inflammation and ulceration. They have been found to reduce blood sugar and a tincture of the seeds is said to raise thyroid function and reduce goitre.

Nettle juice applied to the skin relieves bites and stings, including nettle sting. The stinging hairs of the fresh nettle contain formic acid and histamine and have been used traditionally to stimulate the circulation and relieve arthritis and rheumatism.

Garlic

Allium sativum

PART USED: Clove

CONTAINS: Volatile oil, vitamins A, B, C, fats, amino acids, mucilage, glucokinins, germanium

KEY USES: Antiseptic, digestive, circulatory stimulant, diaphoretic, expectorant, decongestant, antioxidant, hypotensive, reduces cholesterol, vasodilator, hypoglycemic, cholagogue, antispasmodic

Garlic is an effective remedy against bacterial, fungal, viral and parasitic infections. Raw garlic when crushed releases allicin, which has been shown to be more powerfully antibiotic than penicillin and tetracycline.

Garlic can be used for sore throats, colds, flu, bronchial and lung infections, infections in the gut and to help re-establish beneficial bacterial population after an infection or orthodox antibiotic treatment. It is an effective remedy for worms as well as for candidiasis, and thrush in the mouth or vagina when used locally. Garlic improves digestion, relieves wind and distension, enhances absorption and assimilation of food. It also enhances the production of insulin by the pancreas, making it an excellent remedy to lower blood sugar in diabetics.

Garlic acts as a decongestant. It is an excellent expectorant remedy for acute and chronic bronchitis, whooping cough and bronchial asthma, as well as sinusitis, chronic catarrh, hay fever and rhinitis. By causing sweating it helps resolve fevers. It can significantly lower blood cholesterol.

Garlic also reduces blood pressure and a tendency to clotting, thereby helping to prevent heart attacks and strokes. It opens up the blood vessels, increasing the flow of blood to the tissues, increasing the circulation, relieving cramps and circulatory disorders. Recent research has shown that garlic acts as a powerful antioxidant and its sulphur compounds have anti-tumour activities, while it is also said to protect the body against the effects of pollution and nicotine.

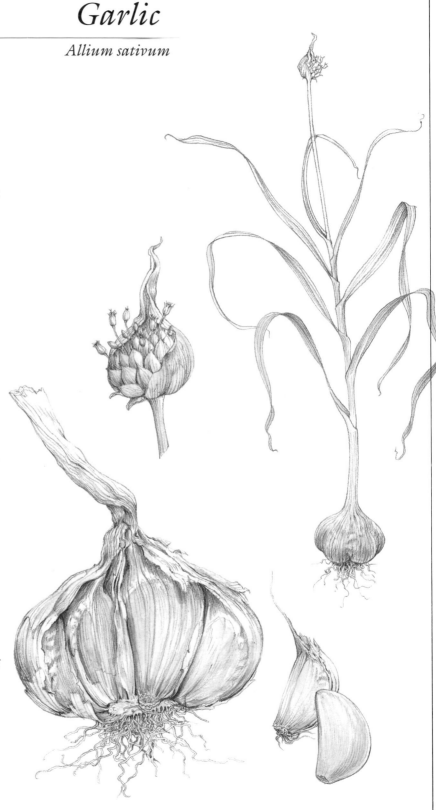

Chamomile

Matricaria chamomilla
Anthemis nobilis

ALSO KNOWN AS: German chamomile, Roman chamomile

PART USED: Flowers

CONTAINS: Volatile oil, flavonoids, coumarins, plant acids, fatty acids, cyanogenic glycosides, salicylate derivatives, choline, tannin

KEY USES: Relaxant, antispasmodic, anti-inflammatory, bitter tonic, antiseptic, diaphoretic, diuretic, analgesic, antihistamine, decongestant

Chamomile is a wonderful relaxant for the nervous system and digestion, and a perfect remedy for babies and children. It relaxes smooth muscle throughout the body. In the digestive tract it relieves tension and spasm, colic, abdominal pain, wind and distension. By regulating peristalsis, it can treat both diarrhea and constipation. It is famous for soothing all kinds of digestive upsets, particularly when related to stress and tension. The bitters stimulate the flow of bile and the secretion of digestive juices, enhancing the appetite and improving a sluggish digestion. The volatile oil has been shown to prevent and speed up the healing of ulcers when used internally and externally, making chamomile an excellent remedy for gastritis, peptic ulcers and varicose ulcers on the legs.

It is highly antiseptic, active against bacteria, including thrush (*Candida albicans*). Chamomile tea helps to bring down a fever and can be given for colds, flu, sore throats, coughs, and digestive infections such as gastroenteritis. Its antiseptic oils soothe an inflamed bladder and cystitis.

It helps relieve nausea and sickness in pregnancy, relax uterine spasm and relieve painful periods, reduce menopausal symptoms, relieve mastitis, premenstrual headaches and migraines, and treat absence of periods due to stress. It can be drunk throughout childbirth to relax tension and lessen the pain of contractions. As a general pain reliever, chamomile can be taken for headaches, migraines, neuralgia, toothache, earache, achiness during flu, cramps, rheumatic and gouty pains. It also helps resolve inflammation in arthritic joints.

Recent research suggests that chamomile acts as a natural antihistamine. It can be used for asthma and hay fever and externally for eczema.

Externally chamomile is an excellent antiseptic healer for wounds, ulcers, sores, burns and scalds. Steam inhalations help relieve asthma, hay fever, catarrh and sinusitis. It can also be used as a cream for sore nipples and a douche for vaginal infections. Sitting in a bowl of chamomile tea is wonderfully soothing for cystitis and hemorrhoids. Chamomile also makes a good antiseptic eyewash for sore inflamed eyes and a lotion for inflammatory skin conditions such as eczema and ringworm.

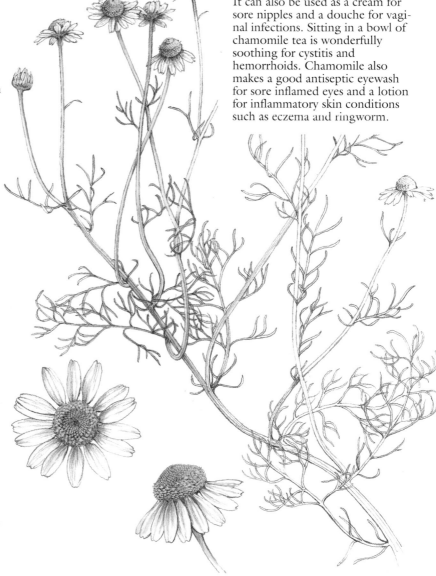

The Essential Oils

Plants contain volatile oils as part of their "essence". These essential oils are extracted from leaves or flowers and have long been used to enhance emotional and physical wellbeing, as aromatherapists do today. You can buy them at health food stores and other suppliers (see Where to Find the Herbs). Throughout this book you will find suggestions to use particular oils as part of a herbal treatment or preventative measure. The two most common uses of the oils are for massage (diluted in a base oil such as soya or grapeseed oil) and undiluted in a warm bath. Many uses recommended here are for ailments outside the scope of this book.

Note Never take essential oils internally.

Basil Migraine, headaches, aches, chest infections, digestive problems, colic, colds, catarrh, fevers. Low libido, depression, painful or scanty periods, tension, engorged breasts, PMS.
Note Avoid in early pregnancy.

Bergamot Coughs, fevers, urinary tract infections, vaginal infections or discharge. Poor appetite and eating problems, acne, boils, cold sores, chickenpox, shingles. Cuts and wounds.
Note Avoid use before exposure to sun or a sunbed.

Black pepper Constipation, colds, flu, weakness. Poor circulation, weak digestion, colic, wind, abdominal pain, muscular pain, stiffness, fatigue, rheumatic and arthritic pain.
Note Dilute well as it can irritate the skin.

Chamomile Insomnia, irritability, colic, gastritis, indigestion, peptic ulcers, diarrhea. PMS, period pains, irritable bladder, fluid retention, cystitis, eczema, boils, skin infections, allergies. Migraine, headaches, children's fevers, teething, earaches. Menopause symptoms, muscular pain, inflamed joints, sprains, burns.

Cinnamon Poor circulation, colds, flu. Rheumatism, arthritis, muscle pain. Weak digestion, colic, wind, nausea, indigestion.
Note Avoid in early pregnancy.

Citronella Repelling insects, weakness, fatigue.

Clary sage Muscle tension, PMS, depression. Uterine tension in childbirth, period pain, asthma, migraine, digestive problems. Night sweats, acne, low libido, sore throats, aches and pains.
Note In early pregnancy, avoid when taking alcohol.

Clove Toothache, headaches, weak contractions in childbirth. Bronchitis, colds, flu, diarrhea, arthritis, rheumatism.
Note Avoid during pregnancy, and on sensitive skin.

Coriander Tiredness, weakness, poor circulation, poor appetite. Digestive problems, wind, neuralgia, rheumatic pain, flu, pain.

Cypress Painful periods, heavy periods. Excessive perspiration (e.g. night sweats, hot flashes, sweaty feet), greasy skin, incontinence, poor circulation, edema, piles, varicose veins. Asthma, repelling insects, cuts and wounds, rheumatism and arthritis, muscular aches, colds, chest infections.
Note Avoid in early pregnancy.

Eucalyptus Colds, flu, catarrh, sinusitis, fevers, bacterial and viral infections, bronchitis, diseases of childhood, e.g. measles and chickenpox. Repelling insects. Urinary infections, fluid retention, cuts and wounds, skin infections, cold sores, burns, shingles. Arthritis, rheumatism, muscular pains.

Fennel Gout, toxic conditions, inflamed joints, alcoholism, wind, colic, hiccoughs, nausea, indigestion, constipation, excessive appetite. Kidney stones, fluid retention, urinary infections, irregular or painful periods, PMS, poor milk flow, menopausal symptoms.
Note Avoid in early pregnancy, in epilepsy and for children under six.

Frankincense Respiratory infections, catarrh, laryngitis, asthma, fevers. Urinary infections, heavy periods, anxiety, tension, hyperventilation, aging skin. Eczema, scarring, sores, wounds.

Geranium Depression, urinary and respiratory infections, sore throats. Greasy skin, eczema, menopausal problems, PMS, irregular periods, fluid retention. Anxiety, over-excitement, mood swings, diarrhea, kidney stones, neuralgia, circulatory problems, repelling insects.

Ginger Catarrh, sinusitis, colds, flu, chest infections, tiredness, depression, low libido. Diarrhea, rheumatism, arthritis, poor circulation, weak digestion, colic, nausea, stomach cramps, period pain, muscular pain and tension, sprains.

Hyssop Viral infections, chest infections, catarrh, sinusitis, sore throats, bruises, rheumatism,

arthritis. Skin problems, mental fatigue, circulatory problems, nervous tension, asthma.
Note Avoid in early pregnancy, and with epilepsy or high blood pressure.

Jasmine Period pain, pain in childbirth, retained placenta, low libido, postnatal weakness or depression, frigidity, tension, anxiety, especially around sexuality, depression, fear, muscle tension. Sensitive, dry skin.
Note Avoid in early pregnancy.

Juniper Toxic conditions, fluid retention, cystitis, vaginal discharge, scanty or irregular periods, piles, acne, poor appetite, rheumatism, gout, arthritis. Exhaustion, hangovers, liver problems, obesity, chest infections.
Note Avoid in early pregnancy, and in cases of kidney infection.

Lavender Depression, anxiety, tension, nervousness, insomnia, mood swings, PMS. Infections, colds, flu, coughs, catarrh, sinusitis, burns, skin infections. Injuries, cuts, wounds. Ulcers, migraine, headaches, muscular pain and tension. Rheumatism, sciatica, arthritis, period pain, scanty periods, vaginal discharge and infection. Pain in childbirth, weak contractions, retained placenta. In children: colic, infections, irritability, insomnia. Palpitations, high blood pressure. Repelling insects, insect stings, bites. Nausea and asthma.

Lemon Infections, fevers, lowered immunity, chest infections, colds, flu, catarrh, sinusitis, sore throats, ear infections and earaches. Cuts and wounds, nosebleeds. Stomach and bowel infections, diarrhea, acid stomach, gastritis, peptic ulcers, gallstones. Rheumatism, gout, arthritis, varicose veins, high blood pressure, arteriosclerosis. Greasy skin, boils and spots, verrucas, warts. Lethargy, tiredness, aging, nervous tension, anxiety.

Marjoram Chest infections, coughs, colds, flu, asthma, catarrh, sinusitis. Insomnia, headaches, nerve pain. High blood pressure, poor circulation, muscle tension and pain. Rheumatism, arthritis, sprains, bruises. Digestive problems, colic, constipation, period pain, cramp. Depression, excess libido, insomnia.
Note Avoid in early pregnancy.

Melissa Skin problems, allergies, asthma, coughs. Menstrual irregularities, period pain, infertility. High blood pressure, hyperventilation, palpitations. Shock, depression, anxiety, lethargy, insomnia. Repelling insects. Stress related headaches, indigestion, colic, diarrhea. Herpes infections, bacterial and fungal infections.

Myrrh Chest infections, colds, flu, catarrh, sinusitis. Sore throats, mouth infections, ulcers, bleeding gums. Digestive problems, diarrhea, poor appetite. Weak contractions, vaginal infections. Cuts and wounds, ulcers, athlete's foot, lowered immunity, candidiasis.
Note Avoid in early pregnancy.

Neroli Depression, insomnia, anxiety, stress, low libido, shock, sexual problems. Scarring, dry skin, aging skin. Digestive problems, colic, diarrhea, palpitations, period pains, menopausal problems.

Oregano Bronchitis, viral infections, fungal infections. Arthritis, rheumatism, muscular aches and pains. Digestive problems. Irregular, scanty periods.
Note Avoid in early pregnancy.

Peppermint Indigestion, colic, wind, diarrhea, heartburn, nausea, vomiting, travel sickness. Colds, flu, poor circulation, lethargy, depression, fevers, catarrh, sinusitis, skin problems. Migraine, headaches, nerve pain, mental fatigue, tiredness, shock. Arthritis.

Pine Catarrh, colds, flu, sore throats. Poor circulation, tiredness, rheumatic pain. Muscular pain and tension. Bladder and kidney infections, fluid retention.

Rose Maroc, or Bulgar Irregular periods, period pain, PMS, prolapse, tendency to miscarriage, gynecological problems, heavy periods, infertility. Poor circulation, allergies, tiredness, debility. Dry, sensitive skin, aging skin.
Note Avoid in early pregnancy.

Rosemary Exhaustion, poor concentration, mental fatigue, migraine, fainting, headaches, anxiety. Raised cholesterol, liver problems, constipation. Colds, flu, catarrh, sinusitis, asthma. Gout, rheumatism, arthritis, muscle tension and pain, sprains. Skin problems, aging skin, problem hair, poor circulation. Pain.

Sandalwood Urinary infections, vaginal infections and discharge, chest infections, sore throats, catarrh. Sensitive skin, acne, rashes, skin infections, fungal and bacterial infections. Low libido, nervousness, anxiety, lethargy, depression, menstrual problems.

Thyme Weak digestion, wind, poor appetite, stomach and bowel infections, diarrhea, worms. Flu, colds, coughs, catarrh, sinusitis, sore throats, asthma. Chest, gum, and mouth infections. Low immunity, thrush, urinary infections, fluid retention. Poor circulation, fatigue, depression, poor concentration and memory, insomnia. Cuts and wounds, rheumatism, arthritis. Insect bites and stings.
Note Avoid in early pregnancy.

Ti-Tree (Tea-Tree) Lowered immunity, colds, flu, childhood infections, fevers, cold sores, shingles, chickenpox. Verrucas, warts, acne, spots and boils, ringworm, burns, athlete's foot, thrush, candidiasis, glandular fever.
Note Dilute well – may irritate sensitive skins.

Ylang-ylang Hyperventilation, palpitations, shock, stress, anxiety, anger, depression, high blood pressure, insomnia, low libido, skin problems, tension, sexual problems, lack of confidence.

2 *The Well Woman*

Women have always played a central role in the health of others, both within the family and the community. Caring for the sick was one of the vitally important domestic skills handed down from one generation of women to another. Caring for others is an innate gift that goes hand in hand with being female, an ability recognized by every woman who has had children and looked after them, physically and emotionally. Women create new life and then protect it, and it often comes naturally to a woman to put the needs of others, especially those of her family, before her own, frequently at the expense of her own energy and health. For this reason, particularly in today's world, caring needs to be a balanced process. A woman needs to care for herself so that she is able to give as much as she wants to others.

At different times in a woman's life, there arise problems specific to being female. In adolescence, emerging body consciousness and sexuality, and the struggle for identity against school and family pressures, can make for very turbulent times. As a woman reaches her twenties and thirties, she may be establishing a career often in a male-dominated, stressful, competitive environment, which can create much pressure. Emotionally, long-term relationships may be established at this time, bringing all the lessons that need to be learned in order to make for harmony between man and woman. Then may come pregnancy and childbirth, making dramatic changes in her life and in her relationship with her partner. These may be deeply satisfying times for a woman, but they can also be traumatic and draining.

Caring for children is an enormous task, and wonderfully rewarding; but to be able to do it satisfactorily a woman needs a wealth of energy, patience, love, wisdom, and understanding. Just when teenage children, with their own emerging problems about sexuality and identity, need particular wisdom and understanding, a woman may be experiencing her own problems related to the menopause. When her children have babies and look to the experience and wisdom of an older woman to help them through difficult times, the caring continues, often against a backdrop of diminishing energy and health.

Many of a woman's roles in life are deeply rewarding but are also stressful.

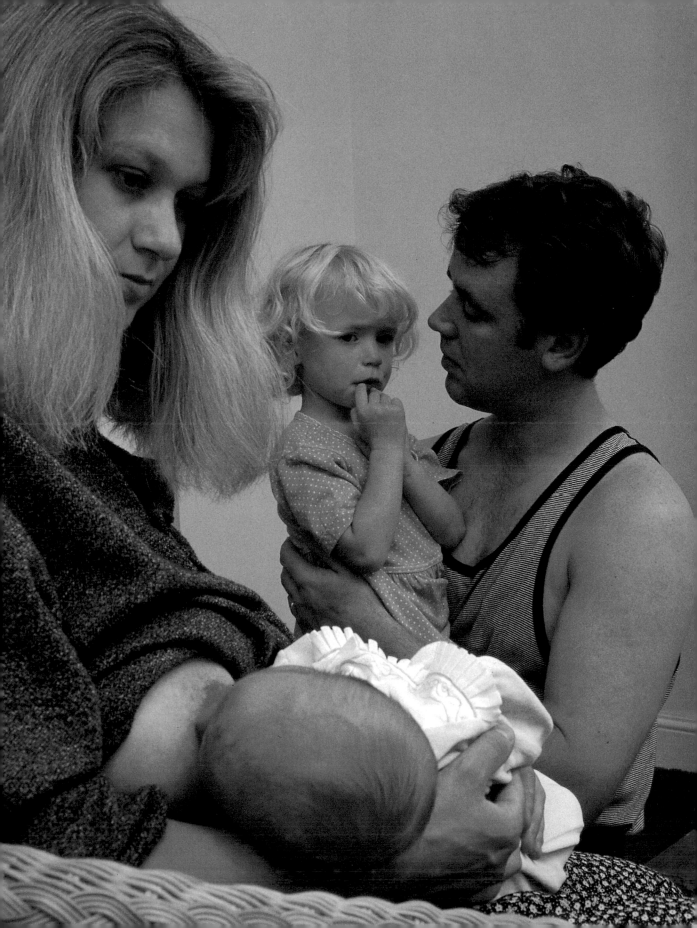

A balanced life

A vital factor in modern life is the balance between stress and relaxation. In the rushed lives of most busy women, the need for rest and relaxation is often forgotten, and as a result stress can start to take its toll.

Stress is a natural, unavoidable part of life, a facet of the human condition; as the stress expert Hans Selye said, "Complete freedom from stress is death". It is also often said that "Stress is not what happens to you – it is how you respond to it." We tend to view stress as an entirely negative force, but it is true to say that stress can be a good motivator, providing it does not get out of hand. The stress of a deadline is a challenge to finish the required work on time; depression (transient rather than clinical) may provide the impetus we need to make necessary changes in our lives. Stress can be a tool, a stimulus for action, a key to transformation.

For stress to be a positive force in our lives it needs to be balanced by calm, relaxation and freedom from stress. Prolonged stress will only serve to deplete our vital energy and lead to exhaustion or illness. It is possible to find calm and peace within ourselves despite the madness of the outside world, and for this we may need help, perhaps through relaxation, meditation, or the release of stress through bodywork such as T'ai chi or yoga, sports or dance. We need to have a haven in our lives where we can be refreshed and find renewed energy to meet the demands of everyday life.

What is stress?

Stress is a normal healthy reaction to the physical and mental demands made on us throughout each day. The physical work we do makes demands on our energy, which has to be produced by continual biochemical reactions in our bodies, even while we are asleep. The greater the physical work, the more energy is required and the more stress there is on the body, which a healthy person can deal with. In more demanding or threatening situations our bodies respond by producing a number of physical changes which speed up our reactions and prepare us for any necessary action.

Our adrenal glands are central to our stress response – they release the hormones adrenalin (epinephrin) or noradrenalin (norepinephrin), or both, into the bloodstream. This can cause increased heart rate and blood pressure, increased blood supply to the muscles and away from the skin – explaining why we may turn pale and have goosepimples if we are anxious or scared – and the release of stored glucose from the liver to provide the energy for this increased physical activity. To maintain an alert state requires a good deal of energy.

After this initial stress reaction, the symptoms should settle down, provided the demands that initiated them have been met. However, if stress is extreme or prolonged, the body may be in this alerted state for long periods of time, depleting our health and energy, and contributing to illness and nervous problems. To prevent this from happening, each woman needs to develop her own way of dealing with the stresses in her life. She needs a strategy which allows her insight into the more positive aspects of stress as a tool for transformation and joyful living.

Most of us tend to perceive stress as something that comes from outside, upsetting our balance of emotions, rather than as an internal matter. However, our emotional or mental condition and attitude influences to a great extent how we respond to what happens around us. What may cause one woman to feel threatened, scared or tense, may amuse another or pass unnoticed by a third.

While some women are prone to interpreting events and circumstances as stressful or difficult, and are chronically tense or anxious, others may consistently respond in a completely different way and remain fairly tranquil. Their metabolic and biochemical processes will be correspondingly different, their thoughts and feelings having a powerful effect on their physiological functions.

What is required is not freedom or escape from the effects of the world around us, but an ability to relax, to let go of psychological conflicts. We need a change of consciousness which allows us to be more at peace with ourselves and less susceptible to our potentially stressful environment.

Stress in women's lives

Today there is a wide range of sources of stress, from outside and inside the home, and outside and inside the body. Not only are there the perennial stresses of poverty, violence, and hardship, there are the modern pressures caused by noise and pollution.

Much has changed in modern society to make these stresses worse. In the days of the extended family there was plenty of help, support, and advice available from other women in the family. Caring for the family was a shared concern. Knowledge about the care of babies, children, and even teenagers was readily available, a free childminder was on hand, and home nursing skills were handed down from one generation to another.

The nuclear family puts a good deal more pressure on parents – women at home often feel isolated, and their anxieties, unshared by their wider family, can grow bigger and more stressful. Bringing up a young family alone can be exhausting and worrying, particularly if a child is ill and your nursing skills are negligible. Then there is the attitude to motherhood and children in a world where a career is paramount, and children are either ignored or considered a nuisance.

In the working world the juggling of a job or career with childcare can be equally stressful, especially if the childcare system breaks down. It is usually women who are made to feel responsible for childcare arrangements. Women also feel it necessary to work harder at their jobs, to prove that broken nights and family demands do not reduce their productivity or efficiency in the workplace, that women can compete on equal terms with men.

Women and their emotions

Women who live as carers play the more sensitive roles in our society; they tend to be more in touch with their emotions than men and experience a range of emotions in response to their lives that is often not acknowledged in the male world. Women's experiences are often misunderstood and undervalued, their responses interpreted as over-sensitivity, their needs considered too demanding or perverse. This may mean that many women, while continuing to support those around them, deny their own emotional needs.

For many women a major problem is a feeling of powerlessness and vulnerability. Women with children are largely expected to take sole responsibility for childcare and are often expected to devote their lives to it. Doing so may lead to financial dependence and may force some women to remain in unrewarding or destructive relationships. It can lead to lack of contact with the outside world, particularly if there are transport problems, to isolation, lack of stimulation, tension and depression. Resentments build up within the family, bringing anger between partners, or a variety of other emotions, so often unexpressed or unacknowledged as valid.

Women and their bodies

There are other sources of stress in women's lives arising from the demands of a woman's bodily rhythms, of menstruation, pregnancy, childbirth, breastfeeding, and the menopause. Added to this, women often feel very negative about their physical selves. We worry about our size or shape, and may feel inadequate sexually, and even ugly. Concern about appearances can lead us to spend precious time and money on changing or improving our looks. We allow ourselves to overemphasize the importance of the outer body while ignoring the value of wisdom and inner beauty.

On top of all the normal demands, there do occur other stresses in life that can stretch a woman to the limits of her endurance – a miscarriage, stillbirth, or cot death; divorce, heartbreak, or bereavement; single parenthood; illness either in herself or her family. It is hardly surprising that sometimes women fail to cope with stress and fall prey to stress-related disorders such as chronic anxiety, tension, depression, nervous exhaustion, or insomnia. They may also be prone to illnesses such as digestive problems, headaches, recurrent infection, and gynecological disorders.

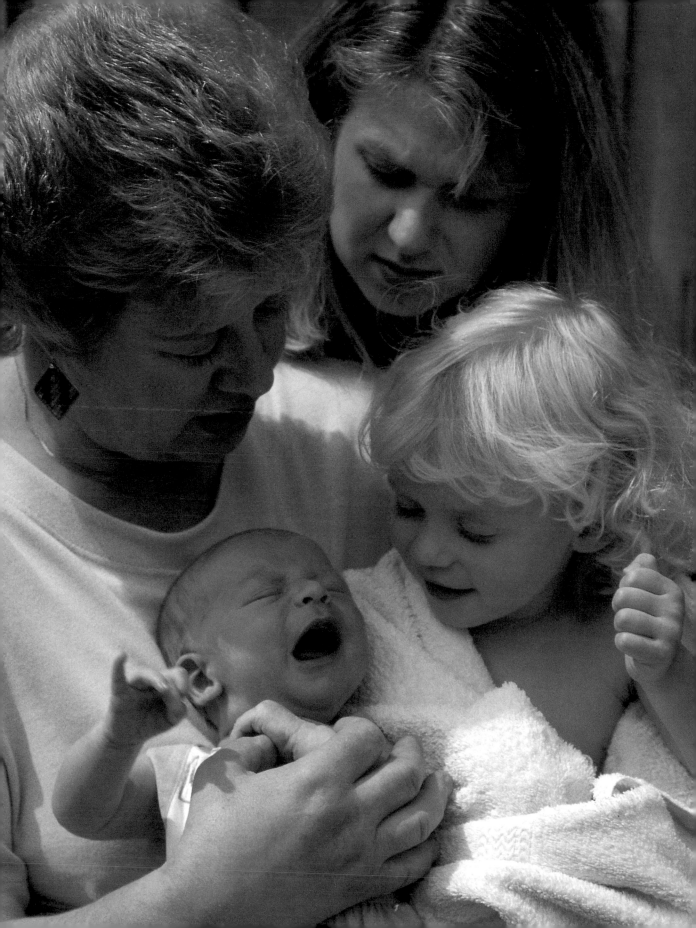

The mind and the body

It is generally understood that because of the strong connection between them, the mind and the body are equally likely to be the origin of an illness. Emotional problems are often manifested physically, while at the same time physical illness affects the way we feel.

Thoughts and feelings create activity in the brain which affects messages sent to the rest of the body. The higher centres of the brain concerned with our senses, creativity, thoughts and memory are connected to another part of the brain called the hypothalamus and are constantly influencing it (see p.187). When we feel stressed, threatened, or scared, messages are relayed to the adrenal glands which spark off the "fight or flight" mechanism.

Adrenaline and noradrenaline are secreted by the adrenal glands producing a variety of changes in the body including:

Increased heart rate or palpitations
Increased respiration
Tightened muscles ready for action
Increased blood pressure
Goosepimples and pallor as blood supply to the skin is restricted to increase blood supply to the muscles
Diversion of blood away from the digestive tract so that the digestive system stops working properly and temporarily shuts down
Drying of the mouth as saliva dries up
Enlargement of the pupils
Mobilization of the liver's energy stores and release of glucose into the bloodstream
Decrease of urine output as blood flow to the kidneys is reduced
Inhibition of the immune system

If the physical changes brought about by adrenaline and noradrenaline are prolonged, they may give rise to symptoms such as:

High blood pressure
Heart problems
Hyperacidity in the stomach
Gastritis and peptic ulcers
Bowel problems such as irritable bowel syndrome, diverticulitis, and colitis
Recurrent infection, candidiasis, ME
Headaches or migraine
Skin problems
Menstrual pain and irregularities
Muscle tension or back problems
Insomnia
Depression, fatigue, poor mental performance
Poor circulation
Sexual problems

It is not hard to see how our thoughts and feelings can profoundly influence our metabolism, our hormone balance and fertility (see also p. 88).

Since it is clear that some women are more prone to these kinds of problem than others, stress is very much a matter of how we respond to a situation rather than the situation itself. If you are prone to feeling stressed there is plenty that you can do to enhance your ability to cope so that it does not deplete you and lead to emotional problems or physical illness.

It is important to eat regularly to prevent falls in blood sugar which can exacerbate feelings of stress. Try not to feel guilty about any of the so-called bad habits such as eating chocolate or drinking coffee. Changes in diet need to be gradual, and an integral part of enhancing general health. They are best made along with other lifestyle changes, such as starting a regular exercise and relaxation routine, seeking support from herbal remedies, and counselling if necessary. Inner and outer changes need to go hand in hand.

Sleep is a wonderful healer and replenisher of vital energy. To sleep well it is best to avoid stimulants such as caffeine and to relax for a few hours before going to bed. Ginseng and B complex supplements taken too near to bedtime may also increase alertness. Magnesium, B6, and zinc are all helpful in relieving insomnia.

Food allergies, or intolerances, or chronic infections such as candidiasis (see p.226) can upset both mind and body, causing emotional symptoms – irritability, depression, mood swings, anxiety, and lethargy – as well as physical problems. Dairy products and wheat are the most common allergens.

It is important to have plenty of fresh air and exercise if only for the sense of wellbeing they give. A brisk walk for half an hour once or twice a day may be quite sufficient; it will help alleviate tension and depression, and encourage restful sleep.

Try to minimize stress in your life whenever possible, even down to small details. By tidying the house or workplace you may gain a sense of order and achievement and by completing any unfinished tasks such as writing letters, returning phone calls, or paying bills, you can relieve the unpleasant feeling of work hanging over you when trying to relax properly.

Having some time to yourself regularly, without interruption, is important in order to replenish your energy. We all need to take time to reflect and get right away from daily pressures and responsibilities. Relaxation, breathing or meditation techniques, prayer, or simply a period of quiet, all enable us to look within ourselves for a while. It is there that our healing ability lies, in the innate wisdom that we all possess which can guide us through our lives and particularly our difficult times. Inner clarity and calm are vital to balance stress, to keep it in its right context and to prevent it from getting out of hand.

It is easy to feel that snatching even a few minutes alone is completely impossible. In this case try to assert your need for this and ask your partner or other members of the family to look after your small children for a little while regularly – preferably half to one hour a day. Make sure that when they are asleep you use the time to look after your own needs.

If your job is stressful or unsatisfying, finding rewarding spare-time activities will help to keep you balanced and make you feel better about your life. If your relationship with your husband or partner is difficult and you feel unsupported, it is important to nourish supportive friendships; those with other women will probably be most rewarding. Women may be better able to empathize and understand your sources of stress. It is important to express and work through any problems you have with your husband or partner, and if you find this impossible you may benefit from consulting a family therapist or counsellor.

If you feel inadequate, either physically or in any context of your life – as a wife, mother, cook, professional – try not to punish yourself or use this negative self-image to push yourself into forever striving to be better. Try to work towards a more positive view of yourself; seek help from other women by talking to them about your feelings. Together you could look at the deeply entrenched attitudes which make you dislike or criticize yourself. Feeling better about yourself will stop you wasting an enormous amount of energy, and will increase your ability to accept things as they are, or else work for change.

It is said that the key to self-healing is compassion – compassion for oneself, affirmation of the life force that flows through us just as it does through every other living thing. A new perception of things as they really are, rather than as how we think they are, can be enhanced by quiet meditative times when we can be in touch with our real selves.

Caring for ourselves using herbs

Herbs can be used to help us to restore balance in our lives, and to enhance our health and ability to function effectively and energetically. Several herbs such as nettles, kelp, oats, horsetail, borage, and dandelion are wonderfully nutritious, and provide us with essential vitamins, minerals and trace elements to supplement our diets. If we have a specific tendency to problems in one physical system or another, be they circulatory problems, respiratory ailments, digestive problems, or joint problems, the world of herbs has a wealth of remedies to offer us, to enhance our own healing abilities and to go hand in hand with other necessary changes in our lives to enhance our health and wellbeing. When stress weighs heavily upon us, and upsets the dynamic balance necessary for health and vitality, herbs for the nervous system can provide enormous support.

Herbs for the nervous system

Herbs work on the nervous system in a variety of different ways. Nervine herbs act as tonics, feeding and strengthening the nervous system and enhancing its healthy functioning. Very often when you are exhausted or debilitated from prolonged or severe stress, a nervine tonic will restore balance in the nervous system and reduce anxiety, ease sleep, relax tension, and lift depression – without any need for tranquilizers or antidepressants.

Oats are a wonderful tonic to the nervous system, supplying many of the nutrients that it may be lacking. They act as food for the nerves, and are recommended particularly for nervous exhaustion, depression, lethargy and weakness. Oats can be taken during difficult times as a preventative and protective herb, to enhance your ability to cope with stress.

Skullcap is probably my favourite nervine, supporting the nervous system, relieving stress and anxiety, tension and spasm, while lifting depression, and increasing energy and *joie de vivre* in those feeling exhausted and run down. It can be relied upon in all problems connected with stress.

Vervain is similarly relaxing, relieving tension and anxiety, easing depression and nervous headaches, and reviving depleted energy. It has the added benefit of acting as a tonic to the liver.

Ginseng has the amazing ability to increase the body's resistance to stress, and can be taken for a period of two to three months by young people who are under stress of exams, or depleted by illness or emotional problems. It is particularly suited to elderly people who feel tired and run down, depleted by stress or illness. It acts as an adaptogen, relaxing tension and anxiety but also stimulating those feeling tired and debilitated, protecting those under stress from fatigue and nervous exhaustion.

Wood betony is strengthening and relaxing at the same time. It is recommended for nervous exhaustion, anxiety, and tension and is particularly useful for headaches and migraines related to stress.

Sage is excellent for nervous exhaustion and can be used to strengthen the nervous system and enhance the ability to cope with stress. It is particularly useful during the menopause.

Relaxants
Some herbs are particularly suited to those who feel in need of calm and peace in their lives, who are tense, fearful, anxious, restless, agitated, and cannot sleep. They can safely be used instead of orthodox tranquilizers and are completely non-addictive.

There are many herbs which have relaxing or sedative properties, including:

lavender	motherwort
blessed thistle	cramp bark
pulsatilla	chamomile
passionflower	lemon balm
rosemary	black cohosh
St. John's wort	hops
skullcap	linden blossom
catmint	

Each of these herbs, as well as relaxing mind and body, has a variety of different actions, and should be chosen according to the affinity they have for particular systems in the body and stress-related symptoms which you may be experiencing. For example, chamomile, lemon balm, and hops have an affinity for stress-related digestive disorders, releasing tension in the gut muscles, enhancing appetite and digestion, soothing colic and spasm, and relieving a range of digestive problems.

Lemon balm and motherwort benefit the heart and relieve palpitations; black cohosh, cramp bark, pulsatilla, and motherwort relax uterine muscles and are excellent remedies for stress-related period pains. Rosemary, lavender, black cohosh, and St. John's wort will help relieve headaches, while linden blossom will reduce high blood pressure. Lemon balm can help people who get worked up to the point of feeling almost hysterical, and for those who feel depressed. It has a calming effect and helps the mind and body to let go and relax. It gives renewed energy to an over-tired system. Taken as tea, lemon balm is delicious; taken at night it relieves tension and induces sleep, taken first thing in the morning it is refreshing and sweeps away tiredness.

Anti-depressant herbs
Several herbs have thymoleptic or "mood elevating" properties, easing depression and debility, or the lethargy associated with it.

These anti-depressant herbs include:

oats	borage
rosemary	St. John's wort
skullcap	vervain
lemon balm	lavender
ginseng	linden blossom
blessed thistle	

Liver remedies
The liver is responsible for filtering the blood and removing wastes, contaminants, or toxins, which might cause damage in the body or interfere with normal functions. If the liver is not functioning properly then toxic materials remain in the bloodstream and can affect the nervous system by interfering with the function of the brain and central nervous system. This can create a feeling of apathy, lethargy and particularly depression. When using herbs for the nervous system and to give support during emotional crises, it is always important to include liver remedies in the prescription – choose from rosemary, calendula, dandelion root, yellow dock root, or burdock.

Tonic herbs
Several of the warming aromatic herbs increase general energy and vitality, and have a beneficial and strengthening effect on the nervous system. Such herbs include ginger and cinnamon, cloves, and cardamon. They lift the spirits, chase away lethargy, depression, and winter blues, to give a feeling of wellbeing. The alkaloid in capsicum stimulates the secretion of endorphins (opiate-like substances in the brain) as does vigorous aerobic exercise, giving a sense of optimism, and a feeling of vitality and good health.

The systems of the body

It is important to understand the body, how we affect it by the way we live, and what the effects are when imbalances occur. Such knowledge will enable us to feel secure in our bodies and more in touch with our ability to heal them. It will help us be aware of the language our bodies use – the symptoms we exhibit which tell us that imbalances require our attention. We can be grateful that our bodily problems have their symptoms, because they can be a wonderful incentive for change.

The digestive system

The digestive system enables our bodies to convert the natural resources of the world around us into the energy we need for our daily lives, and for the continuous biochemical reactions that go on within us.

The digestive tract is a tube which runs for about 36 feet (11 metres) from the mouth to the anus. Because it opens at both ends to the outside world and yet travels right through the middle of us, it makes for constant interaction between our inner and outer environments.

Some say we are what we eat, others say we are what we digest and assimilate. Either way, our health and vitality both depend on how efficiently our digestion makes available to us the vital nutrients from our food. The digestive tract is lined with a mucous membrane which serves to protect it, and to secrete digestive juices containing enzymes that are necessary to break down food into a form we can absorb. Other digestive enzymes are supplied to the digestive tract by the liver, pancreas and gallbladder.

The digestive tract itself requires energy to do its work. If our digestive energy is depleted, problems arise, which produce symptoms such as stomach aches, diarrhea or constipation. A weak digestion also affects our health and energy generally, resulting in lethargy, irritability, poor concentration and sleep problems, nutritional deficiencies, and allergies. Aromatic herbs such as ginger, cinnamon, thyme, rosemary, garlic, and fennel will all enhance digestive energy and ease digestion and absorption.

For our digestive tracts to remain healthy we need to evacuate food residues and the waste products of metabolism from the bowel. Otherwise, a toxic bowel state can result, and in this state the bowel is prone to infection and the spread of toxins into the rest of the body. Regular bowel movements require sufficient fluid as well as roughage in the diet so that food is pushed down the alimentary canal. The health of the bowel and the regularity of bowel motions also depend on the bacterial population living in it. A diet high in meat and refined carbohydrates will encourage a proliferation of putrefactive bacteria at the expense of the beneficial bacteria encouraged by eating plenty of fresh fruit and vegetables. Live yoghurt, olive oil, and garlic will help maintain the right bacterial population in the gut, while yellow dock, root, golden seal, dandelion root, licorice and burdock will all ensure regular evacuations.

The circulation to and from the digestive tract, and the secretion of digestive juices, are regulated by the autonomic nervous system. Stress can have a disrupting effect on the digestion – for example it can cause excess acidity in the stomach which can irritate and inflame and eventually ulcerate the lining of the stomach or intestine. Absorption of food depends upon its being broken down by digestive enzymes and this process is very susceptible to the effects of mind and emotion, personality, and constitution. Herbs such as chamomile, lemon balm, rosemary, catmint, and lavender will relax mind and body, and ease digestive problems related to stress.

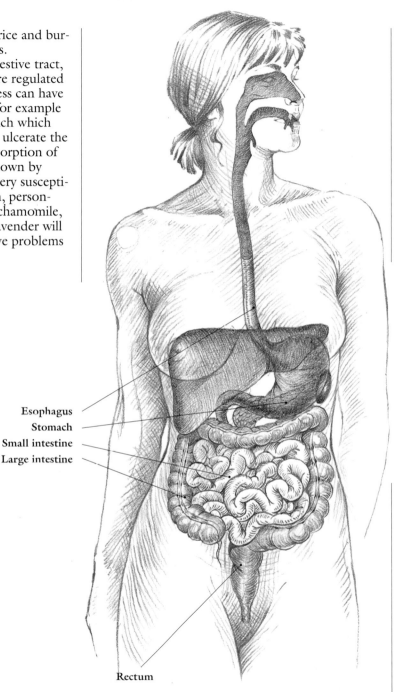

Esophagus
Stomach
Small intestine
Large intestine

Rectum

Digestion starts in the mouth where our food is partly broken down by chewing and mixing with digestive enzymes in saliva. Once passed down the esophagus into the stomach, the food is further broken down by digestive juices, including hydrochloric acid, and then moves into the small intestine. Here it is mixed with more digestive enzymes as well as bile from the gallbladder, and most of the nutrients are then absorbed into the bloodstream and carried to the liver. The undigested and indigestible parts of our food pass into the large intestine where most of the water and some nutrients are absorbed into the bloodstream, while the remainder passes to the rectum where it awaits evacuation.

Rosemary

Rosmarinus officinalis

PART USED: Aerial parts

CONTAINS: Volatile oil, flavonoids, phenolic acids, carnosic acid (rosmaricine) triterpenic acids, tannins, bitter principle, resins

KEY USES: Diuretic, antiseptic, circulatory stimulant, rejuvenating tonic, antioxidant, expectorant, decongestant, digestive, bitter tonic, astringent, relaxant, carminative, antispasmodic, antidepressant

Rosemary contains volatile oils which are antiseptic, with antibacterial and antifungal properties and which enhance the function of the immune system. By increasing circulation to the skin rosemary causes sweating and makes a good remedy to bring down fevers. Its warming and stimulating properties help to clear phlegm from the head and chest, useful for relieving colds, flu, catarrh, coughs, wheezing, bronchitis and whooping cough. Its additional relaxant effects help relieve spasm in the bronchial tubes as in asthma.

Rosemary is a wonderful tonic, particularly to the heart, brain and nervous system. By increasing the flow of blood to the head, it stimulates the brain and heightens concentration. It has been used for anxiety, tension, exhaustion, lethargy, depression, insomnia and as a tonic during convalescence and for the elderly. Rosemary makes an excellent remedy for preventing and treating migraines and headaches. It improves vitality and stimulates digestion, relieves flatulence and distension, enhances the appetite and increases the flow of digestive juices. It helps move food and wastes efficiently through the system, removes stagnant food, improves sluggish digestion and helps absorption of nutrients. Its bitters stimulate liver and gallbladder function, increasing the flow of bile and aiding digestion of fats. Rosemary is famous as a rejuvenating tonic and is said to slow the aging process. It is a powerful antioxidant, preventing damage by free radicals.

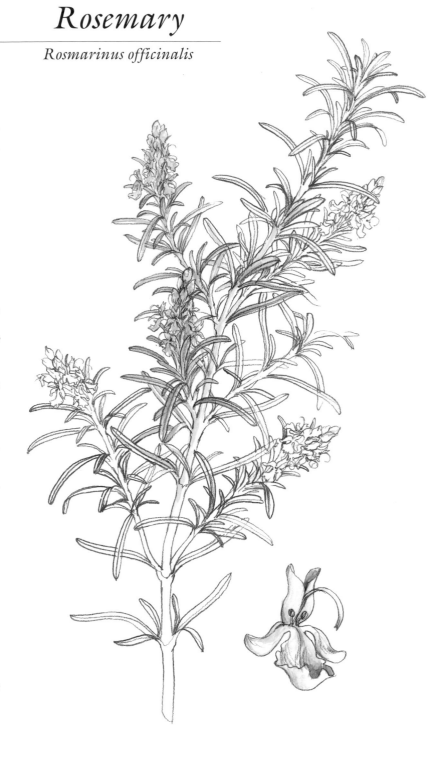

The urinary system

The urinary system performs the vital task of producing and excreting urine, so cleansing the body of waste products and toxins. It also helps to maintain a constant internal environment by governing the water and chemical composition and the acid-alkali balance of the body.

The two kidneys collect chemicals and fluid from the blood flowing through them. They regulate the amount of water and determine which chemicals are passed out as urine and select those to be reabsorbed back into the bloodstream for our bodily requirements. If much water is lost through other channels, particularly from the skin in sweat during exercise or hot weather, less is excreted in the urine. In cold weather, when less is lost in sweat, the urine flow is more abundant. If we drink large volumes of water, the kidneys will excrete a correspondingly greater amount.

Along with water, the kidneys collect the waste products of metabolism, such as urea from the breakdown of protein, as well as salts including sodium chloride, and nitrogen-containing substances such as uric acid. Valuable substances such as glucose and amino acids will be reabsorbed, while substances the body does not need will be voided as urine. It is important to drink plenty of fluid, around four pints (2 l) daily, to flush these out in the urine, otherwise they can concentrate in the kidneys and cause irritation. This in turn can lead to infections such as cystitis, and the formation of stones and gravel.

Healthy adults pass about three pints (1½ l) of urine daily, while another two pints (1 l) of fluid is passed out through the lungs, skin and bowels. Herbs that enhance urination are a useful part of any cleansing regime – these include mild diuretics such as corn silk, meadowsweet, cleavers, chamomile, plantain, and dandelion leaves.

The kidneys have other important functions. Through a hormone produced in the kidneys called renin they can cause constriction of arteries in the body, causing a rise in blood pressure. A kidney imbalance can therefore be one of the reasons for persistently high blood pressure. The kidneys also produce erythropoietin, a substance that stimulates the formation of red blood cells in the bone marrow.

Kidney tonics such as cinnamon, borage, horsetail, plantain, dang gui, corn silk, and saw palmetto will help maintain kidney energy.

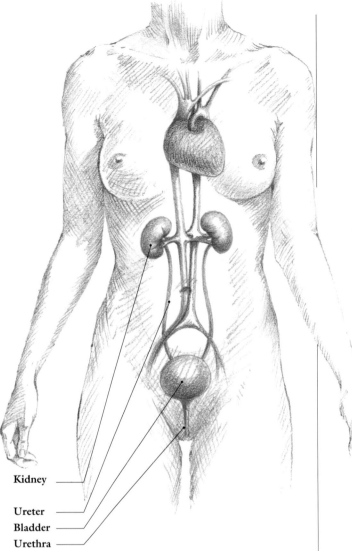

Kidney

Ureter

Bladder

Urethra

Urine collects in the pelvis of the kidney from which it passes out by a slender tube, the ureter, into the bladder. The bladder resembles a muscular bag, which stretches as it slowly fills the neck of the bladder, which connects to the urethra. It is normally kept closed by rings of firmly contracting muscles which we learn to control in early childhood. Once the bladder is fully distended, a stimulus is sent to the brain telling us it is time to empty it. During urination, urine is passed out of the bladder through the urethra.

The respiratory system

While the digestive system breaks down the food we eat, the respiratory system is responsible for deriving energy using the air we breathe. Through respiration we take in oxygen from the atmosphere, the vital ingredient for the metabolism of each cell in the body.

We can live without food and water for a few days, but without air we cannot survive for more than a few minutes. In many cultures and religions the use of the breath is central to spiritual practices such as yoga and meditation, and traditional movements like T'ai chi and Qi Gong. Correct breathing is also vital for our nerves and muscles because it permits relaxation as well as keeping the mind clear and alert. The value of deep breathing is recognized for helping to counter stress, to ensure sleep, and during childbirth to enhance normal uterine contractions and help with pain control. Herbs such as lavender, chamomile, and rosemary and essential oils such as frankincense, neroli, and clary sage will calm the nerves and relax muscles, and also slow down and deepen the breathing.

Most adults breathe in and out between 10 and 15 times each minute, but this can be increased enormously, by up to 15 times, when taking exercise, because a greater supply of oxygen is needed to maintain exertion. The amount of air that we take in on each breath is important to our health – if we breathe shallowly and take little exercise, our bodies will be trying to function with inadequate oxygen.

The origin of respiratory problems can lie in the respiratory system itself, for it is open to the atmosphere at the nose and mouth and therefore vulnerable to airborne infection. Troubles can also arise when the respiratory system becomes overloaded with toxins. It works alongside the skin, bowels and urinary system as an organ of elimination, and excess toxic waste in the body can cause extra work for the respiratory system.

Normal function of all body tissues is maintained so long as the blood carries adequate nutrients and oxygen to each body cell and carries waste products away. To ensure sufficient oxygen is taken in, we need to take plenty of fresh air and exercise and to breathe properly. Is the air we breathe really fresh? Even when we breathe properly, the air we breathe may be smoky, and polluted with carbon monoxide and lead from car fumes. The pollution in our lungs is then carried in the blood all around the body.

Poor diet, particularly one high in meat, refined carbohydrates, and dairy produce, will contribute to a toxic state of the body, congested bowels and nutritional deficiencies. These can give rise to congestion, allergies and infections affecting the respiratory system. Herbs such as garlic, thyme, sage, chamomile, rosemary, ginger, cinnamon, and lemon balm taken regularly will help prevent accumulation of catarrh and infection.

The lungs are covered by a thin membrane, the pleura, which is doubled back to line the chest walls forming an airtight cavity, the thorax, to house the lungs. At either side of the lungs lie the ribs and intercostal muscles and diaphragm. On an inward breath, the rib cage lifts upwards and outwards, depressing the diaphragm, and air rushes in through the nose and trachea to fill the space created in the lungs. On an outward breath, the intercostal muscles and diaphragm relax back into place, the lungs deflate and the carbon dioxide and water in them are released into the atmosphere.

Our respiratory systems consist of the nose, throat, larynx, trachea, bronchi, and lungs. Air is breathed in through the nose and mouth and passes into the trachea, which divides into two tubes, the bronchi, which pass into the left and right lungs. Each bronchus divides into smaller and smaller tubes called bronchioles, which finally expand into the air sacs or alveoli, which have elastic tissue enabling them to be stretched as they fill with air. Surrounding the alveoli are networks of capillary blood vessels and between these and the alveoli occurs an exchange of vital gases.

Hemoglobin in the blood has a great affinity for oxygen which thus passes from the alveoli into the bloodstream, while the blood releases carbon dioxide produced by tissue respiration and metabolism into the alveoli to be expelled into the atmosphere.

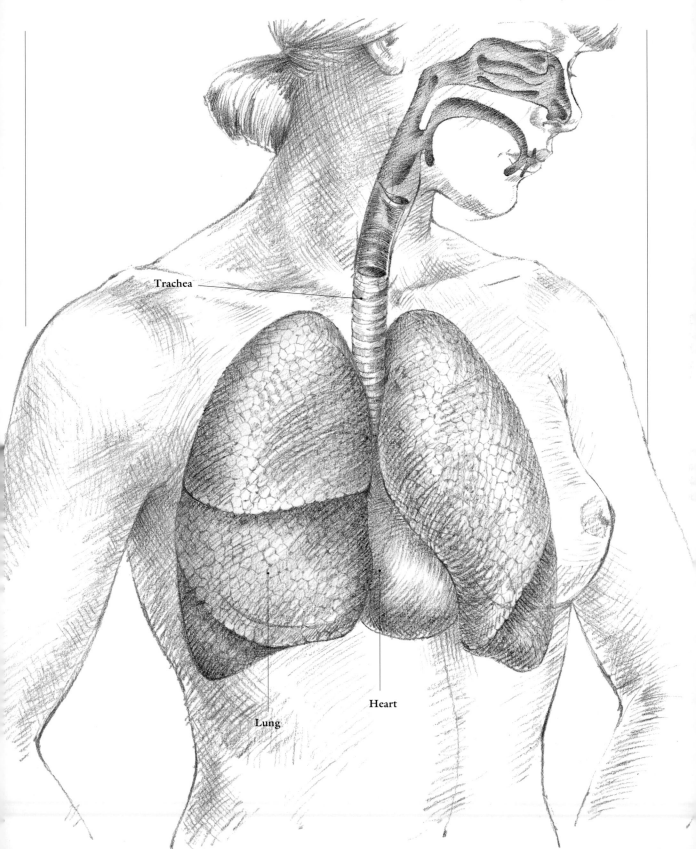

Trachea

Lung

Heart

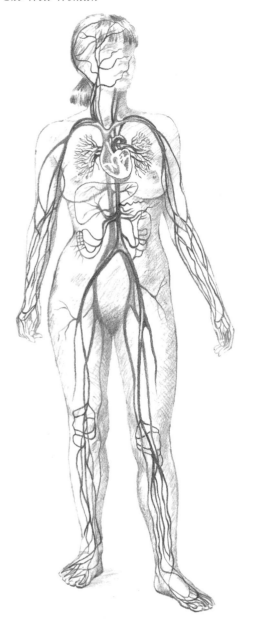

The circulatory system

The heart and blood vessels comprise the vital transport system of the body, carrying essential nutrients to every cell in the body and removing the waste products of metabolism. In the adult body there are eight to ten pints (4-6 l) of blood, made up of a clear yellow fluid, plasma, in which are floating millions of red and white blood cells and platelets. The red blood cells contain hemoglobin which picks up oxygen from the lungs and carries it around the body. The white blood cells form a vital part of the immune system, engulfing disease-carrying microbes and producing antibodies to neutralize them and the toxins they produce. Platelets are involved in the clotting mechanism of the blood. Plasma makes up more than half the volume of blood and contains proteins, salts, glucose, and substances in transit from one part of the body to another, either nutrients or waste products.

So that this transport system works healthily and efficiently it is important to take good care of our heart and blood vessels. In the West, cardiovascular disease, including coronary heart disease, high blood pressure, heart attacks, and strokes, causes more than half of all deaths. It is related to inadequate exercise, stress, smoking and poor diet – all of which we can remedy.

Herbs such as hawthorn, linden blossom and yarrow help to reduce high blood pressure. Hawthorn is a wonderful tonic to the heart, horsetail helps to strengthen the blood vessels and protect against fatty deposits in the arteries, while cayenne and ginger stimulate the circulation and help to warm those prone to poor circulation and feeling the cold. Ginkgo helps to guard against the effects of aging in the arterial circulation.

The blood is pumped round the body by rhythmical contractions, or beats, of the heart, normally occurring around 72 times a minute and more than this during exercise. The heart is made of muscle which never tires. From the lungs oxygenated blood passes through the pulmonary vein into the left side of the heart from where it is pumped into the aorta, the main artery in the body, and is distributed through the arteries throughout the body. The arteries divide into smaller and smaller arteries and then into arterioles and microscopic capillaries which carry blood right amongst the cells where the oxygen is used in respiration. The capillaries then join together to form small veins, which again join to form larger ones which carry deoxygenated blood from the cells back to the right side of the heart from where it is pumped into the lungs to release its carbon dioxide and water and pick up more oxygen. On its way round the body the blood picks up nutrients from the diet from the liver and intestines and water and wastes are filtered from it by the kidneys.

Vervain

Verbena officinalis

PART USED: Aerial parts

CONTAINS: Glycosides (verbenalin, verbenin), alkaloid, bitter principle, volatile oil, tannin

KEY USES: Nervine, tonic, antispasmodic, diaphoretic, galactagogue, hepatic, sedative, astringent

Vervain is a wonderful tonic to the nervous system, calming the nerves and easing tension. It used to be held as sacred, as a holy herb for sacrificial rites, revered by the druids as highly as mistletoe. It was dedicated to Isis, the goddess of birth, and was a famous ingredient in love potions. It can be taken to relieve anxiety, to lift depression and for stress-related problems such as headaches and migraines as well as nervous exhaustion. The bitters stimulate the liver and enhance digestion, making vervain useful for problems related to a sluggish liver, including lethargy, depression, headaches and irritability. It has been used for liver disorders and gallstones, and to increase energy during convalescence. In hot infusion it acts as a diaphoretic, increasing sweating, and can be used for bringing down fevers.

During lactation vervain increases the flow of breastmilk and because it brings on menstruation and stimulates uterine contractions is best avoided in pregnancy. It can be used during the birth to enhance contractions. Its diuretic properties make it useful for fluid retention and gout.

The tannins in vervain make it a useful astringent for bleeding gums and mouth ulcers when used as a mouthwash, and for sores and wounds and insect bites when used as a skin lotion.

Note Avoid in pregnancy.

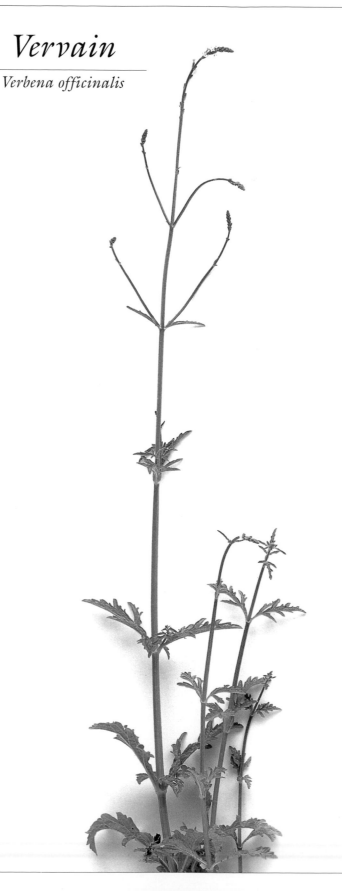

Calendula

Calendula officinalis

ALSO KNOWN AS: Marigold, marybud, bull's eyes

PART USED: Flowers

CONTAINS: Carotenoids, resin, essential oil, flavonoids, sterol, bitters, saponins, mucilage

KEY USES: Antiseptic, astringent, anti-viral, diaphoretic, detoxifying, antispas-modic, estrogenic, anti-inflammatory, bitter tonic, diuretic

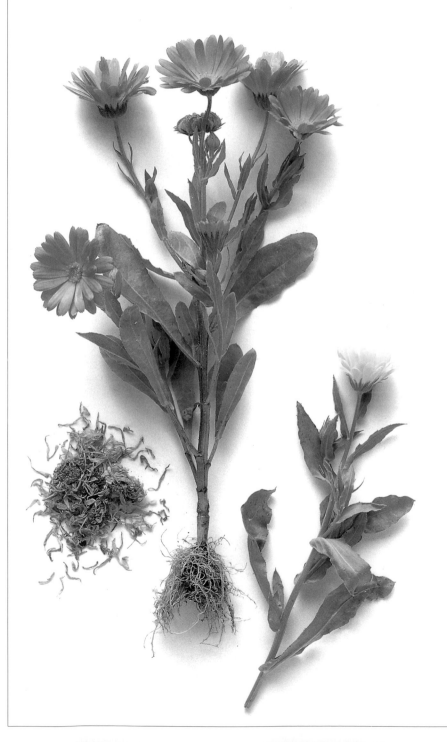

Calendula has antiseptic and astringent properties, stimulating the immune system and helping the body fight against infections such as flu and herpes viruses. It reduces lymphatic congestion and swollen lymph glands. It is antibacterial, and is one of the best plants for treating fungal infections such as thrush. It has been used for pelvic and bowel infections, including enteritis, dysentery, worms and amebae, and for viral hepatitis.

In hot infusion calendula stimulates the circulation and promotes perspiration, helping the body to deal with toxins and eruptions such as measles and chickenpox.

Calendula has an affinity for the female reproductive system, regulating menstruation and relieving menstrual cramps. Its estrogenic effect helps at menopause and reduces breast congestion. Its astringent properties help reduce excessive bleeding and uterine congestion. It has a reputation for treating tumours and cysts. During childbirth it promotes contractions and delivery of the placenta.

In the digestive tract calendula makes a wonderful healing remedy for gastritis and peptic ulcers, for inflammation and irritation of the lining of the stomach and bowels. It checks diarrhea and stops bleeding. By enhancing the function of the liver, calendula helps to cleanse the body of toxins.

Calendula has pride of place as a first aid remedy for cuts, abrasions, and as an antiseptic healer for sores and ulcers.

Note Calendula should not be used internally in pregnancy.

The reproductive system

The female reproductive tract is wonderfully suited to carrying out its supreme function – to bear children. The uterus or womb is perhaps the most important of the reproductive organs for it is here that the fertilized ovum is developed, nourished and protected until it is ready to enter the world and carry on a separate existence.

The fallopian tubes are passages joining the ovaries to the uterus, along which a mature ovum or egg cell passes each month and where it may or may not be fertilized. The ends near the uterus are very narrow but the tubes open out towards the ovaries into frilly, fringe-like fingers which reach down and curl over the ovaries to aid the entry of the egg at the time of ovulation.

The two ovaries consist of a number of egg cells or ova, which in response to hormonal messages from the pituitary gland are one by one developed to maturity and released once a month in the middle of the menstrual cycle, ready for fertilization by a male sperm.

The healthy functioning of the reproductive system is predominantly governed by hormonal messages. For a full account of these hormones see p.86. The relationship between the female hormones is delicately balanced to ensure optimum fertility and smooth functioning of the reproductive system. For a correct hormone balance to be maintained, both body and mind need to be healthy. If the diet is faulty, the circulation poor, if stress is causing muscle tension or there is anxiety or other emotional problems, the hormone balance will be upset and the menstrual cycle disrupted. There is now a wealth of information on the effects of diet on the reproductive tract and the menstrual cycle, and healthy eating, often combined with nutritional supplements, will help correct many such imbalances. Medicinal herbs which have been used effectively since ancient times to provide a range of remedies which correct hormonal imbalances and ensure the normal healthy working of the whole reproductive system.

The womb or uterus is shaped like a flattened pear and is kept in position in the lower abdomen by a sling-like band called the broad ligament. The top of the uterus is joined to the two fallopian tubes and it is connected below to the vagina. The neck of the womb is the cervix. The uterus is mainly composed of muscle which can be stretched extensively, large enough to hold a full-term baby (or two or three), and also contract effectively to expel the baby from the womb during the birth.

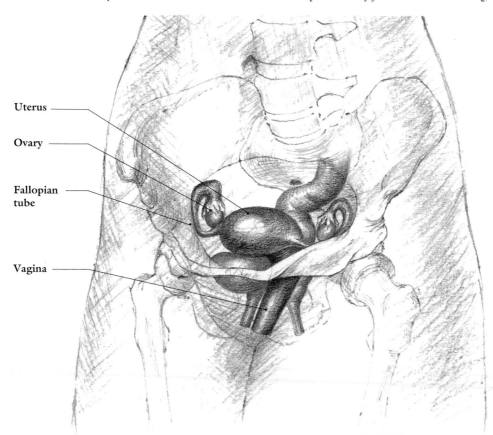

Uterus

Ovary

Fallopian tube

Vagina

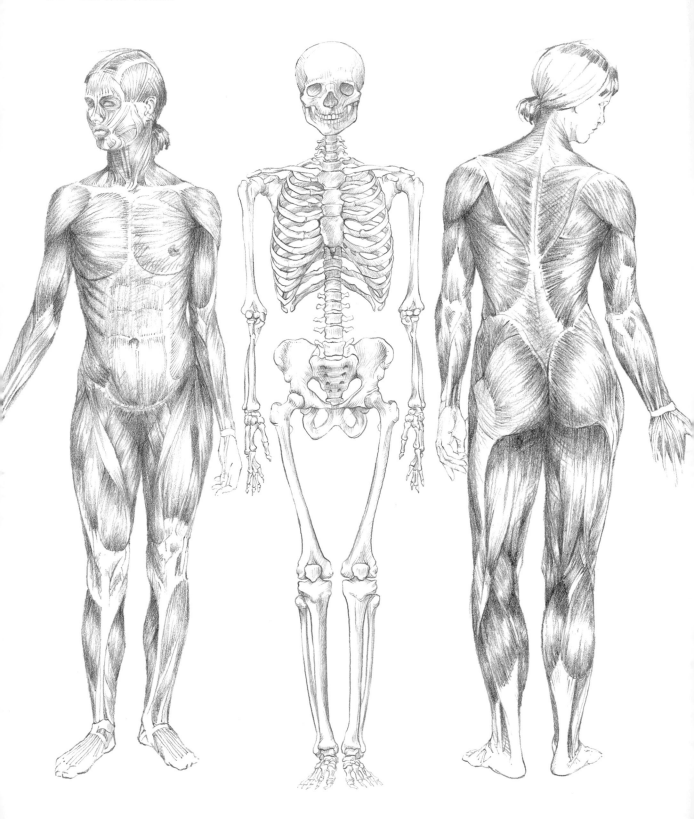

The musculo-skeletal system

Muscles and nerves together control the movements of the body, enabling it to carry out the skilled movements that characterize humans. To allow these to take place the body has a jointed framework, the skeleton, without which the rest of the body would fall into a soft shapeless mass.

The central pillar of this framework is the spinal column, or backbone, to which all other bones are directly or indirectly attached. Where bones meet, joints are formed, some of which are moveable. Each moveable joint consists of a smooth-lined cavity supplied with cushions of cartilage, or gristle, and fluid to enable the bones to glide easily over one another.

In order that the bones are sufficiently rigid to provide support, they contain a high percentage of calcium. They are amply supplied with blood vessels and from the blood they obtain materials for their formation, growth, and maintenance such as calcium, phosphorus, and sodium. For laying down of firm bones, vitamins A, D, and C are vital.

Bones are hollow in the middle and in this space is found bone marrow, a substance very rich in fat and in some bones the source of new red blood cells. The fact that bones are hollow makes them lighter but does not lessen their strength. The strength of bones largely depends on how much we use them. The more weight-bearing exercise we take, such as walking, jogging or dancing, the more active are the bone-forming cells and the more thick and strong the bones grow.

Muscles, which enable us to move, are composed of bundles of fibres which possess the power of contraction. There are three kinds of muscle – voluntary, involuntary, and cardiac. Voluntary muscles are attached by strong ligaments to the bones of the skeleton and act as levers. Voluntary muscles differ from involuntary ones in that we can exert control over them. Involuntary muscles are found in hollow structures such as blood vessels, the uterus and the digestive tract; while cardiac muscle makes up the greater part of the wall of the heart. The function of a muscle is to exert force and do work, the energy for which is produced by the "burning" of sugar in the body, giving off heat and carbon dioxide. So muscles have the vital function of helping to maintain the body at the temperature essential for its proper functioning.

Like bones, the size and strength of our muscles depend on the amount of work they are called upon to do. Regular exercise is important, for if muscles are not used enough they will become unhealthy and permeated by fat. Loss of muscle strength is not an inevitable feature of later life, it is very much related to how much we use our muscles. This in turn has a significant effect on the strength and density of bone. Adequate muscular exercise can therefore help prevent the onset of osteoporosis.

At the same time the health of our musculo-skeletal system is affected by our diet and metabolism, assimilation and elimination, as well as by our posture, and how we physically use our bodies. A healthy diet, with plenty of B vitamins, calcium, magnesium, and potassium, is vital in allowing proper relaxation of our muscles. Stress and negative emotions play an enormous part in the way we use them. Unexpressed emotions may cause chronic muscle tension, while negative emotions are often expressed in our muscles – our posture, our freedom of movement, our facial expressions, our body language. Relaxation is also very important to the health of muscles and the whole body.

Remedies such as cramp bark, skullcap, passionflower, lavender, and linden blossom will relax nerves and reduce tension in muscles. Nutritious herbs such as oats, horsetail, and nettles will provide valuable nutrients for bone formation and repair, for cartilage elasticity and muscle relaxation.

Circulatory stimulants including cayenne, ginger, cinnamon, and garlic will all enhance blood flow to the muscles and bones to ensure their proper function, formation, and repair.

Where an accumulation of toxins in the tissues contributes to joint problems such as arthritis and gout, or to muscular rheumatism, alterative herbs such as burdock, yellow dock, nettles, echinacea, and poke root will help to cleanse the system.

Diuretics such as borage, meadowsweet, and celery seed are also helpful. Certain herbs with anti-inflammatory properties will be beneficial for painful inflamed joints – echinacea, meadowsweet, licorice, wild yam, and feverfew can all be used.

Supplements of evening primrose oil with marine oils, as well as the antioxidants selenium and vitamins A, C, and E are useful adjuncts to herbal treatment.

The immune system

The defensive system of the body is such that despite the millions of potentially disease-producing microbes, such as bacteria, viruses, fungi, and parasites that surround and inhabit us, we only occasionally fall prey to infection.

We have several intricate mechanisms which prevent the entry of disease-carrying organisms into our bodies, among which are:

Eyes with antiseptic tears

Nose with sticky mucus, and hairs to trap microbes

Sneezing which expels dirt and microbes forcibly

Mouth with antiseptic saliva

Chest with mucus and hairs trapping organisms and pollutants to stop them from reaching the lungs

Coughing which expels them forcibly

Stomach with acid that destroys organisms

Intestine with bacteria that hold unwanted organisms in check

Bowels which excrete them along with toxins

Bladder which flushes out organisms and toxins through the urine

Vagina with acid that destroys organisms

Skin which secretes sebum and antiseptic oils

Acid mantle in the skin which holds infective organisms in check

A waterproof outer layer of skin to protect underlying tissues

If any of these defence mechanisms fails and microbes invade the body, the immune system calls into action two different systems of attack, one to deal with all types of invaders, the other with more specific responses to certain organisms.

When microbes invade the body, through a cut in the skin for example, an inflammatory response occurs which will repel the invasion and heal the damaged tissues. Extra blood flow to the area brings white blood cells as well as certain chemicals and plasma proteins to the rescue. If the infection is not cleared, more powerful white blood cells (monocytes) move in to attack and destroy microbes, and should this not work, the lymphatic system is called into the fray. The lymph picks up debris and microbes and carries them to the lymph nodes where there are concentrations of white blood cells, including macrophages, which engulf the microbes. There are also lymphocytes there which produce antibodies to the invading organisms. Should these measures not repel a highly infectious invasion, specific immune responses come into effect. Molecules on the surface of the infecting organisms (antigens) stimulate lymphocytes to produce antibodies to combine with each specific antigen. These antibodies have a memory, so that should the same infection recur, the antigens are recognized so rapidly that the body is able to deal effectively with the organisms in the lymphatic system and bloodstream before an infection develops. When this happens, one is said to have immunity.

Once bacteria and viruses have been destroyed in these ways, the debris needs to be cleared from the system, and this involves the work of the liver. The liver has an intricate system of tiny blood vessels lined with white blood cells which destroy unwanted matter brought in the bloodstream. Other matter such as dead cells, drugs, hormones, toxins, and substances such as pesticides and food additives are rendered harmless by various enzymatic reactions.

For the immune system to function efficiently it requires certain raw ingredients, including plenty of proteins, essential fatty acids, vitamins, minerals, and trace elements. These include vitamins A, B, C, and E, copper, iron, magnesium, selenium, and zinc. Certain food substances actually act against the immune system, including sugar, salt, saturated fats, refined oils, preserved and processed foods, fried foods, and caffeine.

Stress has far-reaching effects on our immunity, causing the body to overuse valuable nutrients required for normal function of our defence mechanisms, and depress antibody function, while calming thoughts and meditation have been shown to activate our immunity and to increase effective function of white blood cells in the blood. Certain herbs have the wonderful ability to enhance our immune mechanisms, including garlic, huang qi, dang gui, licorice, borage, wild yam, echinacea, ginseng, and myrrh.

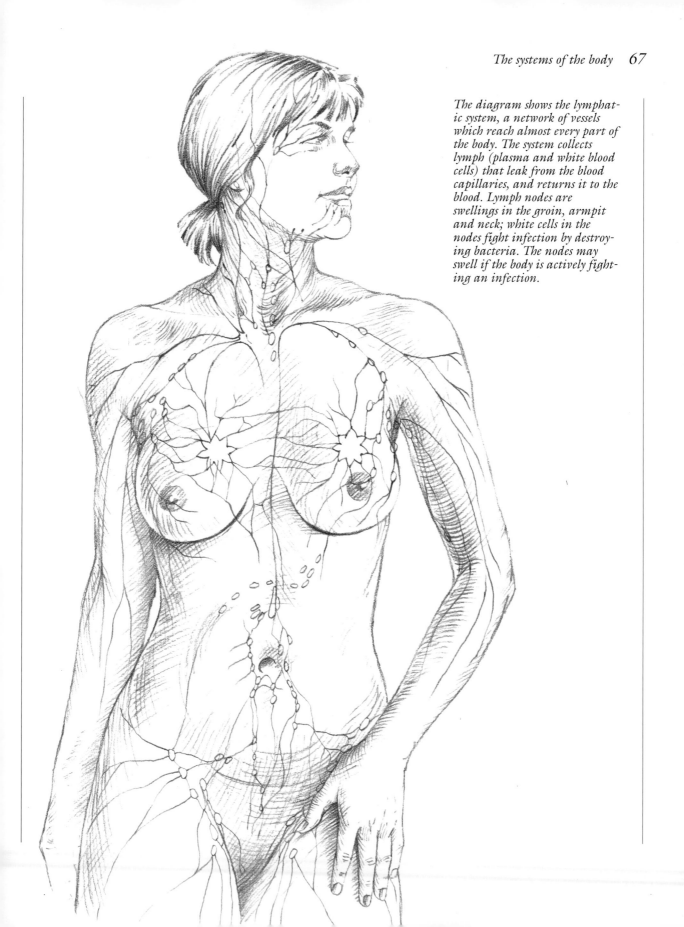

The diagram shows the lymphatic system, a network of vessels which reach almost every part of the body. The system collects lymph (plasma and white blood cells) that leak from the blood capillaries, and returns it to the blood. Lymph nodes are swellings in the groin, armpit and neck; white cells in the nodes fight infection by destroying bacteria. The nodes may swell if the body is actively fighting an infection.

Good nutrition

Diet, the mind, and the emotions have an interdependent relationship. How we feel psychologically affects what we eat, how it is digested, absorbed, and assimilated, and how the body uses it. In turn, our nutrition affects our psychological health.

People vary widely in their psychological composition, and so also in their nutritional requirements. Research has shown that serious psychological trauma can hugely increase the need for certain nutrients such as vitamins B and C, and that unless some of the resulting inner disturbance and conflict is resolved, this will continue indefinitely. If the necessary nutrients are taken, this will aid enormously the ability to cope with and resolve conflict and stress. If not, nutritional deficiency will develop and considerably diminish vital energy and resilience to stress.

A healthy diet, with plenty of fruit and vegetables, nuts and seeds, and whole grains, should provide most of these nutrients. However, it is important to take extra, in the form of supplements, during times of stress. This could be a preventative measure, or as part of treatment for stress-related problems, such as tension, anxiety, depression, debility, or insomnia.

Sugar

Stress tends to cause a craving for sugar, which unfortunately can in turn further increase stress. The reason for this is that sugar consumption can upset the balance of our blood sugar – when it rises we may experience a surge of energy but it then drops and we may feel weak, anxious or irritable, and crave something sweet to eat again.

The liver should regulate the amount of sugar going into the bloodstream but if it is not working efficiently it will fail to do so, and there will be peaks and troughs in blood sugar levels. Alcohol can upset the liver and cause it to function sluggishly; a high protein diet, the use of drugs, and pollutants in food all further limit its efficiency.

Low blood sugar (hypoglycemia) imposes stress on the body because if the blood sugar drops too low the nervous system does not work properly. Low blood sugar is interpreted by the body as a danger signal and the adrenal glands respond to this by secreting adrenaline, putting into action the "fight or flight" mechanism described on

p.50. This has the effect of mobilizing glucose stores from the liver to raise the blood sugar, but it also causes fear, palpitations, shakiness, cold and clammy hands, and breathlessness – which are often interpreted as misplaced anxiety.

These mood swings, indicating changes in blood sugar levels, seem to aggravate any existing stress and decrease our ability to cope with it. They make extra demands on the adrenal glands, increase the amount of adrenaline in the system and serve to deplete our vital energy. They could also contribute to stress-related illness.

When trying to understand why some people are more prone to hypoglycemia than others, the role of the pancreas must also be considered. The pancreas secretes insulin which causes sugar in the blood to enter the body's cells, and also glucagon which helps to regulate the release of stored sugar from the liver into the bloodstream.

Stress may be a major factor in the regulation of both insulin and glucagon secretion from the pancreas, and resultant imbalances of blood sugar. However, regular consumption of refined sugar may also cause the pancreas to function erratically, causing poor sugar control, which becomes even worse under stress. In this way a vicious circle is created, and under even minimal stress we may fly off the handle for no apparent reason, be overly sensitive, or overreact to stress.

Vitamins and minerals

The greater the demands that stress imposes on our energy and physical processes, the greater the need for nutrients to support them. There are certain nutrients which are vital to normal function of the nervous system and of which we need an adequate supply at all times. Unless they are in plentiful supply during times of stress a deficiency may arise, further exacerbating any stress-related problems. It is apparent that some people naturally require more of certain nutrients for the nervous system than others, and these people more easily become deficient, making them particularly prone to stress, anxiety, depression and psychiatric problems. Many of the important vitamins and minerals are described on the Diet chart on p.70-73, giving their sources and their functions in the body. Vitamins and minerals are both involved in neurotransmitter production, and the transport of vital blood components to the brain, so that the nervous system works properly.

Vitamins B and C are considered to be the most important vitamins in the battle against stress. A diet high in sugar, refined carbohydrates, junk foods, and carbonated drinks may cause a deficiency of vitamin B, which can upset the nervous system, causing symptoms such as insomnia, anxiety, agitation, nightmares, fatigue, night sweats, poor appetite, bowel problems, depression, and recurrent infections.

Vitamin B3 may be deficient in people with a low protein diet particularly if they have a high alcohol intake. It can cause irritability, fatigue, anxiety, headaches, insomnia, poor memory, emotional instability, and skin problems. There may be diarrhea and a sore tongue in some extreme cases.

Vitamin B6 deficiency can cause anxiety, depression and personality changes – often experienced before a period as premenstrual syndrome. It can be a result either of poor diet or of taking the contraceptive pill.

Vitamin B12 deficiency can give rise to depression, fatigue, nervousness, and anxiety. It may arise during stressful periods because gastric acidity, necessary for proper B12 absorption, is reduced in some people with emotional problems.

Vitamin C (ascorbic acid) has been researched widely for its ability to enhance resistance to stress and its use as a treatment for nervous and psychiatric problems. It has been found for example that schizophrenics can require 70,000 mg of vitamin C before their body reaches saturation, while others may only need 4,000 mg. Emotional stress and strain causes the body to use much more ascorbic acid.

Essential fatty acids are vital to normal function of the nervous system. Make sure you have plenty of unrefined vegetable oils in your diet and eat nuts and seeds and fatty fish to boost your intake.

Zinc deficiency has been shown to be related to depression, irritability, mood swings, tearfulness, sullenness, as well as schizoid behaviour. Zinc requirements increase considerably during pregnancy and lactation, and deficiency at these times may well lead to postnatal depression, and hormonal problems after childbirth. Zinc is required for normal hormone balance.

High copper levels – often found in women on the pill – upset zinc balance in the body, and have been associated with irritability, mood swings, and senile dementia.

Potassium deficiency can occur from excess losses of potassium in the urine, resulting from taking diuretics, or drinking too much tea, coffee or alcohol, or from diabetes. It is associated with lethargy, debility, depression, and mental apathy.

Calcium and **magnesium** are essential for proper relaxation of nerve tissue. Deficiencies can cause cramps, muscle tension and twitching, headaches, PMS, poor appetite, apathy, debility, tiredness, anxiety, panic attacks, hyperactivity, insomnia, and depression.

Iron deficiency is linked to lethargy, tiredness, depression, anxiety, heart palpitations, and poor concentration.

Refined carbohydrates – white bread and pasta, white sugar, polished rice, and junk food should all be avoided. Not only do they contribute to constipation, giving

rise to a toxic system which predisposes to a range of illnesses, but also they lead to nutritional deficiencies, notably of magnesium, calcium, and B vitamins. They also upset your sugar balance. While alcohol can have a relaxing effect, ideally it should be kept to a minimum or avoided completely. It creates high urinary loss of magnesium and destroys vitamins B and C, zinc, and potassium.

Caffeinated drinks such as cocoa, cola drinks, chocolate, tea, and coffee should be avoided, as caffeine is well known to exacerbate the effects of stress by potentiating adrenalin. It also causes loss of vitamins B and C. Tea and coffee substitutes such as dandelion coffee, instant chicory, and herbal teas are preferable. Bear in mind that caffeine withdrawal can lead to lethargy and headaches for a few days.

Smoking destroys vitamin C and puts further stress on the body. It is obviously best avoided, but if you are a smoker and feel you depend on cigarettes to relieve tension, it is important to provide yourself with alternative support, such as herbal nervines and tonics, before you try to kick the habit to prevent causing yourself further stress.

Diet chart

This chart summarizes our main nutrients, their sources in our diet, and their functions in the body. The result of deficiencies in some nutrients is described on p. 69.

Nutrient	*Function*
Protein	
Complete proteins: meat, poultry, fish, eggs, milk, yoghurt, cheese, soya products **Incomplete proteins**: nuts and seeds; beans and pulses; grains Protein consists of twenty-three amino acids, most of which we manufacture in the body, but eight of which (nine in children) we obtain from our food. **Complete protein** foods contain all these amino acids; there are also three groups of **Incomplete protein** foods, items from which can be combined in order to make complete protein	*Proteins are the basic building blocks of all body tissues, so they – and their constituent amino acids – are essential for growth and repair. They are particularly important, therefore, in the diet of babies and children. Antibodies, enzymes, and hormones are proteins, too, so protection against infection, body metabolism, and coordination of tissue function depend upon a full and regular supply of all 23 amino acids* *Extra protein is needed during pregnancy and breast-feeding, after illness and for those who do heavy manual work or heavy exercise* *The body cannot store excess protein*
Fats	
Polyunsaturated fats: fish and fish oils, nuts and nut oils, vegetable oils	*Polyunsaturated fats are needed to help the body absorb trace elements and fat-soluble vitamins A, D, E, and K from food. They are involved in making adrenal and sex hormones, and maintaining a healthy population of bacteria in the gut, healthy skin and circulation*
Monounsaturated fats: nuts, seeds, olive oil	*Monounsaturates are good substitutes for saturates*
Saturated fats: dairy produce, meat, processed fats, refined oils, coconut oil, palm oil	*Saturates provide concentrated energy, as well as insulation and protection. Should be kept to a minimum as excessive amounts may lead to cardiovascular disease, obesity and many other problems*
Essential fatty acids (in polyunsaturates): seeds, nuts, pulses, beans, unrefined vegetable oils, oily fish, fish liver oils	*EFAs are vital to the normal development of nervous and immune systems. With proteins, they form the major structural part of the cell wall in every cell in the body*

Carbohydrates

Starch: whole grains, rice, pasta, bread, potatoes, nuts, seeds, pulses, beans

Starch or complex carbohydrate is our prime source of energy. Unrefined carbohydrates are good sources of protein, vitamins, and minerals

Sugar: fruits, milk

Sugar is a simple carbohydrate, and is also an energy source. Refined sugar is a source of calories but no nutrition

Fibre: vegetables, seeds, pulses, beans

Fibre is essential for healthy bowel function and protects against bowel disease and gallstones, and reduces cholesterol levels

Vitamins

Vitamin A (fat soluble): fish oils, milk produce, (organic) liver, egg yolk, carrots

Carotene is a source of vitamin A, found in green, yellow and orange vegetables, orange and yellow fruits, dandelion leaves, parsley, watercress

Builds resistance to infections, promotes growth, healthy hair, teeth, skin and gums, and helps repair tissues. Necessary for healthy eyes, bone formation, red and white blood cell production, and foundation of hormones involved with reproduction and lactation

Vitamin B1 (thiamin, water soluble): whole grains, oatmeal, (organic) liver, legumes, yeast, milk, nuts, lentils, seeds, eggs

Essential for turning complex carbohydrates into glucose or fat, and for energy production

Vitamin B2 (riboflavin): milk, cheese, butter, yoghurt, cereals, meat, brewer's yeast, green leaf vegetables, peas, beans, eggs, wheatgerm

Involved with the formation of liver enzymes and the use of oxygen in the metabolism of carbohydrates, fats, and proteins stored in the liver

Vitamin B3 (nicotinic acid/niacin): whole grains, milk, milk products, meat, fish, brewer's yeast, green vegetables, nuts, eggs

Involved in forming the enzymes needed for carbohydrate metabolism. Affects cholesterol metabolism and helps reduce the level of fats in the blood

Vitamin B5 (pantothenic acid): cow's milk, breast-milk, eggs, cereals, meat, brewer's yeast, green vegetables, mushrooms

Involved with the metabolism of carbohydrates, fats, and amino acids. Vital to the normal function of the adrenal glands. Helps maintain the immune system

Vitamin B6 (pyridoxine): fish, meat, egg yolk, whole grains, nuts, seeds, green vegetables, brewer's yeast, bananas, avocados, molasses, mushrooms

Involved in the metabolism of proteins and amino acids, sugars, fatty acids, and some minerals. Assists the manufacture of red blood cells, antibodies, hormones, and enzymes

Vitamin B12 (cyanocobalamin): meat, liver, kidneys, fish, eggs, milk, milk products, beansprouts. Also manufactured by intestinal bacteria

Vital for the normal development of red blood cells, for iron metabolism, and for a healthy nervous system

Vitamins *continued*

Vitamin C (ascorbic acid): fresh fruit, fresh vegetables, potatoes, leafy herbs, berries	*Vital for healthy skin, bones and muscles, as it is involved with producing the protein collagen. Also vital for healing and protection from the effects of viruses, toxins, drugs, allergies, and foreign bodies. Necessary for cholesterol metabolism and the production of cortisol by the adrenal glands. Enhances resistance to infection and iron absorption, and is an effective antioxidant*
Vitamin D: milk, milk products, eggs, fatty fish, fish oil Sunlight triggers its synthesis in the skin	*Vital for normal calcium formation, and the growth and health of bones and teeth. Increases absorption of calcium and phosphates from food*
Vitamin E: nuts, seeds, eggs, milk, milk products, whole grains, wheatgerm, unrefined oils, leafy vegetables, avocados, seaweeds, soy beans, breastmilk	*Important to the metabolism of essential fatty acids, absorption of iron, and for red cell manufacture. An antioxidant, it protects the circulatory system, cells and cell membranes, and slows the aging process. Increases fertility and protects against development of fetal abnormalities and miscarriage*
Vitamin K: green vegetables, milk, milk products, molasses, apricots, whole grains, cod liver oil, sunflower oil Synthesized in the intestines	*For the production of blood clotting factors, notably prothrombin*
Folic acid: brewer's yeast, green vegetables, eggs, whole grains, meat, nuts, milk	*For red blood cell formation in bone marrow. For metabolism of sugar and amino acids, and the manufacture of antibodies. Crucial to the normal function of the nervous system and for production of genetic material*

Minerals

Sodium: most vegetables, salt	*Vital for the maintenance of fluid balance and blood pressure, and normal nerve and muscle function*
Calcium: milk, milk products, green vegetables, eggs, nuts, seeds, dried fruit, soya beans, bony fish, cereals	*For healthy bones and teeth, normal function of heart muscle, blood clotting mechanisms, conduction of nerve impulses, and muscle function*
Iron: egg yolk, liver, meat, molasses, soya beans, whole grains, green vegetables, fish, dried fruits, cocoa, wine	*Used in production of hemoglobin, vital for transport of oxygen in the blood. Important for the production of energy and for cellular respiration*

Minerals *continued*

Magnesium: green vegetables, nuts, seeds, whole grains, milk, milk products, eggs, seafoods, "hard" water	*For energy production, protein metabolism, the manufacture of enzymes, nerve and muscle function, and bone and teeth formation*
Phosphorus: whole grains, seeds, nuts, meat, fish, eggs	*Vital for healthy bone formation and for heart and kidney function. Important for nerve conduction and vitamin metabolism*
Potassium: fresh fruit, fresh vegetables, whole grains, nuts, soya beans, seafood	*For nerve conduction and muscle function, and to regulate the blood's acid-alkali balance and water balance*
Copper: green vegetables, liver, seafoods, whole grains	*For formation of myelin sheath around nerves, iron absorption, enzyme production, development of brain, bones, and (with B6) of connective tissue. Acts as an antioxidant. Essential for the function of vitamin C*
Zinc: oysters, herrings, yeast, liver, eggs, beef, peas, seeds, fruit, vegetables, nuts, poultry, shellfish	*A component of about 90 enzymes. Vital for protein metabolism. Helps prevent free radical damage of the eyes, prostate gland, seminal fluid and sperm. For normal immune function and hormone production, and healthy bones and joints. Required for the release of vitamin A from liver stores*
Cobalt: brewer's yeast, fruit, vegetables, whole grains, nuts	*A component of vitamin B12. Enhances copper absorption, and magnesium and sugar metabolism*
Manganese: green vegetables, seeds, whole grains, pulses, brewer's yeast, eggs, fruits, tea	*Important for energy metabolism, healthy bones, thyroid function, and the function of both the nervous and reproductive systems*
Iodine: vegetables grown on iodine-rich soils, fruits, seafoods, garlic, parsley, iodized salt	*Vital to the production of thyroid hormones which are responsible for regulating metabolism and physical and mental development*
Chromium: fruit, vegetables, meat, molasses, whole grains, wheatgerm, brewer's yeast, organic foods	*Vital for fat and carbohydrate metabolism, and the production of energy*
Selenium: garlic, whole grains, eggs, meat, brewer's yeast	*Antioxidant, vital for normal functioning of the liver and connective tissue, and the formation of sex hormones*

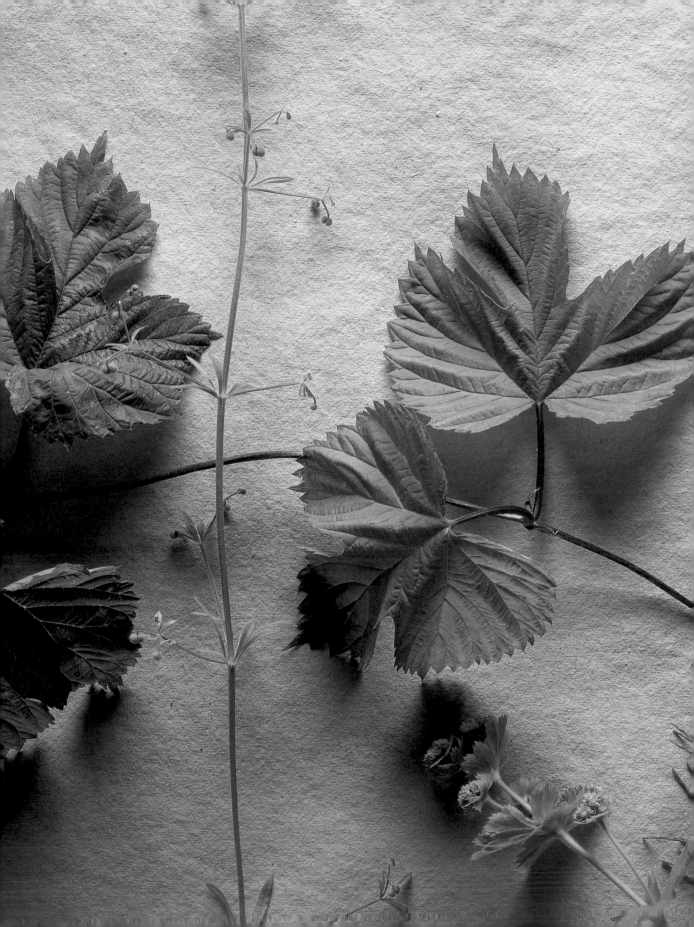

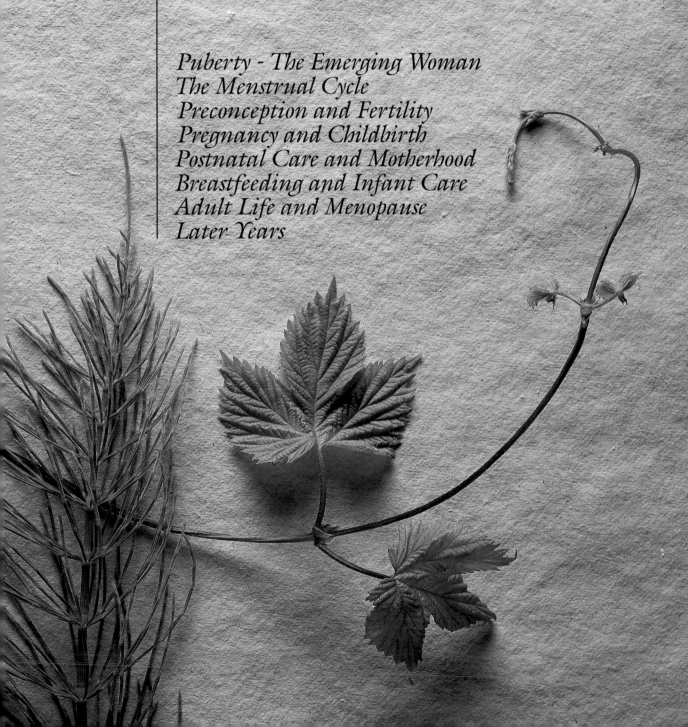

PART TWO

The Seasons of Womanhood

3 Puberty – the Emerging Woman

The changes that herald the transition from childhood to womanhood generally start around the age of ten or eleven. A girl's body will develop more rounded contours; the breasts begin to emerge, the vulva becomes more pronounced and pubic and underarm hair begins to grow. The first period, announcing the physical capacity for motherhood, is known as menarche and usually occurs between the ages of twelve and thirteen. Onset of menarche depends very much on physical development; specifically the amount of fat deposited around the body. It is quite normal for menarche to occur any time between the ages of eleven and fourteen – girls tend to follow a pattern inherited from their mother.

Adolescence is a time not only of great physical change but also of intellectual and emotional development. The metamorphosis from girl to woman can often bring inner and outer conflict while the adolescent tries to establish a balance between independence and dependence. She feels a need to be free of parental control and yet depends on her parents' care and guidance; she is torn between parental values and those of her peer group, and between developing romantic emotions and sexual feelings and the moral codes of conduct held by parents and teachers.

Unless an open relationship exists between a teenager and her parents, puberty can be a painful, lonely time, causing rifts between one generation and another as lack of understanding grows on both sides. Teenagers are said to be moody, resentful, difficult, and rebellious during their struggle to assert themselves as developing adults. In this struggle they may burst into tears easily, complain bitterly – and truthfully – of being misunderstood, and use rebellion, hostility or secrecy to achieve a sense of self.

With the establishment of sex education in schools, one might assume that these days a girl will have been told, either at home or at school, about the coming changes in her life. However, too frequently a girl may start her periods in total ignorance, and become easy prey to those perpetuating myths and superstitions about menstruation. She may be alarmed by her unexpected loss of blood and feel it is something to hide or to be ashamed of. These feelings will lead her to deny her emerging femininity, which is a bad start in a woman's adult life.

Cleavers

Galium aparine

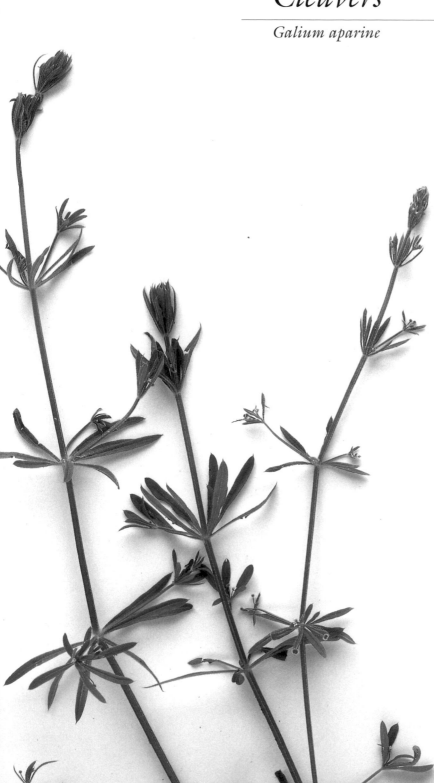

ALSO KNOWN AS: Clivers, goosegrass, gripgrass, stickywillie, catchweed, hedgeburs

PART USED: Aerial parts

CONTAINS: Tannins, rubichloric, citric and galitannic acids, asperuloside, saponins, coumarin

KEY USES: Diuretic, alterative, anti-inflammatory, astringent, antineoplastic, tonic, refrigerant

Cleavers is a common hedgerow weed that is a wonderful cleansing remedy, clearing toxins from the system and reducing heat and inflammation. It has a diuretic action, aiding elimination of wastes, and also acts to enhance the lymphatic system, promoting lymphatic drainage of toxins and wastes so that they can be excreted via the urinary system. These actions combine to make cleavers excellent for fluid retention, skin problems including eczema, psoriasis, acne, boils and abscesses, urinary infections, urinary stones and gravel, arthritis and gout. It can be used for lymphatic problems, such as lymphatic congestion and swollen lymph glands, congestion of the breasts, and is said to have anti-tumour activity, particularly when in the skin or breasts, and the lymphatic system.

Cleavers has cooling properties, reducing fevers and resolving eruptive infections such as measles and chickenpox. It cools heat and inflammation in the body, seen in conditions such as cystitis, arthritis, inflammatory skin problems and digestive problems. Its bitter properties stimulate liver function and enhance digestion and absorption. A cooling drink made of cleavers was traditionally given every spring to "clear the blood".

The fresh leaves can be applied to cuts or wounds to check bleeding and speed healing. The juice or an infusion can be used to bathe varicose ulcers, or the fresh leaves can be made into a poultice. It will soothe and cool burns, sunburn, inflammatory skin problems such as eczema and acne, and clear the skin of blemishes.

Witch hazel

Hamamelis virginiana

ALSO KNOWN AS: Spotted alder, winterbloom, snapping hazelnut

PARTS USED: Leaves and bark; as distilled witch hazel water

CONTAINS: Tannins (including gallotannins, condensed catechins, proanthocyanidins), saponins, resins, flavonoids, choline, volatile oils (in the bark)

KEY USE: Astringent

Witch hazel is well known as a remedy for scalds and burns, swelling and inflammation of the skin and to stop bleeding. Its main action is astringent due to the high levels of tannins that occur in the plant, making it an excellent remedy for internal and external bleeding. It has been used traditionally to stop bleeding from the lungs, stomach, uterus and bowels. It can be put to good effect for excessive menstruation and uterine blood stagnation, with a feeling of fullness, heaviness and discomfort around a period.

Externally either a decoction, tincture or distilled witch hazel can be applied to cuts and wounds, used as a mouthwash for bleeding gums and as a lotion or in an ointment for bleeding piles. The tannins also speed healing, reduce pain, inflammation and swelling and protect wounds against infection.

Witch hazel makes an excellent remedy for diarrhea, dysentery, mucous colitis and respiratory catarrh. It has been used for uterine prolapse and a debilitated state after miscarriage or childbirth to tone up the uterine muscles.

Witch hazel is used externally as a lotion or ointment to relieve the pain and swelling of varicose veins and phlebitis, the itching of hemorrhoids and to speed healing of varicose ulcers. A poultice or compress will relieve burns, swollen or inflammatory skin problems, engorged breasts, bed sores, bruises, sprains and strains. As a lotion it can be applied to soothe mosquito bites and stings, to relieve tender aching muscles, as a toning skin lotion to tighten the tissues and reduce broken capillaries. Mixed with rose water it makes a refreshing eye bath. A lotion, decoction or tincture can also be used as a douche for vaginal discharge and irritation, or as a gargle for sore throats and infections.

Attitudes to the female body

The emotional environment surrounding an adolescent girl is important in determining her attitude to her sexual development, and this may in turn influence the balance of her hormones and their effect on menstruation.

If menstruation is considered by a girl's mother as a regular ordeal, an unfair burden, a curse, an interruption to her normal ordered life, then the girl may resent her periods and her physical changes and dread the inevitable monthly cycles. This may contribute to problems with her periods, – irregularity, pain, heavy bleeding or PMS may result.

In many cultures menarche is a time of celebration when the girl is joyfully initiated into womanhood. It is normal and healthy to go through these changes, and to be standing on the threshold of womanhood and potential motherhood is an exciting time.

In other cultures, however, the negative idea of menstruation being the monthly curse has been more common. The ancient Jews, for example, considered women to be "unclean" during their periods as well as during childbirth; after menstruation Jewish women have been requested to undergo ritualistic cleansing. In some parts of the world the presence of a menstruating woman was – and often still is – believed to turn milk or wine sour, to blight crops, to dull mirrors, to extinguish fires, to break clocks, to cause fruit on trees to rot and seeds not to germinate.

Menstruating women were often expected to take to their beds, or isolate themselves from the rest of their community, only to be seen by other women. In India women would go into purdah at these times. During the Middle Ages the Christian church declared that since menstruation signified women's sinfulness and inferiority, they were not allowed into church or to take communion while menstruating.

More positively, in some primitive cultures, men could not comprehend how a woman who was bleeding did not bleed to death, and her ability to withstand her ordeal so stoically meant that menstruating women were often credited with supernatural powers. This included being able to stop whirlwinds, thunder, lightning and hailstorms. Menstrual blood itself was highly valued for its ability to protect men in battle, put out fires and cure headaches.

Whether it is treated as a curse or a blessing, menstruation is certainly seen as a tangible symbol of woman's essential nature. As in so many cultural taboos, it is the thing we do not understand that we come to fear.

Menstruating women have traditionally isolated themselves, perhaps simply to retreat from everyday demands and responsibilities at a particularly sensitive time of their monthly cycle. Such a retreat gives them an opportunity for quietness and reflection. This segregation has been interpreted by some traditions as a reason for devising rigid prohibitions for menstruating women, keeping them from lovemaking, seeing the sun, preparing or touching food, or even washing their hair.

Menstrual blood is nothing more than a harmless mixture of blood, cells, and mucus – normal constituents of every male and female body. However, the myth that menstrual blood is unclean still appears to be very much alive, and the thought of lovemaking with a menstruating woman is repellent to many men.

Many women are made to feel ashamed of their bleeding, and worry about the smell of the blood, or fear that the odd spot may stain the bedclothes or their clothing. There is pressure to deny menstruation, to hide it even from ourselves. The world of commerce and advertising would provide us with more and more sophisticated and sanitized "protection" so that we can carry on functioning in the mechanized, rushed, unrelenting world of business as if nothing is happening. Women are not even very explicit when referring to their periods amongst themselves; we use euphemisms like "the time of the month", "the curse", "aunty", or "coming on".

These conflicting attitudes towards menstruation provide another stumbling block for the girl during puberty. Her developing body, especially the part from which blood emerges, may be seen as something to fear, or resent. It seems to be related to things that are unclean, secret and cursed. At the same time, a girl's body begins to have the capacity to feel sensual, sexually aroused, and seems to be very attractive to members of the opposite sex.

If we continue to feed girls at puberty with conflicting messages, these sensual feelings of theirs will seem to them dirty, smutty, and most of all to be hidden from parents and others of that generation, causing further rifts in understanding. This can lead to denial of womanhood, sexuality and femininity, creating not only menstrual disorders such as dysmenorrhea, but also eating disorders such as anorexia. By starving the body of food, it drops below the weight at which menstruation can be sustained and periods stop.

Whatever myths and taboos may surround us, it is important to dismiss any ideas that cause misery and shame about our female bodies and their natural processes. Education and information about the female body and how it works, including the changes that occur at puberty, go a long way to dispelling myths.

The body's changes

From the age of about ten or twelve, a girl's secondary sex characteristics emerge. These changes occur over a period of about two years. They include breast development, skin and circulatory changes, growth of hair on the pubis and in the armpits and changes of body shape into a more rounded female figure. Ovulation and menstruation (menarche) occur near the end of puberty, normally at the age of 12 or 13, once a girl has achieved a weight of 105 lb (47.5 kg) and about a quarter of that weight is fat. Periods continue until about the age of 48, although some women have periods until their mid-fifties, after which the menopause occurs.

The development of secondary sex characteristics, ovulation, menstruation and the menopause are all determined by hormones. These chemical messengers trigger a variety of different responses in the body. The levels of sex hormones are low in childhood and rise during puberty. During menstruation they fluctuate throughout each monthly cycle in such a way that, in the right circumstances, the wonderful process of conception can occur.

To understand menstruation it is best to acquaint yourself with the anatomy and physiology of the reproductive tract (see p.63) and to get to know your body by examining yourself. This can be done using a mirror and exploring the crevices and openings gently with clean fingers.

The ovaries are equipped at birth with about 400,000 follicles, like bags of cells, each containing an egg. Out of these immature eggs, 300-500 will mature into developed eggs capable of uniting with a sperm at conception.

Each month at the beginning of the cycle messages are sent from the pituitary gland (known as the master gland) via a follicle-stimulating hormone, to the ovaries, which cause several of these follicles to develop. One follicle creates a fully mature egg, as well as the hormone estrogen.

Toward mid-cycle this follicle moves to the surface of the ovary and the egg is discharged at ovulation from the ovary into one or other of the fallopian tubes. At ovulation some women may experience twinges of pain or cramp in the lower abdomen. Over the next few days the egg travels down the fallopian tube, propelled by muscular contractions in the tube. If, within 24 hours of ovulation, the egg meets a sperm in the fallopian tube, conception can occur, and the united sperm and egg travel down to the uterus together, to implant in the uterus.

After ovulation, the empty egg follicle is known as the corpus luteum, and under instruction from luteinizing hormone from the pituitary gland, it produces progesterone, as well as estrogen. These hormones work together to maintain a pregnancy, should conception occur, by creating certain conditions in the uterus. If there is no pregnancy, the follicle degenerates.

During the first half of the cycle, estrogen causes the blood supply to the uterus to increase and the lining of the uterus, the endometrium, to thicken. In the second half of the cycle, progesterone causes further thickening of the endometrium and the secretion of substances to nurture the developing embryo if a pregnancy has occurred. If no pregnancy exists, the estrogen and progesterone from the ovary begin to dwindle and as a result the lining of the uterus starts to break down and slough off. This causes menstruation. Bleeding normally occurs once a month, and lasts on average from four to six days. The normal amount lost is about an eggcupful, or four to six tablespoonsful; the flow stops and starts throughout the period, tailing off towards the end.

Menstrual fluid is composed of mucus, vaginal secretions, cells and blood, and does not really smell until it is in contact with the air, and bacterial decomposition occurs. There is nothing unclean about it, as it is merely the lining of the uterus being shed. It should be bright red.

One of the first signs of emerging puberty is an increase in vaginal secretions. This is perfectly normal and occurs generally before menarche. It consists of a white, creamy secretion which keeps the vagina healthy and slightly acidic. It changes according to the phase of the cycle once menstruation begins, and increases when we are sexually aroused, and at ovulation time when we are fertile. When girls first start their periods it is not uncommon for the cycles to be irregular. There may be anything from three to seven weeks between periods. This is due to the gradual establishment of the hormonal cycle and it may be two years before ovulation occurs regularly. Irregular periods at this stage are nothing to worry about; they should soon settle down. Periods can be accompanied by pain and they can often be heavy. (For further information see p.88.)

The key to trouble-free periods lies very much in developing a positive attitude towards your emerging femininity and your inevitable monthly changes. Try to let go of any preconceived ideas you have of what menstruation represents. If you feel unhappy or worried about your periods it would be best to discuss them, if you feel able to, with your mother, older sister or other relations, or with friends who are experiencing similar feelings. It is largely your feelings about your periods,

and the maintenance of a healthy hormone balance, that will determine their character. Your diet, lifestyle, the amount of exercise you take and the balance of work and relaxation in your life are all vital to your hormone balance. If you take care of yourself in this way, you are doing all you can in order to have trouble-free periods. (For more information on maintaining a healthy hormone balance, see p.86.)

Skin changes

With the change of hormones at puberty, the glands in the skin become more active, producing more sebum from the sebaceous glands and more sweat from sweat glands. Skin care and the use of deodorants become more important from now on.

Overactive sebaceous glands make the skin more oily, particularly on the face, back and chest. This production of oily sebum and the increased growth rate of cells in the facial skin can cause some hair follicles, containing sebaceous glands, to become clogged. If this happens they can become inflamed, and often infected, forming raised red spots or pus-filled pimples. Sebaceous glands may also become blocked just by excess sebum forming a dark plug known as a blackhead. A skin condition characterized by blackheads and red spots is known as acne vulgaris. In severe cases the inflammation in a sebaceous gland follicle can be so extensive as to cause a cyst, which is more likely than a spot to leave a scar.

Physical development
The diagram illustrates the changes in shape and height of the average girl as she develops into a young woman. The horizontal lines are placed at intervals of six inches (15 cm), so between the ages of 11 and 18 she only gains another 6 in (15 cm) in height, from 5 ft to 5ft 6 in (from 1.52 m to 1.67 m). Other physical changes are more significant. She will gain 49-56 lb (22-25 kg) in weight, the face becomes fuller, hips broaden and breasts develop. Pubic and underarm hair grows, and the voice becomes deeper, though not as deep as in boys. Menstruation usually begins between the ages of 12 and 13.

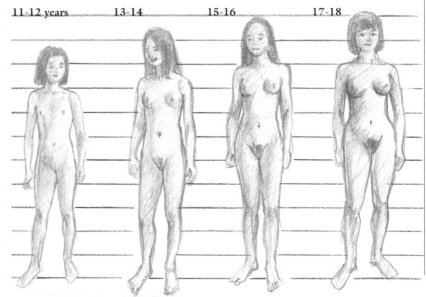

11-12 years   13-14   15-16   17-18

Burdock

Arctium lappa

ALSO KNOWN AS: Great burdock, great bur, clotbur, cockle bur, beggars buttons, lappa, cockle buttons

PARTS USED: Roots, seeds, leaves

CONTAINS: Roots: up to 50% inulin, volatile acids, tannin, polyphenolic acid. Seeds: 15-30% fixed oils, bitter glycoside (arctiin), chlorogenic acid. Leaves: Arctiol, fulcinone, taraxasterol

KEY USES: Alterative, diuretic, bitter tonic, digestive, mild laxative, antibiotic, diaphoretic, hypoglycemic

Burdock is a wonderful blood cleanser and detoxifying remedy, hastening the elimination of toxins from the body. The roots, leaves and seeds are all bitter, stimulating digestion and liver action and activating the pancreas. They can be used to strengthen a weak digestion, relieve wind, distension and indigestion and as a mild laxative. Burdock is an effective remedy for bacterial and fungal infections and to help re-establish normal bacteria in the gut.

Burdock has mild diuretic properties, aiding elimination of toxins via the urine. It can be used for cystitis, water retention, stones and gravel. Taken as a hot decoction, it also helps to clear toxins from the tissues via the skin as it causes sweating. It can be used to bring down a fever and can be taken at the onset of any infection with feverishness. The seeds are effective for treating sore throats, tonsilitis, colds and coughs.

Burdock helps to bring out eruptions and thus speed recovery from infections such as measles and chickenpox. By pushing toxins into the bloodstream, burdock makes an effective remedy for chronic inflammatory conditions such as gout, arthritis and rheumatism. It is excellent for treating skin disease as it improves the action of the sebaceous glands. Burdock also helps to lower blood sugar in diabetics. The root stimulates the uterus, helping to regulate periods and has been used traditionally for prolapse and to give strength before and after childbirth.

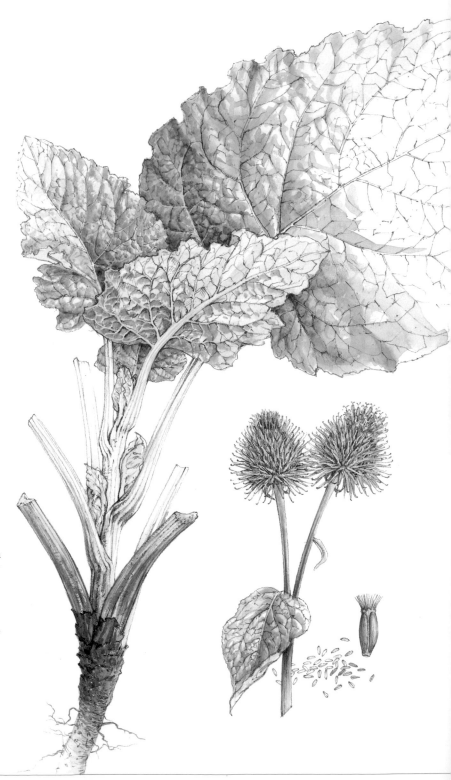

Acne vulgaris is most common between the age of 12 and the early 20s by which time the hormones should have settled down. Besides hormones, there are several other factors which contribute to acne, and which can be remedied if acne becomes a problem.

Diet is important, so make sure you eat a healthy diet, high in green vegetables, carrots, brassicas and fruit. Eliminate fatty foods as much as you can, notably dairy products and animal fats, as well as sugar, caffeine, alcohol, refined carbohydrates and junk foods.

To make up for possible nutritional deficiencies which can upset hormone balance, take supplements of evening primrose oil, zinc, vitamin B complex, B6, and vitamins C, E and A.

To ensure adequate kidney and bowel function, drink plenty of fluids. Sweetened or fizzy drinks are out – stick to pure spring water, add a little lemon juice if you like, and drink about 3-4 pints (2 l) a day.

Food allergies can be to blame, particularly allergies to dairy produce, wheat and yeast. Candidiasis may be involved (see Thrush on p.226). This infection can cause leakage of toxins into the system from the bowels. Seek treatment if you have the symptoms.

Over-hot baths and showers can upset the function of the skin and cause congestion of the circulation in the skin through dilation of the blood vessels. Washing in warm water is better.

Certain drugs such as steroids, and anti-epilepsy drugs can aggravate acne, as can excess iodine, often from iodized salt. Avoid these if possible.

Lack of exercise makes the circulation sluggish, and the skin needs to sweat to excrete toxins. Take regular vigorous exercise, such as jogging, bicycling, or dancing, that makes you sweat.

Stress will allow toxins to gather in the system, and creates a great need for nutrients, which the diet may not meet. Stress also disturbs hormone balance. All these effects will add to the risk of acne. Fresh air, sunshine and sea bathing will help remedy acne, and should help relieve stress.

Puberty, as we know, can be a difficult time, when we may feel over-conscious of the way we look. Embarrassment about physical development, our developing sexuality, awareness of the opposite sex and shyness can all be amplified by the presence of a few spots.

Although acne manifests itself on the skin it is caused by internal imbalance rather than anything external. Healing needs to come from within. It is best to leave your face alone as much as you can; all the washing in the world will not stop acne. Avoid creams, lotions and make-up, and wash your face in cold or tepid water, or with rose water, rather than soap.

Herbal treatment for acne

Hormone balancing herbs should be used, and since an excess of progesterone or a lack of estrogen may well be to blame, the following herbs should prove useful.

Choose from:

chaste tree	*motherwort*
calendula	*false unicorn root*
wild yam	

Add remedies for the liver and bowels to improve elimination, such as burdock, dandelion root, yellow dock or rosemary.

To improve skin function and relieve congestion in the skin, use warm teas of yarrow, plantain, calendula, poke root or cleavers.

To ensure proper elimination through the kidneys you can use diuretic herbs such as corn silk, dandelion leaf, nettles and cleavers.

Herbs which are antiseptic and support the immune system can be taken to reduce infection in the sebaceous glands. Echinacea, myrrh, thyme or sage are all useful.

Relaxants are helpful where stress is involved. Choose from chamomile, vervain or skullcap to add to your prescription.

External treatments To help reduce excess oiliness and infection in the skin, use tepid or cold infusions of plantain, calendula, elderflower, chamomile or distilled witch hazel.

In areas where spots are not active but there is residual scarring, use comfrey, chickweed, calendula, aloe vera gel, lavender or vitamin E oil regularly to heal the skin.

A facial steam once a week will help to clear out the clogged sebaceous glands. Use elderflower, chamomile, lavender or calendula. (See also Herbs for Beauty.)

4 The Menstrual Cycle

Many of the earth's natural processes are characterized by cyclical change: the seasons, the climate, the rock and water cycles for instance. Our physical femininity reflects this in the cycle of our hormones, bringing with it a waxing and waning of energy, feelings and desires. Perhaps this is a reflection of the cyclical patterns of the moon's phases and the sea's tides. Although, when hormone imbalances arise, these changes may be perceived negatively as moodiness, lethargy, discomfort from headaches, or clumsiness, change is part of life. A healthy hormone balance involves cyclical change – ebb and flow, activity and passivity. Such changes are natural and necessary. We need to tune in to them and live our lives accordingly, not expect ourselves to behave like machines. It is our female hormones that give us our femininity, contributing to our receptive and flexible natures. Our ability to feel, to nurture and care for others, to understand intuitively, and to perceive the world in a particular way are attributes to be treasured and certainly not to be scorned.

Events in every woman's life will affect the balance of her hormones, and vice versa. Our hormone balance can affect our reserves of physical energy and our general sense of wellbeing, our emotional state, efficiency at work, concentration when driving, the way we care for our children and so on. The health of our hormones is in turn affected by diet, the everyday demands on our energy and resources, pollution in the air, water and food, and the stresses caused by the speed at which we live.

Hormonal imbalance produces problems such as irregular, painful or heavy periods, premenstrual syndrome (PMS), impaired fertility and eventually menopausal problems. Such difficulties are so widespread that many women actually believe it is normal to have them. There is generally a solution to hormonal imbalance in safe treatment using herbs, as well as adopting a better lifestyle, which serves to offer a better quality of life in the long term.

Instead of cursing our hormones, we need to understand them, and learn what is necessary to keep them balanced. In that way we can enjoy our femininity to the full, and free ourselves from the symptoms of what used to be called "women's problems", avoiding the risk of medical intervention or surgery.

Pulsatilla

Anemone pulsatilla

ALSO KNOWN AS: Pasque flower, wind flower, prairie or meadow anemone

PART USED: Dried aerial parts

CONTAINS: Glycoside (ranunculin in fresh plant which is poisonous, producing anemonin on drying), tannin, saponins, resin

KEY USES: Anodyne, antispasmodic, emmenagogue, nerve tonic, relaxant, sedative

Pulsatilla is a beautiful plant with silky purple flowers. As a nerve tonic, it is recommended for nervous exhaustion, depression, insomnia, neuralgia and tension headaches. Debilitated women and children who feel depressed and irritable, and who weep easily, will benefit most from it. It promotes sleep and rest and thereby facilitates recuperation by preventing unnecessary expenditure of nervous energy by those already nervously run down.

Pulsatilla has a particular application to spasm, pain and inflammation of the reproductive system, both male and female. It relieves premenstrual tension, period pains, scanty or suppressed periods, uterine colic, and inflammation and pain in the ovaries.

The analgesic properties are useful during childbirth and other qualities of the plant help to promote and facilitate birth. It is recommended for sluggish, ineffectual and weak labour pains, and for peevishness and irritability in labour. After the birth, it may be useful for any kind of over-excitement, postnatal depression and anxiety about the birth or the new baby.

This plant may be used to good effect in small doses: 1-2 ml of tincture, or half a teaspoon of herb to a cup of boiling water as tea, taken three times daily when necessary. During the birth, it may be taken as sips of the tea or a few drops of tincture at frequent intervals.

Note Never use this plant fresh, as it is poisonous. Do not store it for more than one year.

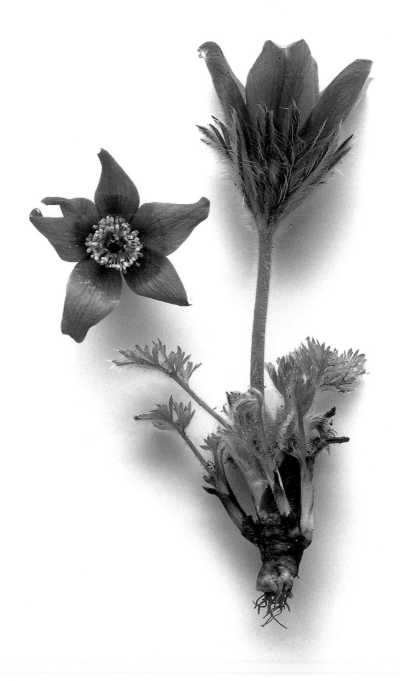

The healthy cycle

In order to understand how the menstrual cycle works, it is important to realize that each monthly event is governed by the action of various hormones.

Understanding our hormones

Our sex hormones, like all the other hormones in the body, are controlled by the pituitary or "master" gland. This is a small gland in the brain connected to the hypothalamus, the part of the brain which influences emotion, weight, water balance, sleep and appetite. The areas of the brain concerned with our senses, creativity, thought and memory are connected to the hypothalamus and are constantly influencing it – so it is not hard to see how the way we think and feel can influence the balance of our sex hormones, and what happens to us from month to month.

Acting on messages sent from the hypothalamus, the anterior pituitary gland produces two hormones which influence the production of sex hormones, follicle stimulating hormone (FSH), and the luteinizing hormone (LH). During the first half of the menstrual cycle, FSH acts on the follicles in the ovaries, causing them to develop from the primordial follicles present in the ovaries at birth to Graafian follicles which contain estrogen.

During each cycle one Graafian follicle ripens, and once fully developed it reaches the surface of the ovary where it ruptures, releasing the ovum (egg) into the peritoneal cavity. The ovum is then picked up by the fimbria, finger-like projections from one of the fallopian tubes, and guided into the tube. It is then wafted along the tube towards the uterus by the action of little hairs, called cilia, on the cells lining the tube.

The rupture of the Graafian follicle is known as ovulation and occurs14 days before menstruation. The follicle then collapses and the little hole in the ovary is plugged by a clot formed by a little blood from the rupture.

The hormone LH, secreted from the pituitary gland, then reaches the ovary via the bloodstream and causes the cells lining the collapsed follicle, the corpus luteum, to multiply and become a hormone-secreting gland. This continues to secrete estrogen as well as progesterone into the bloodstream.

If the ovum becomes fertilized by a sperm around ovulation, then the corpus luteum grows. If not, it degenerates. Meanwhile the lining of the uterus, the endometrium, is acted on by estrogen and progesterone from the ovary. Estrogen in the first half of the cycle causes the endometrium to thicken and its glands to grow longer. The packing between the glands, the stroma, becomes larger and more loosely packed and many more blood vessels appear.

After ovulation, progesterone and estrogen together continue this process, preparing the lining of the uterus for implantation of the egg, should it be fertilized. The lining becomes thicker, and the glands grow so long they start to zigzag; the cells lining the uterus secrete a substance containing glycogen, the stroma become more loosely packed and the blood vessels become longer and more tortuous.

If the ovum is not fertilized and the corpus luteum degenerates, no more progesterone is secreted, and the blood vessels supplying the upper layers of the endometrium go into spasm. This stops the blood supply to this area, the cells die from lack of blood and the blood vessels break down. Gradually the whole new surface of the endometrium is stripped off – this is menstrual bleeding, a period.

The time between the first day of bleeding to ovulation is known as the first half of the cycle, when FSH develops the follicle containing the egg. It takes about 14 days. The time from ovulation to menstruation is always 14 days.

There is a third hormone secreted by the pituitary gland called prolactin which can influence the amounts of estrogen and progesterone secreted through the month.

Nutrition and hormones

An excellent diet, providing the whole range of nutrients, protein, carbohydrates, essential fatty acids, vitamins, minerals and trace elements, is vital for proper hormone balance. Some specific nutrients are particularly important and it is crucial to ensure that your diet is rich in all of them.

• B vitamins are vital for normal metabolism and energy production. Vitamin B6 is vital for normal function of the nervous system. A deficiency is linked to anxiety, depression, insomnia and PMS.

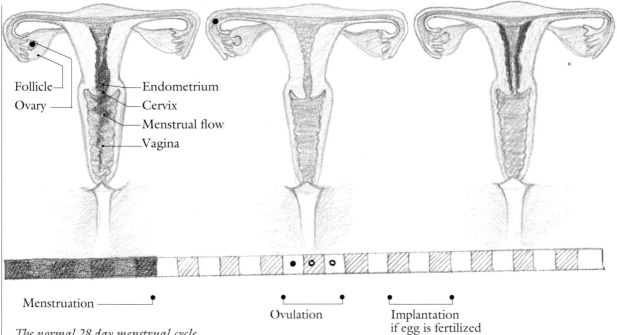

Follicle
Ovary
Endometrium
Cervix
Menstrual flow
Vagina

Menstruation

Ovulation

Implantation
if egg is fertilized

The normal 28 day menstrual cycle

Taking the contraceptive pill, drinking alcohol, and smoking increase your daily requirements.
• Vitamin C is involved in production of sex hormones. It has been shown to help women who have heavy periods. Smoking, infections and pollution increase your requirements. Vitamin E is vital to fertility and normal hormone balance.
• Magnesium has been shown to relieve PMS, tender breasts and painful periods. It is vital for energy production, for the metabolism of vitamin B6 and for maintaining hormone balance. Modern farming methods have led to a deficiency in many foods of natural magnesium – eating organic food will help remedy this.
• Potassium is involved in normal function of the nervous system and the maintenance of the fluid balance in the body. Increasing potassium in your diet will often help relieve fluid retention. It works together with sodium, which we tend to overeat; the more sodium in our diet, the less potassium we have, particularly as potassium is easily lost from vegetables and fruit through cooking and processing.
• Chromium is important for balance of blood sugar, and is helpful for women who tend to suffer from low blood sugar before a period, producing

sugar craving, tiredness and irritability. The more sugar you eat, however, the more chromium is eliminated from the body, so it is important to cut out sugar as much as possible.
• Monthly periods cause women regularly to lose iron (contained in blood) from their bodies, and of course this is accentuated in women with heavy periods. Interestingly, iron deficiency can not only be caused by heavy periods, it can cause them.
• Zinc is essential for normal hormone balance in both men and women. It is also vital for normal growth, cell division, tissue repair, healthy skin and bones and the prevention of osteoporosis. Iodine stimulates the thyroid gland to produce thyroid hormones, chiefly thyroxin. Normal thyroid hormone balance is vital to sex hormone balance, and an underactive thyroid is closely linked to excess estrogen in the body contributing to PMS, breast and endometrial cancer.
• Essential fatty acids are involved in the production of prostaglandins which regulate the effects of sex hormones. Deficiency is related to period pain, breast tenderness and PMS which can improve dramatically when you increase your intake of them, and when taking evening primrose oil, which contains gamma linoleic acid (GLA).

You can ensure that your diet is rich in most of the above nutrients by eating plenty of nuts and seeds, whole grains and wheatgerm, organically grown fresh fruit and vegetables and seafood. Because of stress, high levels of activity, metabolism and individual biochemistry, some women require unusually high amounts of these nutrients, and may need to take supplements to maintain proper hormone balance. Adding wheatgerm, kelp tablets and evening primrose oil to your diet may be sufficient. You could also take a good multimineral and vitamin supplement.

Disturbances of the normal cycle

The menstrual cycle can be disturbed by many factors, mostly related to hormone balance. This section deals with the causes and symptoms of the more common disorders of the menstrual cycle, giving suggestions for self help and herbal treatments.

We have already seen how a good diet can maintain the balance of hormones. There are other factors, however, which affect the hormones, and cause their disruption.

A high consumption of saturated animal fats can interfere with essential fatty acid metabolism. When unrefined cold-pressed vegetable oils, nuts and seeds, fatty fish, beans and pulses are eaten the essential fatty acids from them are then transformed into a usable form, gamma linoleic acid (GLA). Saturated fats block this transformation, as do processed oils. Moderate to high consumption of alcohol and deficiencies of zinc, magnesium, and vitamin B6 also reduce GLA formulation. Diabetes, certain viral infections, radiation, and the aging process are other factors which could also block GLA.

Caffeine in tea, coffee, cocoa and chocolate can interfere with hormonal balance by inhibiting the liver's breakdown of hormones once they have done their work. Tea interferes with the absorption of iron and zinc, particularly if it is drunk with meals, and along with coffee has been shown to increase the tendency to PMS and breast problems, including fibrocystic breast disease (painful, lumpy breasts).

Stress affects hormone production by the pituitary gland by its connection with the hypothalamus; it also causes our bodies to secrete a range of other hormones that interfere with our sex hormones. Caffeine, by increasing the effects of adrenaline, increases the effects of stress and aggravates symptoms such as anxiety, tension, irritability and hypoglycemia. Alcohol increases the body's needs for B vitamins, magnesium, zinc and calcium, creating deficiencies of these nutrients which upset the hormone balance. Added to this, alcohol damages the liver which may in turn interfere with hormone metabolism. Chemicals such as phosphates and polyphosphates (E544, E545, E450 in Europe) in food products such as soft drinks, processed meats, and cheeses, can interfere with the absorption of nutrients.

Sugar depletes nutrients in the body, particularly B vitamins, and also reduces hormone transport around the body. Women who eat a lot of sugar tend to suffer more hormonal problems than those who don't. Eating sugar also increases the tendency to hypoglycemia (low blood sugar) particularly premenstrually. This gives rise to sugar cravings, lethargy, weakness, irritability and headaches.

Smoking can contribute to hormonal problems by increasing the need for vitamins and minerals to detoxify all the different poisons in tobacco smoke. This reduces the amount of nutrients available for hormone production.

Your weight influences your hormone balance. The ratio of fat to lean in the body is critical in the initiation and continuation of the ovarian cycle. If you fall below a certain weight, the pituitary hormones stop sending their messages to the ovaries, and ovulation and menstruation stop.

Exercise is a factor. Athletes and those training vigorously and regularly have a tendency to upset their hormone balance and lose their periods. It is related to weight balance and also to nutrition. The physical demands of the training may use up so many vitamins and minerals that there are insufficient to maintain hormone production.

Food sensitivity or allergy can disrupt hormone balance, and it may be that either eliminating certain culprit foods, or increasing your nutrition to make up for deficiencies causing allergies, or both, will help the body to regain its balance.

Chronic illness can also upset our hormones. Chronic candida, or candidiasis, for example, is well known for causing hormone imbalances giving rise to a whole range of menstrual and gynecological problems. Prescribed drugs such as steroids and the contraceptive pill, particularly when taken over a long period, cause severe disruption of vitamin and mineral balance in the body. Sex hormones are inevitably affected by this. Synthetic hormones in the pill increase the need for nutrients such as vitamin B6, and by suppressing the body's natural hormone production, cause confusion in the body. After ceasing to take the pill, it may take some while for your own hormones to settle down and find their own rhythm. The pill increases the tendency to allergies and liver problems, which can also affect hormone balance.

Low levels of thyroid hormone have been related to estrogen excess in the body which gives rise to a whole range of menstrual and gynecological problems, including PMS and endometriosis.

Premenstrual syndrome

Premenstrual syndrome (PMS), also known as premenstrual tension (PMT), describes a wide range of symptoms that occur up to about 14 days before a period, and soon disappear once the period starts. These symptoms – which can be both physical and emotional – are very common, particularly in the thirty to forty age group, where about 75 per cent of women are prone to them.

Symptoms of PMS

water retention: weight gain, bloating
swollen and tender breasts
headaches and migraine
low libido
general aches and pains, backache
hypoglycemia: cravings for sugar and chocolate
constipation or diarrhea, nausea or vomiting
fatigue, dizziness, fainting, lethargy
palpitations
insomnia
poor co-ordination, clumsiness, physical tension
nervous tension, anxiety, mood swings, panic attacks
irritability, aggression, self-loathing, vulnerability
depression, crying, desperation
confusion, forgetfulness, poor concentration
period pains, dragging sensation in the lower abdomen
increased tendency to sore throats, boils, styes, herpes
aggravations of chronic problems, or allergies such as asthma, epilepsy, cystitis, rhinitis

Some women suffer so badly from PMS that they feel agoraphobic or claustrophobic, and may panic so much about normal everyday things, like collecting children from school, driving the car, relating to other people, that they stay at home and can feel very isolated. Irritability and bad temper may be so extreme as to cause physical aggression, which when directed towards loved ones often causes guilt and depression. Depression can sometimes be so severe that it leads to suicidal thoughts.

Factors contributing to PMS

PMS is primarily caused by an imbalance of hormones, mostly an excess of estrogen in relation to progesterone.

This is related to:

hereditary disposition
age – especially being over 30
stress and emotional problems
low thyroid function
a sluggish liver
deficiency of essential fatty acids and B vitamins
deficiencies of magnesium, zinc, vitamin C
 chromium deficiency, calcium deficiency
high salt intake
constipation
over-consumption of caffeine and alcohol
over-consumption of sugar and refined carbohydrates
lack of exercise

PMS is often precipitated by hormone changes occurring at puberty, after pregnancy, or when ceasing to take the pill, and when restarting periods after a break due to illness, loss of weight, or sterilization.

Self help for PMS

• Cut out or drastically reduce consumption of sugar, alcohol, salt, coffee, tea and chocolate to help balance your blood sugar, water balance and hormone balance. Do not smoke. Make sure your diet is excellent, with plenty of (preferably organic) fresh fruit and vegetables, whole grains, nuts and seeds, beans and pulses, and unrefined, cold pressed vegetable or seed oils.
• Tackle any constipation by changing your diet, eating plenty of fibre in whole grains, fruit and

vegetables. Avoid fatty meats, processed fats and deep fried foods. Avoid additives, preservatives and other food pollutants as far as possible.

• Treat systemic problems such as candida (see p.226). If you suspect you have food allergies, it is advisable to seek help from a qualified practitioner. Avoid taking steroids and the pill.

• Take plenty of exercise and fresh air. Make sure you put time aside to rest and relax. If you need help with this try relaxation exercises, music, meditation, regular massage or aromatherapy, T'ai chi or yoga. If there are specific emotional problems that are causing you stress, it may help to visit a counsellor or psychotherapist.

• Talk to your family or those you are living with about your PMS and explain why you can be irritable, depressed or "difficult" at certain times. Ask them for patience and understanding; assure them that it is your hormones that are causing you to behave differently, not them. Be careful not to miss meals, particularly in the two weeks before a period as this will increase the tendency to low blood sugar. If you do suffer from symptoms associated with low blood sugar, such as sugar cravings, increased appetite, faintness, irritability or headaches before a meal, eat some unrefined carbohydrate about every two hours.

• Take supplements for a few cycles to correct any nutritional deficiencies. Take 50 mg of vitamin B6 once or twice daily in the second half of the cycle, but stop if you become pregnant. Take 500 mg of evening primrose oil once or twice daily, and both 100-300 mg of vitamin E and 200 mg of magnesium daily. A multimineral and vitamin pill will supply added essentials such as chromium and zinc.

Herbal treatment of PMS

Use hormone balancing herbs to help restore normal levels of both estrogen and progesterone. Chaste tree acts directly on the pituitary gland to balance sex hormone production. By reducing follicle stimulating hormone (FSH) and increasing the production of luteal stimulating hormone (LSH), the relative excess of estrogen to progesterone can be remedied. Chaste tree may also help where there is thyroid hormone imbalance.

False unicorn root also has a balancing effect upon estrogen and progesterone and acts as a tonic to the ovaries. Wild yam and black haw are also hormone balancing. Several herbs have estro-

gen-like properties, so if blood tests show low estrogen levels, these could be helpful. Try sage, motherwort, hops and black cohosh, all of which are estrogenic.

Other herbs can be added to your prescription depending on your particular symptoms.

For tension, anxiety, or depression use:

skullcap	*vervain*
wild oats	*chamomile*
wood betony	

To lift the spirits use:

rosemary	*St. John's wort*
cinnamon	*ginger*
oats	*lemon balm*

For extreme tension use:

valerian	*passionflower*

For fluid retention, bloating, or breast tenderness use diuretics such as:

corn silk	*dandelion leaf*
burdock	

Breast swelling and tenderness is relieved by:

cleavers	*calendula*
poke root	

All prescriptions for PMS should include remedies to stimulate the liver into functioning efficiently, and to help it in its work of detoxification. They should include herbs which will also help to balance blood sugar levels. Use either burdock, dandelion root, wormwood, yellow dock, rosemary or calendula.

If you suffer from constipation or digestive problems, use yellow dock, burdock root or licorice to regulate the bowels. For nausea or vomiting, or both, take chamomile, lemon balm, cinnamon, ginger and peppermint. Licorice is a useful remedy for minimizing the effects of stress on the body by affecting the adrenal hormones.

Essential oils of lavender, rosemary, melissa, rose and bergamot can be used for massage or for adding to a relaxing bath.

Dandelion

Taraxacum officinale

ALSO KNOWN AS: Lion's teeth, fairy clock

PARTS USED: Root, leaves

CONTAINS: Root: Inulin, sterols, triterpenoids, bitter principle, taraxacin, sugars, pectin, glycosides, choline, phenolic acids, asparagine, potassium. Leaves: Lutein, violaxanthin and other carotenoids, bitters, vitamins A, B, C, D, potassium, iron

KEY USES: Cholagogue, diuretic, antirheumatic, laxative, tonic, nutrient, detoxifying

The whole plant can be used as a medicine and is highly nutritious. The roots are best harvested in early spring and late autumn and the leaves should be picked when young in spring and early summer, when you can eat them as a bitter tonic to cleanse the body of wastes from the heavy clogging food and more sedentary habits of winter. Dandelion is most famous as a gently detoxifying bitter tonic, increasing elimination of toxins, wastes and pollutants through the liver and kidneys, cleansing the blood and tissues.

The bitters in both root and leaf activate the whole of the digestive tract and the liver, increasing the flow of digestive juices, enhancing the appetite, easing digestion, and cleansing the liver. Dandelion root has been used traditionally for liver disease, jaundice, hepatitis, gallbladder infections, to dissolve gallstones and for problems associated with a sluggish liver, such as tiredness and irritability, skin problems and headaches. Its stimulating effect extends to the pancreas, where it increases insulin secretion, helpful in diabetes. The root is also mildly laxative. Dandelion, particularly the leaves, is an effective diuretic, useful in water retention, cellulite, urinary infections and prostate problems. A decoction of root and leaves has been used for dissolving urinary stones and gravel. While diuretic drugs leach potassium from the body, dandelion has a high potassium content, replacing that lost through increased urination.

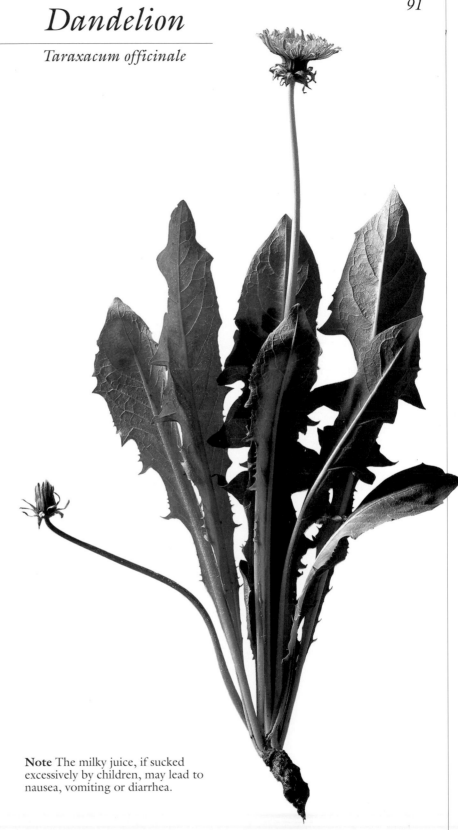

Note The milky juice, if sucked excessively by children, may lead to nausea, vomiting or diarrhea.

Bach Flower Remedies can be very helpful for negative attitudes towards menstruation that could be contributing to PMS.

Allow yourself the space and time needed to relax, be quiet and introspective, or to be creative. Learn to listen to the messages that femininity manifests in all of us – they may show us that what is creating much of the inner tension is really a suppression of our innate selves.

Menstruation and the days leading up to it can be a specially creative and very positive time, if we will allow it.

Painful periods (dysmenorrhea)

The discomfort experienced by women with painful periods varies in intensity from a heavy, dragging sensation in the low abdomen or back, to intense cramp for up to three days, so bad as to require painkillers.

Primary dysmenorrhea

Primary dysmenorrhea is characterized by sharp, cramping pain or dragging aches in the lower abdomen, back, or both, occurring around the beginning of the period and lasting up to two or three days. The pain or aching can affect the thighs. There may be associated headaches, diarrhea, frequency of urination, and nausea, vomiting or fainting if the pain is severe. The pains tend to start after the first four periods or within the first three years of menstruation. As women reach their twenties and thirties the pain tends to lessen and then disappear.

The tendency to painful periods is very often remedied by the birth of a baby. Young women who have these kinds of painful periods suffer from uterine contractions, that are both too strong and too frequent, when the uterus attempts to shed its lining. The resulting tension in the uterus impedes blood flow to the uterus, which in turn causes more cramping.

Causes of primary dysmenorrhea

genetic predisposition
emotional problems often related to sexuality and femininity
embarrassment or shame about periods
fear of pregnancy
poor circulation
muscular tension
smoking
lack of exercise
tight clothing impeding blood flow to the uterus
stress, overwork, tiredness, leading to muscle tension
caffeine in tea, coffee, cocoa and chocolate, exacerbating tension
bad posture and shallow breathing, inhibiting blood supply to the uterus
hormone imbalance
deficiency of essential fatty acids, magnesium, vitamin B6, zinc, vitamin C and niacin
iron deficiency

Secondary dysmenorrhea

Secondary dysmenorrhea tends to start later in a woman's life than the primary kind, usually in the twenties or thirties. If symptoms occur in a young woman who has been menstruating regularly for more than three years, it should be considered as secondary dysmenorrhea.

It is characterized by pain which begins three to four days – or even up to a week – before menstruation, and it may either be relieved or continue after bleeding begins. Pain can be associated with heavy bleeding, and sometimes large clots are passed. The pain can be mild to severe, but tends to have a less colicky nature than primary dysmenorrhea. There is often a dull, aching sensation of dragging down in the lower abdomen, which can extend to the lower back and thighs. The pain is more related to congestion in the uterus than to tension and spasm there.

Causes of secondary dysmenorrhea

hormone imbalance
infection or inflammation in the pelvis
adhesions caused by endometriosis
fibroids
an IUD causing congestion
a recent operation or investigation in the abdomen
a sedentary lifestyle
stress and tension causing pelvic congestion
poor posture, lower back problems
tight clothing, wearing high-heeled shoes
constipation
genetic predisposition

Before seeking treatment for your period pains, consult your practitioner. It may be that there are structural abnormalities or a problem which requires specific treatment.

Self help for dysmenorrhea

• Follow the advice on diet, dietary supplements and exercise given for PMS on p.89.
• Practise regularly these exercises which direct blood circulation to the pelvis. Use them particularly when you are in pain.

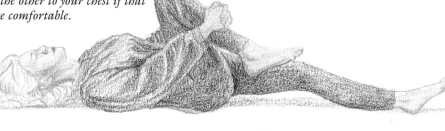

1 Lie flat on your back, bring your knees up to your chest and clasp them with your arms. Maintain this position for a few minutes. You can leave one leg outstretched on the floor and bring the other to your chest if that is more comfortable.

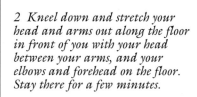

2 Kneel down and stretch your head and arms out along the floor in front of you with your head between your arms, and your elbows and forehead on the floor. Stay there for a few minutes.

3 Lie on your back with your legs in the air and rest for a few minutes. You can rest your legs against a wall if that is more comfortable.

• If your bowels are sluggish or you are prone to constipation, make sure your diet is good and that you have plenty to drink (see p.121). Exercising regularly should help your bowels.

• Make sure you keep warm, as cold will increase tension in the muscles. Wrap up well in cold weather, and when you have pain, keep a hot water bottle by your abdomen to release the spasm and stimulate the circulation.

• Allow yourself to relax. It is important to put some time aside in your busy life to enjoy yourself and let go of accumulated tension.

• If you have specific emotional problems which you are unable to solve alone you may find that therapy such as counselling or psychotherapy is necessary.

• If you suffer from lower back pain or you know your posture could be improved, some gentle manipulation may be necessary, and the Alexander Technique could help you.

• If you are aware that you breathe shallowly from the top of your chest, practise diaphragmatic breathing every day for a few minutes to increase blood flow to the pelvis and relax tension.

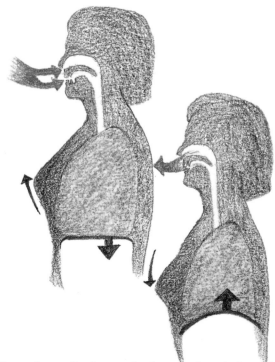

Expand your diaphragm slowly as you breathe in and let it relax as you breathe out.

• If you have an IUD it may be best to seek alternative contraception, though preferably not the pill.

• Take supplements of calcium, magnesium, EFAs in evening primrose oil, edible linseed oil, borage or blackcurrant seed oil, vitamin B complex, vitamins C and E and zinc.

• Take cold sitz-baths for a few minutes each morning. They may sound very unpleasant, particularly in the winter, but can significantly improve circulation in the pelvis.

Herbal treatment for painful periods

There are several herbs which help to relax tension in the uterus and cervix. You can choose from: pulsatilla, wild yam, blue cohosh, cramp bark, black haw, partridge berry and motherwort. For intense pain try black cohosh.

Add herbs that increase the circulation to and from the uterus which will relax spasm and clear congestion. Choose from: cayenne, ginger, dang gui, or rosemary.

For secondary dysmenorrhea where there is congestion and stagnation of blood, use herbs such as: false unicorn root, lady's mantle, calendula, dang gui and raspberry leaves

Where there is general tension and stress add relaxing herbs such as: skullcap, lemon balm, chamomile, lavender, or vervain. For more extreme tension you can try valerian. Add hormone balancing herbs such as shatavari, chaste tree or false unicorn root.

Liver remedies will help to detoxify the system, particularly useful in secondary congestive dysmenorrhea, and also help correct the hormone balance. Choose from: burdock, yellow dock, dandelion root, rosemary, calendula, or golden seal.

Any prescription you prepare can be taken throughout the month, three times daily. As your period approaches, before the pain starts, take hot teas made from ginger or cinnamon to stimulate the circulation, and add spices to your cooking. Infusions made of any of the above herbs can be added regularly to the bath, or to either cold or warm sitz-baths.

Massage of the back and lower abdomen using dilute essential oils can help relieve tension and pain. Use essential oils of either lavender, geranium, clary sage, ylang ylang, chamomile, lemon balm, ginger or rosemary.

Heavy bleeding

The amount of blood lost during a period varies between women; what may be normal for one is heavy bleeding for another. If your periods are so heavy that they are interfering with your normal life, are making you worry about going out, or they change from their normal pattern to suddenly become heavier, then you need to seek treatment.

Blood loss is very often heavier during the first 24-48 hours, as the period becomes established, and then tails off. If you are having to change your protection (tampon or pad) every two hours or more frequently, then your bleeding is on the heavy side. If you have large clots, flooding, have to use double pads and cannot get through the night without changing, it would certainly be considered as too heavy. If the rate of blood loss is not as high as this, but your periods continue longer than the average five days, then they could be considered as heavy, because overall blood loss may be excessive.

Causes of heavy bleeding

genetic predisposition
hormone imbalance, particularly leading up to
    menopause
rare problems with blood clotting mechanisms
fibroids, polyps, endometriosis
stress
infections and inflammation in the reproductive tract
IUDs
low thyroid hormone
obesity
endometrial cancer
nutritional deficiencies

What is necessary to control bleeding and prevent hemorrhage is adequate contraction of the muscles in the uterine arteries, proper hormone balance, and substances necessary for repair of the endometrium.

If you have heavy periods, particularly if your periods are heavier than normal for you, it is important to establish whether there is any underlying cause which requires treatment. Often there is no apparent cause and the condition is known as dysfunctional uterine bleeding. This kind of heavy bleeding often accompanies anovulatory cycles (where no egg is produced) and is most likely in the first few years of menstruation and after the age of thirty-five.

Self help for heavy bleeding

Good diet is vital for maintaining normal muscle contractions in the tiny arteries in the uterus, to control bleeding, and to enable the uterus to repair itself. Protein, essential fatty acids, B vitamins, bioflavonoids, zinc, vitamin E, potassium, calcium and magnesium are all essential. Poor diet, stress, kidney problems, chronic diarrhea, the use of drugs such as cortisone and diuretics, and malabsorption can all cause deficiencies. Avoid caffeine, alcohol, smoking and fatty foods.

Often women who have low thyroid function have a tendency to heavy bleeding. Signs of low thyroid include lethargy, dry skin, feeling cold and a low temperature (below 97.8°F or 36.6°C under the arm). Food rich in iodine will help maintain thyroid hormone balance.

A relationship exists between fat and estrogen; those tending to be overweight are more likely to have excess estrogen in the system stored in fat tissue. This will upset the normal hormone balance. Take regular exercise, and make sure you get plenty of rest and relaxation. Deal with any stress (see p.51 for stress management). Make sure you put time aside for yourself and your own needs, away from the demands of work and family. Rest during your period as over-exercising stimulates bleeding.

Herbal treatment for heavy bleeding

To correct hormone imbalances use chaste tree or false unicorn root. Add uterine astringents – beth root, or oak bark. Uterine tonics will increase the energy in the uterus and improve its tone and function – use false unicorn root, raspberry leaves or partridge berry. Add a liver remedy to your prescription to aid the metabolism of hormones. Choose from calendula, rosemary, dandelion root, golden seal, or yellow dock.

Tonics to the mucous membrane will help control the shedding of the uterine lining – golden seal is best for this. Where there is uterine congestion, which interrupts the normal control of bleeding as the muscles cannot contract properly, use herbs to drain the area, such as cleavers, calendula, golden seal, raspberry leaves, or lady's mantle. Where stress may be related to hormonal imbalance, add herbs to support the nervous system, such as skullcap, lemon balm or vervain.

Amenorrhea: lack of periods

Missing periods is, of course, perfectly natural if you are pregnant or breastfeeding. If you are approaching forty it could be the start of an early menopause, particularly if your menarche was late. There are two types of amenorrhea – primary amenorrhea when periods have never started, and secondary amenorrhea when periods cease.

Causes of primary amenorrhea

late menarche (onset of periods) after the age of 16
low weight
hereditary disposition
illness, stress, emotional upset
poor diet
hormone imbalance
low vital energy
rare congenital abnormalities
low levels of thyroid hormone
an imperforate hymen

Causes of secondary amenorrhea

low weight, especially from over-dieting
nutritional deficiencies, anemia
excessively high or low levels of thyroid hormones
other hormone imbalances
obesity – upsetting the body's estrogen balance
ceasing to take the pill
diabetes, liver disease or chronic illness
drugs such as morphine, and those taken for high blood pressure and cancer
stress, overwork, fatigue
radiotherapy
poor circulation
shock or emotional upset
physical disruption, such as travel
rarely, a tumour of the pituitary or adrenal glands, or the ovary

Note It is important to consult your practitioner for a clear diagnosis if your periods stop.

Self help for amenorrhea

Once you have excluded pregnancy and menopause and ruled out other illness as possible causes, there are several things you can do to correct your hormone balance.
• Improve your diet: make sure you have all the nutrients necessary for normal hormone balance (see p.86), including B vitamins, particularly B6, folic acid, vitamin E, zinc, magnesium, calcium, and EFAs. Common causes of amenorrhea are deficiencies of B6 and zinc, indicated by white spots on the fingernails, slow healing, poor resistance and a tendency to stretch marks. You may need to take supplements for a few months – take evening primrose oil, B complex and a multimineral and vitamin supplement.
• Do not allow your weight to drop below 112 lb (50 kg) and if you have a tendency to underweight make sure you eat properly. Do not adopt extreme diets to lose weight but ensure your diet contains plenty of protein and unrefined carbohydrate as well as EFAs. If you have eating problems such as anorexia, you should seek help. Digestive disorders may cause deficiencies of vital nutrients and should be treated promptly.
• Take regular exercise, especially if you are otherwise sedentary, though without going to extremes. It is particularly important to take regular exercise if you tend to feel the cold, and to wrap up warmly in chilly weather. If your circulation is poor add spices to your cooking and avoid cold foods and drinks. If you suspect your coldness could be related to low thyroid hormone (a blood test will indicate this) take kelp.
• If you feel stress is the cause of your amenorrhea, it is important to reduce your commitments and allow more time for yourself. If you have specific emotional problems you may need professional help to resolve them. Massage, yoga, relaxation and meditation are also of great benefit. It may be that certain feelings that you have about your body, your femininity or your sexuality, or unconscious anxieties relating to these, are upsetting your hormone balance.
• If you suspect anemia could be the problem, indicated by tiredness, breathlessness, palpitations or pallor, a simple blood test will show it. You may need to take iron, and you should increase iron-containing foods in your diet and vitamin C containing foods to aid iron absorption.

It is important to treat amenorrhea if it continues for more than a few months, as one long-term effect is an increased tendency to osteoporosis. Treatment may need to continue for several months before menstruation resumes.

Note Amenorrhea does not necessarily indicate infertility so if you want to avoid pregnancy, continue using contraception.

Motherwort

Leonurus cardiaca

ALSO KNOWN AS: Lion's tail, lion's ear

PART USED: Aerial parts

CONTAINS: Alkaloids, including leonurine and stachydrine, bitter glycosides, including leonurin and leonuridin, tannins, resins, vitamin A

KEY USES: Antispasmodic, carminative, cardiotonic, emmenagogue, relaxant, nervine, gentle uterine stimulant

Motherwort is predominantly a womb remedy, for painful, delayed or suppressed periods, and also to prepare for childbirth. If taken two to three times daily, in the last few weeks of pregnancy, it encourages more co-ordinated contractions of the uterus when otherwise they could be painfully spasmodic or insufficient. The name motherwort could also come from its traditional reputation for soothing stress and tension during pregnancy, childbirth and motherhood.

Both alkaloids in motherwort induce uterine contractions, stachydrine doing so particularly at the end of pregnancy when the nature of uterine muscles changes and Braxton-Hicks contractions begin in practice for labour. This stimulating effect is coupled with an appreciable sedative and relaxing effect, contributed by bitter glycosides, useful for anxiety or tension about the coming birth. This combination of relaxant with uterotonic effects gives motherwort a useful role both as a partus preparator and during labour to facilitate the birth. It has a reputation for preventing miscarriage and relieving false labour pains.

Motherwort has other cardiotonic properties, making it beneficial to the heart. It strengthens the heart, especially useful during pregnancy and childbirth when more stress is imposed on the heart. It may also be used for irregularities such as arrhythmias and palpitations which are associated with anxiety and tension. The glycosides have been observed to have a short-term ability to lower blood pressure.

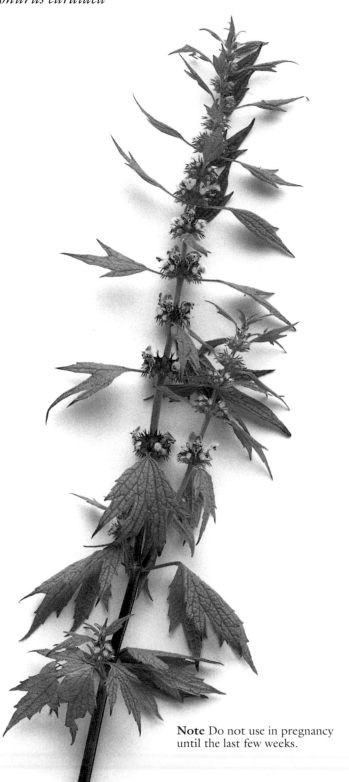

Note Do not use in pregnancy until the last few weeks.

Herbal treatment for amenorrhea

Use the hormone balancing herbs chaste tree or false unicorn root. Shatavari is a nourishing tonic to the reproductive system, supplying ingredients for hormones, and is particularly useful where there is deficiency and debility. Add tonics to the uterus and ovaries to bring blood to the area and stimulate normal function. False unicorn root, sage, motherwort, dang gui, calendula, blue cohosh, yarrow and wormwood are all helpful.

If you feel the cold and suffer from poor circulation, add warming herbs such as ginger or cinnamon. Use liver remedies to ensure normal metabolism of hormones in the liver. Choose from wormwood, rosemary, calendula, dandelion root or yellow dock root.

If you feel stress is related to your lack of periods add supportive herbs such as rosemary, lavender, chamomile, skullcap, vervain and wild oats. Choose the appropriate Bach Flower Remedies (see p.246–7) to help with any emotional problems. Essential oils such as clary sage, rose, melissa and lavender can be used in the bath or in massage oils to help relieve stress and tension and to help restore normal hormonal balance.

Irregular periods and abnormal bleeding

A healthy woman generally has regular cycles, even if they are slightly less or more than 28 days, and bleeds roughly the same amount each month. If you never know how long your cycle is going to be as it varies so much from one period to another, or if you miss some months altogether, then you clearly have irregular periods.

Causes of the hormonal imbalance contributing to irregular periods

failure to ovulate regularly; approaching menopause
low thyroid function
drugs, such as antibiotics
dietary deficiencies, particularly iodine, vitamins B6, C, E, manganese and chorine, essential fatty acids, zinc, calcium, iron and magnesium
overweight or underweight
trauma, stress, tiredness
chronic illness such as candidiasis
lifestyle changes, travel
allergy

Bleeding or spotting between periods

A slight loss of blood between periods is frequently caused by hormonal changes which can occur in teenagers just starting their periods, and in women approaching menopause. Many women in their thirties have light spotting at ovulation time when estrogen levels drop.

Other causes of spotting:

the pill
IUDs
pelvic inflammatory disease
ectopic pregnancy
cervical erosion or polyps
cancer of the cervix or uterus
chronic cervicitis
endometriosis

In post-menopausal women abnormal bleeding can be caused by ERT, vaginitis, endometrial polyps or cancer. If you suffer from abnormal uterine bleeding it is important to obtain a clear diagnosis from your practitioner and for treatment to be aimed at the underlying cause. Providing there is no pathology found, treatment is aimed at balancing the hormones – follow the suggestions for self help and herbal treatment to regain normal hormone balance in amenorrhea and PMS (p.89).

Herbs should be used to balance hormones and increase energy and circulation to the reproductive area. Chaste tree, false unicorn root, partridge berry, motherwort, calendula, lady's mantle and raspberry leaves are all helpful.

Menstrual headaches and migraine

These tend to occur during the premenstrual phase or during a period. It may be hard to distinguish between a bad headache and a migraine, although migraines tend to have warning signs – visual disturbances such as tunnel vision, seeing an "aura" around things, nausea and vomiting. Both headaches and migraine can persist for a few hours or a few days.

These pains frequently accompany premenstrual syndrome, the main cause of which is hormone imbalance. All the advice given on PMS (see p.89) will be relevant. These hormonal imbalances may combine with other "triggers" to give headaches and migraine.

These triggers include:

stress, physical or mental
tiredness, overwork, eyestrain
spinal problems, particularly in the neck
neck and shoulder muscle tension
the pill and drug side effects
lack of, or too much, sleep
extremes of temperature
caffeine and caffeine withdrawal
dietary triggers: alcohol, especially red wine, sherry,
    port, cheese and other dairy products, citrus fruits,
    pickles, chocolate, bananas, fried or fatty foods, pork
    and red meat, yeast extract, brewer's yeast, peanuts,
    onions, seafood, sugar
poor circulation, lack of exercise
food allergies, especially to any of the trigger foods
low blood sugar (hypoglycemia); missing meals
digestive disorders, sluggish liver, constipation
smoking and pollution, such as gas leaks

Self help for headaches

• Do not miss meals and avoid refined carbohydrates and sugar particularly before your period. Eat only whole grains and unrefined foods, and to keep your blood sugar up before a period it is best to eat little and often.
• Avoid caffeine, alcohol, and smoking. Avoid any of the common migraine and headache triggers, especially in the second half of the cycle.
• You may need to consult a chiropractor, osteopath or masseur to correct spinal problems or muscle tension in the neck and shoulders. Alexander Technique may also be helpful.
• Follow the advice given for PMS on p.89–90 about relaxation, exercise, stress and diet.
• Avoid using the contraceptive pill.

Herbal treatment for headaches

There are many herbs which have been used for centuries to treat headaches and migraine.

They include:

pulsatilla	*rosemary*
wood betony	*chamomile*
lemon balm	*dandelion root*
lavender	*feverfew*
peppermint	*ginger*
skullcap	*valerian*

Take your herbal remedy over several cycles, not just when you have the pain.

Where you feel that tension and stress are playing a part, use relaxing herbs such as:

pulsatilla	*chamomile*
linden blossom	*vervain*
skullcap	*wood betony*
lavender	*rosemary*
passionflower	*hops*

If you tend to feel cold easily and have poor circulation, you can use herbs that increase the circulation, particularly to the head.

These include:

ginger	*cayenne*
rosemary	*thyme*
wood betony	*feverfew*
peppermint	

You may find that liver remedies help, especially if you suffer from digestive problems or sluggish bowels.

Choose from:

dandelion root	*yellow dock root*
burdock	*wormwood*
rosemary	*feverfew*

Hormone balancing herbs should always be included in your prescription. Take either chaste tree or false unicorn root or both. Some herbs contain natural salicylates (contained in aspirin) and can help to relieve head pain. These include black cohosh and meadowsweet. Feverfew has been researched widely for its application to migraine. Regular use of feverfew will help to prevent migraine. Pick one leaf straight from the plant and eat it in a sandwich every day. Chewing the leaves alone can cause mouth ulcers in some people.

Essential oils can be applied directly to the head to relieve head pain – rosemary oil is the best known for this purpose. You could also use chamomile, lemon balm, lavender or peppermint oil. A few drops of essential oil can be added to the bath, or used in a massage oil to relieve tension in the neck and shoulders.

5 Preconception and Fertility

A child's pattern of health begins with its parents at the time of conception. Upon them depends the health of the sperm and egg which contain the genetic blueprint for the child's future; the stronger and fitter they are, the healthier the fetus. It is vital for parents to prepare positively for parenthood, to give their offspring the best possible chance for optimum health and vitality. Our responsibilities to our children begin some time before conception, and not simply once the baby is born. It is in the preconceptual months that preventative medicine is really important.

The four months prior to conception are the most vital for the normal development of sperm and egg, and thus the baby formed from their union. Both ova and sperm can suffer the effects of poor nutrition, toxic metals, environmental chemicals, viruses and some drugs before conception. These adverse factors have the potential for causing harm in the form of infertility, fetal abnormalities, miscarriage, stillbirth, perinatal death and low weight babies. They can also arrest the baby's development.

It is therefore important to strive for optimum health before you conceive. Now is the time for a good general check-up to give yourself time to correct any imbalances, allergies or illness which could be potential risk factors. Before you actually plan to conceive, find time to address any tendency you have to infection, and to raise your immunity using diet and herbs.

The time to pay attention to diet, and if necessary change it for the better, is several months prior to conception and not when pregnancy is confirmed. Most women who are pregnant do not realize it until they are six to eight weeks pregnant, by which time it is a little late to start changing the diet. Much of the crucial development of the baby occurs during the first eight weeks, when the nutritional and toxic state of the mother can largely determine the normal development of the embryo. Mineral and vitamin imbalances, which might go unnoticed in a child or adult, may have a disastrous effect on the developing baby, because the rapid rate of growth of the embryonic cells causes an exaggerated response to pathogenic factors. If these imbalances interfere with the growth or metabolism of these developing cells, it can result in malformations or impaired function of organs and tissues.

The ovum will unite with just one sperm to form a new life.

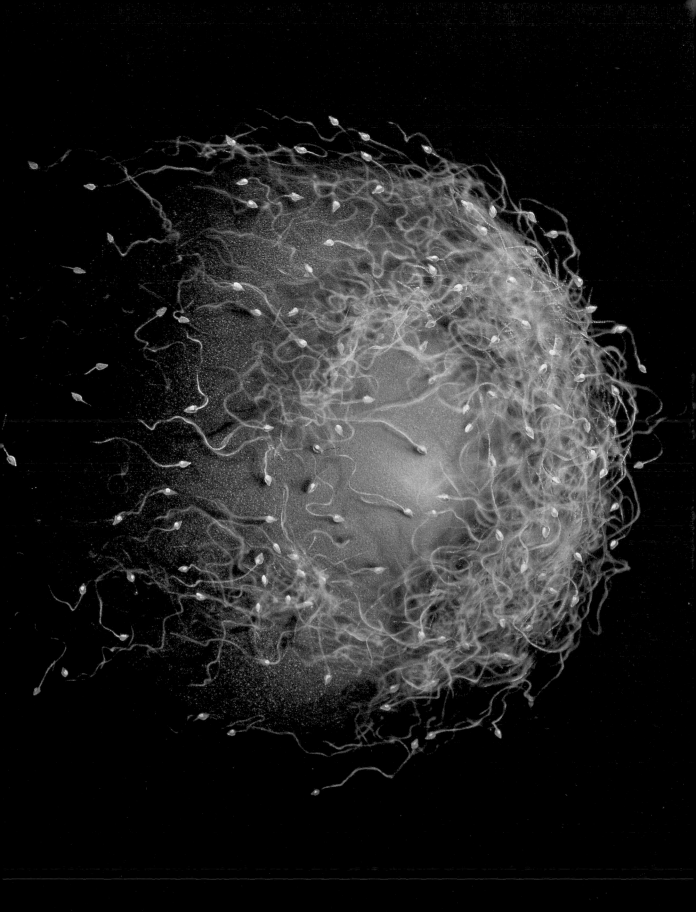

Conception

Each month at ovulation, an egg is released from one or other ovary and trapped by the finger-like projections of one of the fallopian tubes, there to begin its journey to the uterus. Conception takes place when a man's sperm unites with the egg in the fallopian tube.

During sexual intercourse, when a man ejaculates, up to fifty million sperm are released into the vagina. They then travel at a rate of about an inch every four minutes, via the cervix, through the uterus and into the fallopian tubes. When a woman is ovulating the cervix softens and dilates, easing the entry of sperm into the uterus; the vaginal secretions, which are normally acid, become more alkaline and thereby more hospitable to the sperm. With the help of muscular contractions and natural hormonal and chemical assistance, the sperm may arrive in the fallopian tube to fertilize an egg within a few minutes of intercourse. It more often takes between one and four hours.

Conception may occur at any time over several days. After it is released into the fallopian tube, an egg can survive for up to 48 hours, although there is more chance of conception in the first 24 hours. The sperm can survive longer than this, for up to three days, though most are able to penetrate and fertilize the egg only during the first two days.

The best chances of conception occur if you have intercourse at the time of ovulation, which is about 14 days before your period. It is also possible, however, to become pregnant by having intercourse up to three days before ovulation and up to three days afterwards.

At about the time of ovulation, the vaginal secretions increase and become thinner. One indication that you are ovulating is that the mucus in vaginal secretion increases. It has a stretchy quality so that it can be strung between two fingers. This change makes it easier for the sperm to swim through the mucus to enter the uterus via the cervix.

Once the sperm and egg have successfully united, the fertilized egg spends the next three days travelling down the fallopian tube, and then arrives in the uterus. After a couple more days it embeds itself in the wall of the uterus. When the sperm penetrates the egg, the nuclei of the sperm and egg fuse, and the process of cell division is initiated. The fused nuclei split first into 2 cells, then 4 cells, then 8 and so on, each containing the 46 chromosomes necessary in a normal, healthy human being.

Fertility and infertility

For conception to occur, the right conditions need to exist for a sperm to successfully fertilize an egg, and for the fertilized egg to implant in the uterus. Both potential parents need to be in good general health for these conditions to prevail. It is important to understand what makes for fertility before looking at ways of overcoming difficulties in achieving it.

Conditions necessary for fertility

Sufficient normal, healthy sperm need to be produced by the man.

The mucus in the woman's vagina and protecting the cervix needs to be thin enough to allow passage of sperm. During much of the cycle it is too thick for sperm to penetrate. Around ovulation the mucus should become more profuse and watery so that the sperm are able to enter the uterus via the cervix.

A fully developed, healthy egg needs to be produced by the woman and released from the ovary into the fallopian tube, where it should move down to meet the sperm. Once they meet the sperm needs to be able to penetrate the surface of the egg to fertilize it.

Once they have fused, they need to be propelled down the fallopian tube into the uterus.

The lining of the uterus should build up sufficiently under the influence of estrogen and progesterone for the fertilized egg to implant and start growing. A high percentage of eggs do not implant properly, as the womb lining often does not develop adequately.

There are several factors which can affect these vital conditions and therefore fertility. They are different in men and women, so if you are trying to conceive you need to be aware of both.

Factors affecting fertility in women

A woman's fertility is governed by a number of factors, some perfectly natural, such as age, and others over which we have some control.

A woman's fertility drops as she gets older, and significantly so over the age of 35.

Mucus produced by the cervix may be too thick or profuse for the sperm to penetrate. The mucus may contain antibodies to the sperm, which kill them. Vaginal infections can make the mucus "hostile" to sperm. The pH of the vagina may be too acid for the sperm to survive. Artificial lubricants, jelly or cream may damage sperm.

One or both of the fallopian tubes may be blocked because of such ailments as pelvic inflammatory disease, scarring from previous surgery or abortion, endometriosis, or sexually transmitted disease. (See Chapter 12.)

There may be damage to the uterus caused by infection or fibroids, preventing successful implantation. One or both ovaries could be affected by ovarian cysts or endometriosis, and fail to produce the balance of hormones needed for ripening the egg follicle and for developing the womb lining. A damaged ovary may not release its ripe eggs successfully into the fallopian tubes.

Hormone imbalances caused by a wide range of factors (see Hormone balance p.86) such as illness, stress, nutritional deficiencies or loss of weight, may affect the ovaries, uterine lining and cervical mucus. They may inhibit ovulation.

The contraceptive pill affects the natural hormone balance, and the menstrual cycle may be erratic for several months after ceasing to take the pill. The use of IUDs can contribute to infection and inflammation in the uterus or fallopian tubes where resultant scar tissue can cause blockage.

Smoking can inhibit normal function of the reproductive system by reducing the blood flow to the pelvis and slowing the action of the finger-like projections, called cilia, in the fallopian tube which propel the egg towards the uterus.

Damage to the cervix from infection, erosion, polyps, abortions or surgery to remove pre-cancerous cells can upset the mucus balance and inhibit the sperm's entry into the uterus.

There may be retroversion of the uterus, or in some cases a congenital defect causing infertility.

Being overweight or underweight can affect the hormone balance and so interfere with ovulation (see Hormone balance p.86).

Caffeine, taken regularly, has been shown to reduce fertility by about four times.

Low thyroid function can affect fertility by upsetting hormone balance. Other endocrine problems, upsetting the function of either the pituitary or adrenal glands which help to regulate the menstrual cycle, can cause failure to ovulate.

Certain nutrients including vitamins B6, C, B2, A, E, B12, zinc, iron, folic acid, essential fatty acids and magnesium are vital to fertility. Deficiencies in such nutrients can cause infertility.

Stress not only upsets hormone balance but also causes contraction of the fallopian tubes, inhibiting the egg's passage and decreasing blood supply to the pelvis. It can inhibit proper development of the womb lining and affect sex by causing spasm in the vagina.

Factors affecting fertility in men

Many of the causes of fertility problems in men are related to lifestyle and general health, and can successfully be overcome without medical treatment or expensive therapies.

A low sperm count will decrease fertility. The average man ejaculates around 300 million sperm, although conception is possible even with a number as low as 20 million. Sperm count is affected by diet and lifestyle. Smoking, X-rays and drugs, alcohol, toxic chemicals, and stress will all lower sperm count.

Overheating of the testes by overhot baths, tight underpants, undescended testes or a varicocele (an enlarged vein around the testicle, like a varicose vein) can impair sperm production. Infection, high fevers, hormone imbalance, caffeine, overweight and underweight, can all reduce sperm production.

Often low sperm counts are associated with a higher number of poor quality sperm. Not only should there be sufficient sperm, but also they need to be able to swim straight and strongly. They need to be both mobile and motile. Sperm quality can also be affected by infection, hormonal imbalance, varicocele, inflammation of the prostate gland, too little or too much semen, and toxic chemicals such as lead and cadmium.

There may be no sperm. Blockage in the tubes bringing the seminal fluid from the testicles, retrograde ejaculation when the semen passes backwards into the bladder, and infections such as mumps or damage to the testes may be the cause.

Sperm may have other problems. Sometimes they stick together in clumps which stops them from being able to swim freely towards the fallopian tubes. This can be due to infection or to the production in the man of antibodies to his own sperm. Some sperm are unable to penetrate the protective barrier around the egg. Normally, to do this, a sperm head sheds its outer membrane and releases an enzyme which helps it to break through into the egg.

Impotence and premature ejaculation are clearly problems for fertility.

Stress can affect hormone balance, and the blood supply to the reproductive system, inhibiting normal function. It can also affect sexual performance.

It is estimated that in 30 per cent of couples who have fertility problems there is a medical problem with the male partner, in 30 per cent one with the woman, and the rest of the time it may well be related to poor diet, toxic chemicals, stress and other factors, simply upsetting hormone balance. It is important for both partners to be thoroughly checked over and a proper diagnosis made before treatment is attempted. If no medical problem is found in either partner, self-help and herbal remedies to enhance fertility may well be the answer.

Diet and herbs to enhance fertility

Dietary measures
To help ensure the correct pH balance of the cervical mucus, you need to eat plenty of alkaline foods. An over-acid vagina will inhibit sperm. Most fruit and vegetables, as well as milk, are alkaline. Meat, fish, whole grains, cheese, eggs, and seeds are acid. Tea, coffee and alcohol acidify the system.

Try to make sure your weight is right for you. Over-exercising, or excess dieting causing low weight, can stop ovulation.

Eat plenty of foods containing essential fatty acids – unrefined vegetable and seed oils, nuts and seeds, beans and pulses, fatty fish and Evening Primrose oil. Linseed oil, blackcurrant, borage seed oil are all good sources. Eat foods containing vitamin E (see p.72) which is vital to fertility, as well as foods containing protein, vitamins A, C, Bs, and minerals, particularly zinc, iron and magnesium. Avoid coffee and alcohol which can cause vitamin B6 deficiency. Supplements of the above nutrients may be necessary to improve infertility.

Avoid any unnecessary drugs (marijuana is known to lower sperm count), junk foods, fatty foods, alcohol and tobacco.

Self help for improving fertility
It is important for both partners to be in as good health as possible – chronic infections should be cleared up and other health problems attended to. Exercise should be taken regularly, but not to the point of excess; overwork and stress should be avoided as far as possible. If you feel tense, tired or run down, it may be necessary to consult a practitioner to help improve your general health and vitality.

Relaxation exercises, hypnotherapy, yoga, T'ai Chi, meditation, counselling or psychotherapy may help where unexplained fertility problems are related to stress or emotional problems. Now is the time to deal with such issues.

Cold hip baths may help low sperm production and menstrual problems as they increase circulation to the reproductive system.

Clearly, the most likely time to conceive is around the time of ovulation. During that week make love only two or three times; any more and you may deplete vital energy and reduce the sperm count. Abstaining for the week leading up to this time will allow sperm and energy to build up and increase fertility.

Men should keep their testicles cool; it is better to wear boxer shorts rather than tight underpants, loose trousers, and avoid hot baths and electric blankets.

Make sure your menstrual cycle is regular so that you can tell when you are ovulating. A temperature chart is often helpful. If you have menstrual problems, use herbs and diet to treat them (see p.88).

The sperm need to be deposited high in the vagina and stay there for at least half an hour after sex. So the penis needs to penetrate deeply and it is best for the woman not to jump up immediately afterwards to wash or pass water. Lie on your back with your knees raised; this is the best way to help the sperm's journey to the fallopian tubes.

Saw palmetto

Serenoa serrulata

ALSO KNOWN AS: Sabal

PART USED: Berries

CONTAINS: Volatile oil, steroidal saponins (including B-sitosterol), alkaloid resins, tannins, fixed oil

KEY USES: Sedative, diuretic, expectorant, tonic decongestant, nutritive, antiseptic

This North American plant was first noted for its beneficial and fattening effect the berries had on animals who fed on them after the summer drought. When used in humans they were found to enhance digestion, improve strength and vitality and increase flesh and weight, and were prescribed as a nourishing tonic particularly for those suffering from wasting diseases. The nourishing and tonic effects of saw palmetto were especially observed in the reproductive system, and it is a well-known remedy for atrophy of the testes, low libido, impotence, prostate enlargement and any inflammation in the reproductive tract. It has also been used as a reproductive tonic for women, increasing sexual energy, fertility and increasing milk flow in nursing mothers, and can be prescribed to relieve painful periods, to regulate the menstrual cycle, and for inflammatory conditions such as salpingitis and ovarian pain.

Saw palmetto also has an affinity with the urinary system, and can be taken to relieve urinary infections and fluid retention, as well as for incontinence and bed-wetting. It relaxes the nervous system, soothes tension and anxiety, and also has a toning action on the mucous membranes throughout the body, useful for treating colds, catarrh, and sinusitis. Its added expectorant properties make it a good remedy for bronchitis and asthma.

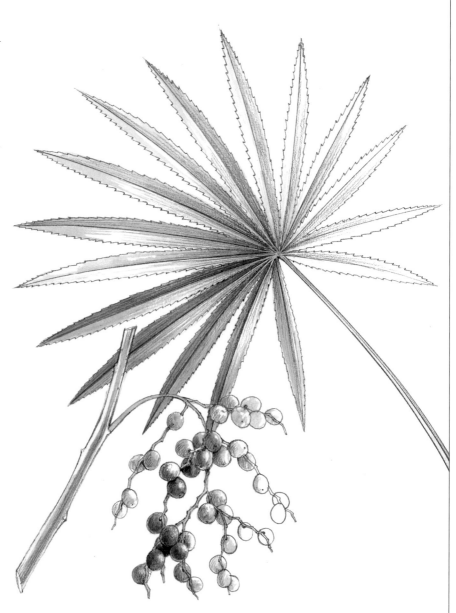

Herbal remedies for improving fertility

For women who need help to correct hormonal imbalances, there are several suitable herbs which can be recommended.

Use the following, singly or in mixtures:

chaste tree	false unicorn root
wild yam	dang gui
shatavari	kelp

Men may also need to balance their hormones.

Men should choose from:

ginseng	ashwagandha
kelp	wild yam
saw palmetto	false unicorn root

There are also herbs which will increase general vitality in both men and women.

Choose from these rejuvenative herbs:

ginseng	shatavari
cinnamon	ginger
ashwagandha (for men)	
dang gui (for women)	

Where there is weakness, debility or stress, which affects both hormone balance and sexual performance, take tonics to the nervous system.

Choose from:

skullcap	vervain
ginseng	lemon balm
wild oats	cinnamon

Combine with them herbs that act as tonics to the reproductive system, notably:

shatavari	wild yam
false unicorn root	ginseng
partridge berry	
dang gui (for women)	
ashwagandha (for men)	

Add a liver remedy to your prescription to help detoxify the body and maintain normal hormone balance – choose from dandelion root, rosemary or yellow dock root. A useful recipe to strengthen women, normalize their cycles and enhance fertility is as follows: equal parts of lady's mantle, false unicorn root, dang gui, ginger, wild yam and raspberry leaves, and half a part of licorice. Take three times daily over a few months until energy is restored and cycles are normal.

Essential oils can be used in massage oils, in baths and to inhale. Lavender, geranium, lemon balm and rosemary will help relieve stress and tension. Ginger, cinnamon, and peppermint will act as tonics, warming the body and increasing the circulation. They are useful where there is tiredness and debility related to sexual weakness or scanty periods and deficiency of vital warmth. Rose has a particular affinity for the female sex organs and is particularly recommended for stress related to the reproductive system.

Other remedies

In Ayurvedic medicine, which is practised mainly in India, there are several simple recipes used for sexual debility.

Equal parts of dried dates, blanched almonds, pistachios and sugar are macerated in ghee for a week. An ounce (25 g) of the mixture can be taken each morning. (Ghee is clarified butter resembling oil, which can be bought from an Indian or wholefood store.)

The juice of white onions, and fresh ginger can be taken together with honey regularly to restore lost virility. To extract onion juice, chop an onion finely and cover with honey overnight. By morning the honey will have drawn off the juice; strain it and discard the onion.

Cooked rice with large quantities of ghee and soup of kidney beans is said to invigorate the body and increase sexual energy.

For depleted conditions of the semen and sperm, seeds of watercress can be taken in decoction. Watercress itself is high in vitamins B and C and zinc, all vital to healthy reproductive function and normal action of the pituitary gland.

The juice of onions with honey or a generous helping of lady's fingers (okra) eaten each morning benefits sperm formation. Cardamons, mace, almonds, clarified butter and unrefined sugar mixed together and taken each morning have similar benefit.

To help invigorate the reproductive organs and increase their efficiency, add asparagus, fenugreek, garlic, raw onions, sesame seeds and licorice to your diet regularly.

Passionflower

Passiflora incarnata

PARTS USED: Flower and vine

CONTAINS: Alkaloids (including harmane, harmol, harmaline, harmine, harmalol), sugar, gum, sterols, flavonoids

KEY USES: Sedative, antispasmodic, anodyne

Passionflower is a wonderfully relaxing remedy and one of the best tranquilizing herbs for chronic insomnia, having no addictive effects and allowing you to awake refreshed and alert in the morning. It has a sedative and antispasmodic action, relaxing spasm and tension in the muscles, and calming the nerves and lessening pain. It can be used for neuralgia, shingles, sciatica, Parkinson's disease, muscle pain, twitching and spasm, anxiety, agitation, stress and any physical problem that is stress-related, such as colic and asthma, as well as high blood pressure. Wherever physical symptoms are related to or aggravated by anxiety or tension, passionflower can be added to your chosen prescription; for example for hot flashes, migraine, headaches, abdominal pain or a tickly cough.

Passionflower exerts its beneficial effects on the nerves by toning the sympathetic nerve centre, and improving circulation and nutrition to the nerves.

The name passion flower gives little indication of its action; it was so called by Spanish explorers and missionaries who saw a resemblance in the flower to the crown of thorns of Christ's passion.

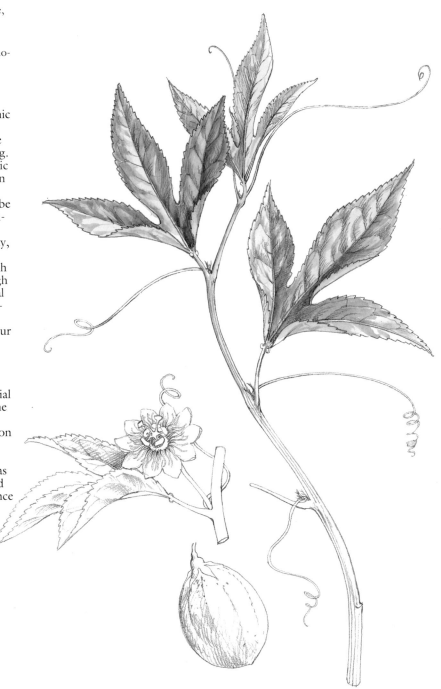

Ashwagandha

Withania omnifera

ALSO KNOWN AS: Winter cherry

PART USED: Root

CONTAINS: Bitter alkaloid somniferin

KEY USES: Aphrodisiac, sedative, astringent, bitter tonic

Ashwagandha is a very important herb in Ayurvedic medicine, held in as high esteem as ginseng is in Chinese medicine, but it is much less costly. It is a famous rejuvenative herb, useful in all conditions of weakness and tissue debility, particularly recommended for weakness in children and the elderly, for those run down by chronic illness, and those suffering from stress, overwork, nervous exhaustion and insomnia. When taken as a milk decoction and sweetened with honey it is said to inhibit aging and build up strength by catalyzing the anabolic processes in the body. It is calming and used to clear the mind, and has been prescribed for general debility, for convalescence, for loss of memory, nervous problems such as multiple sclerosis, rheumatism, skin problems, anemia and loss of muscular energy.

Ashwagandha has a particular affinity for the reproductive system in both men and women. It is good for weak pregnant women and is said to stabilize the embryo. It acts as a tonic to the hormonal system, and is recommended for sexual debility, low sperm count, infertility, impotence, weakness of the back and knees, to improve the condition of the semen and promote conception.

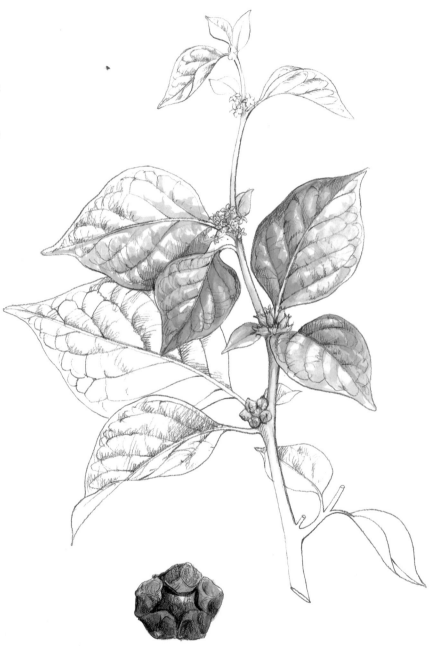

Shatavari

Asparagus racemosus

ALSO KNOWN AS: Tian men dong

PART USED: Root

KEY USES: Diuretic, demulcent, galacta-gogue, expectorant, tonic

Shatavari is the most important rejuvenative tonic for women in Ayurvedic medicine. It is prepared as a milk decoction with ghee, raw sugar and honey. Its main action is on the female reproductive tract and it is used for sexual debility, infertility, and to balance hormones. It increases milk production in nursing mothers and is an excellent remedy for women during the menopause as it supplies many steroidal precursors, building blocks for production of sex hormones. It is said to nourish and strengthen the reproductive system. It increases semen production in men.

Shatavari means "who possesses a hundred husbands" as its tonic and rejuvenative action on the female reproductive organs is said to be considerable.

It has soothing qualities and is used for dry, inflamed mucous membranes throughout the body. It soothes and heals gastritis and peptic ulceration, relieves hyperacidity as well as diarrhea and dysentery. It also soothes irritated conditions of the urinary system and respiratory tract.

Shatavari is nourishing and also detoxifying – it is recommended during convalescence, and for infections such as herpes and chronic fevers. It is calming and helps relieve anxiety and stress.

In Ayurvedic medicine Shatavari is used to increase spiritual awareness and compassion.

It is used externally to help relieve painful swollen joints and muscle tension.

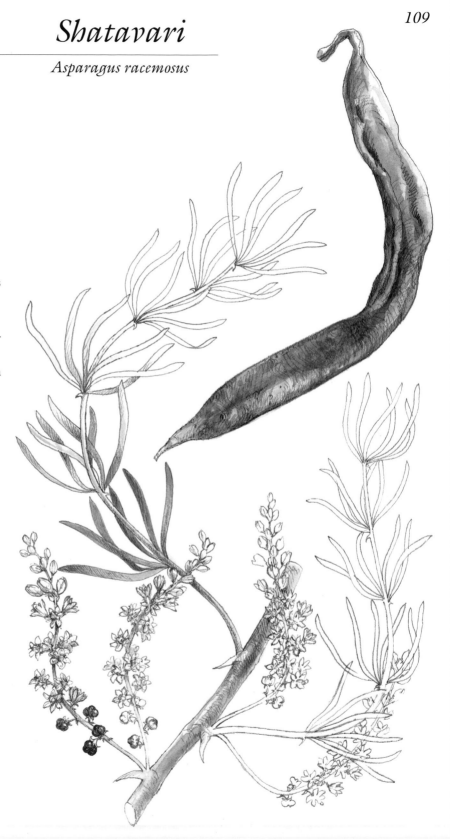

Lady's mantle

Alchemilla vulgaris

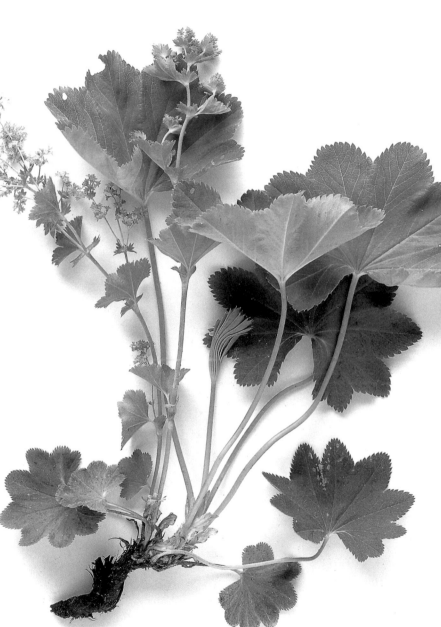

ALSO KNOWN AS: Lion's foot, bear's foot

PART USED: Aerial parts

CONTAINS: Tannins, salicylic acid, saponins, volatile oils, bitters, phytosterols

KEY USES: Astringent, emmenagogue, uterine stimulant, anti-inflammatory, vulnerary, diuretic

Lady's mantle is said to resemble the Virgin Mary's cloak, and has an affinity for the female reproductive tract. Its astringent tannins help to reduce heavy periods, particularly useful around the menopause, while as a uterine stimulant and emmenagogue it stimulates menstrual flow and can be used to stimulate contractions during childbirth. It can be used to relieve period pains and to regulate periods, and was a traditional remedy for inducing sleep.

The astringent properties are useful for treating diarrhea and gastroenteritis, while the salicylic acid reduces inflammation in the digestive and reproductive systems.

Lady's mantle can be used externally as a douche or lotion (mixed with rose water if you wish) for vaginal discharge, irritation and infection. It also makes a good skin lotion for rashes such as eczema, cuts and wounds, sores and insect bites. As a mouthwash or gargle it can be used for bleeding gums, mouth ulcers and sore throats.

Note Avoid during pregnancy.

Miscarriage and its prevention

For those who have suffered miscarriage in the past, trying to conceive again is both stressful and worrying. Herbal remedies may well prove effective in preventing another miscarriage, but only in cases where the outlook for the pregnancy is good. Herbs support the body's own systems, they cannot oppose them, and if the body's purpose is to terminate the pregnancy herbal treatment cannot prevent it. If the fetus is normal and your general health, both physical and emotional, is good when you next conceive, herbal treatment will help and support you.

Miscarriage is far more common than we may suppose. It is estimated that one in two very early pregnancies miscarry, appearing as a late or heavy period, and that one in six women who have a positive pregnancy test suffer miscarriage. It is also estimated that about half of "threatened miscarriages" can be prevented. Where a "missed miscarriage" occurs, the baby dies in the womb but may not be expelled from the womb for up to a few weeks. After the 24th week of pregnancy, the death of the baby is called a stillbirth rather than a miscarriage. Miscarriage is defined as losing a baby before 24-26 weeks.

In most cases the causes of miscarriage are:

fetal abnormality
structural problems in the uterus (such as fibroids)
viral infections (such as flu, herpes)
cervical incompetence
hormone imbalances – notably low progesterone
debility, chronic illness or nutritional deficiency

Repeated miscarriage can be caused by the presence of tiny clots in the placenta which are caused by an imbalance between the two substances which dilate blood vessels.

Abnormalities in the male's sperm may also be to blame for recurrent miscarriage.

Immunological problems might also be a factor in repeated miscarriage. The body should be programmed to recognize that a developing fetus is not a "foreign body" which requires rejection, despite the fact that it develops partly from "for-eign" tissue – the sperm from your partner. In some cases, this programming does not work.

Women who conceive while on fertility drugs have a higher chance of miscarriage as their own hormone balance may not be able to sustain the pregnancy.

A faulty egg may cause placental failure, as the placenta develops from the egg. It may also be due to impaired circulation to the placenta.

Some medical disorders can increase the risk of miscarriage, including underactive thyroid, diabetes, kidney problems and lupus. It is important to seek treatment for any medical condition before conceiving. Some, such as diabetes, may not be curable but can be managed. Others, such as an underactive thyroid and some kidney problems, are quite treatable.

If you have a history of high blood pressure it is very important to check it before conceiving and seek treatment if it is raised. Once pregnancy is confirmed, your blood pressure will be checked regularly.

Check your blood group before trying to conceive – you will need careful monitoring through pregnancy if you or your partner are rhesus negative and the other is positive.

Threatened miscarriage

Watch for bleeding, particularly with bright red blood, clots and mucus.

Abdominal pain rather like cramping period pain, or back pain, or both, may occur.

Note Extreme abdominal pain, with or without bleeding, may indicate an ectopic pregnancy. Consult your practitioner.

Some women have spotting during pregnancy, or light periods once a month so that they may not be aware they are pregnant. Spotting such as this does not indicate a threatened miscarriage. A miscarriage will be inevitable if the cervix opens and bleeding continues. In such cases the uterus sometimes empties completely and then the cervix closes, but more usually the uterus empties only partially and the miscarriage is "incomplete". A dilation and curettage (D and C) is required to clear away remaining tissue. At the first signs of bleeding or cramping in the abdomen call your practitioner immediately.

This is what you can do to help yourself:

Lie down and rest totally – only get up to use the lavatory

Keep warm, relieve any backache with a hot water bottle but do not put it on your abdomen

Try not to panic

Call your partner, a friend or relation to give you emotional support

Use deep breathing, relaxation exercises or meditation to calm you if you feel the need

Think as positively as you can – distract any nagging thoughts or panic by talking, reading, or listening to music. It may help to sleep

Herbs for threatened miscarriage

Take false unicorn root in decoction and sip it every few minutes, taking about 1 cupful every 15-60 minutes depending on the severity of the symptoms. This is said to work best in women who feel a dragging sensation in the uterus.

You can combine your false unicorn root with equal parts of cramp bark which relaxes the uterus, soothes cramp and helps to prevent miscarriage and the stress and tension related to it.

Black haw and cramp bark can also be used together to avert miscarriage. They relax the uterus and the system generally, and help ensure rest and relaxation while you take bed rest. Sip the tea through the day at the outset of symptoms.

Wild yam can be taken for tension and stress and cramping pains. You can enhance its effects by adding a little ginger and drinking it as hot tea.

Other tonic herbs used to prevent miscarriage include raspberry leaves and partridge berry.

For stress and tension you can add relaxing herbs to your mixture, such as lemon balm, skullcap, vervain or valerian. The Bach Flower Remedies rock rose and mimulus or Rescue Remedy can be taken frequently through the day.

After a miscarriage or termination

If you have recently suffered a miscarriage or have had a termination you can use herbs to aid recovery, to support you through an unhappy time and to help regain normal hormone balance.

Use hormonal balancing herbs such as chaste tree or false unicorn root.

Add tonics to the reproductive system to help aid recovery – either raspberry leaves, partridge berry, false unicorn root, wild yam, dang gui,

shatavari or lady's mantle.

Use herbs to support the nervous system such as rosemary, vervain, skullcap, wild oats, lemon balm or St. John's wort.

Where there is bleeding you can use beth root or raspberry leaves to aid healing of the uterus. Add antiseptic herbs such as echinacea, thyme or calendula to help prevent infection.

Essential oils such as lemon balm, geranium, ylang ylang, bergamot and lavender will help relieve stress and tension. Rose oil is particularly recommended where there is sadness related to the reproductive system.

Self help after miscarriage

Follow guidelines for re-establishing hormone balance (see p.106). Give yourself a chance to grieve, even though others around you may not appreciate how upsetting a miscarriage or termination can be. Talk to supportive friends, relations or your partner as much as you can so that you express your grief. Counselling may be helpful.

Avoid sex for at least two weeks afterwards, otherwise you may introduce infection. Do not use tampons until after your first proper period.

Make sure you give yourself a chance to recover. Take time off work and other responsibilities and allow time to indulge yourself and really relax.

If your miscarriage or termination is fairly late on in pregnancy you may produce colostrum (first breast milk). Leave your breasts alone and it will soon dry up. Drinking sage tea will help.

The Bach Flower Remedies may help during the emotional crisis that follows miscarriage or a termination. Feelings of grief, helplessness, anger, resentment, shock, or depression may be eased by the appropriate remedy (see p.246–7)

If you want to conceive again do not concern yourself overmuch and cause yourself stress. Statistics show that women who have had one miscarriage have the same chance of having a successful pregnancy next time round as women who have never had a miscarriage.

If you have suffered an early miscarriage it is important to try and ascertain the cause, if one can be recognized, so that you can undertake any necessary treatment before conceiving again. Where miscarriage is "unexplained" it is very important for both partners to build up their general health for 6–12 months before trying again.

Herbs to prepare for pregnancy after miscarriage

Hormone-balancing herbs should be included in all prescriptions: choose either chaste tree or false unicorn root. Add tonics to the reproductive system such as wild yam, shatavari, partridge berry, dang gui or lady's mantle. Use remedies for the liver to help detoxify the body and ensure proper hormone metabolism. Either dandelion root, burdock, yellow dock root, or rosemary are indicated. To ensure adequate circulation to the uterus use cinnamon or ginger in your prescription. To support the nervous system and relax tension, or to help resolve anguish or grief related to miscarriage, add vervain, skullcap, lemon balm, rosemary or rose.

Bach Flower Remedies would also be helpful (see p.246–7). Essential oils of lemon balm, geranium and lavender can be used in massage oils or added to bath water to relieve tension and stress. Oil of rose has a particular affinity to the reproductive system and is recommended for helping to relieve sadness related to it. Where tension is expressed through upset in the menstrual cycle, particularly where there is spasm and dysmenorrhea (see p.92) add relaxants specifically for the reproductive system, such as wild yam, blue cohosh, motherwort, lemon balm or cramp bark.

If you have a history of miscarriage, it is helpful to take a cupful of equal parts of false unicorn root and cramp bark every day for the first 14-16 weeks after you have conceived.

Preparation for pregnancy

The months spent preparing yourself for pregnancy can be spent very positively. You will have time to study your diet and lifestyle and discover what is required to enhance your health and put it into practice.

This is your opportunity to resolve certain problems and correct any imbalances, be they hormonal imbalances, kidney problems, chronic infections, stress, debility, overwork, lack of exercise, poor diet, faulty digestion or a general toxicity of the system.

Make sure your diet is excellent and provides everything that is required for normal function of the reproductive system (see Fertility p.104) and hormone balance (see p.86), notably vitamins C, E, and B, particularly B6, zinc, folic acid, bioflavonoids, magnesium and protein.

Take regular outdoor exercise for at least an hour three or four days a week. Make sure you get plenty of rest and relaxation, and balance your hours of work and responsibility with fun and leisure.

Avoid alcohol which can increase the risk of miscarriage by causing chromosome abnormality in the egg. Smoking should be cut out – it is estimated that it can double the risk of miscarriage.

Stop taking the pill at least six months before planning to conceive.

Be careful not to have any contact with cat feces which can cause toxoplasmosis with a risk of miscarriage or damage to the baby. Raw meat can also spread toxoplasmosis – handle only with gloves and wipe surfaces well that have been in contact with it. Cook all meat thoroughly.

Avoid foods which could cause listeriosis or salmonella. The most risky ones are soft cheese, paté, pre-cooked chilled food or prepared chilled food, soft ice cream, and soft eggs.

Avoid all drugs and check any prescription you have to take with your practitioner in case it is contraindicated in pregnancy.

Avoid caffeine in coffee, tea, cocoa and chocolate as this increases risk of miscarriage when taken regularly.

Be watchful of the various chemicals in your environment. Check which substances you are using daily at home in your kitchen, and at work, and if possible exchange any potentially toxic substances with safer substitutes. Your drinking water could contain over-high levels of lead, aluminium or copper, so filter all tap water for internal use or buy bottled water to avoid any such risk. Avoid insecticides and herbicides by eating, where possible, food that is organically grown. Hazardous substances at work such as carbon monoxide, mercury, aniline, lead, radioactive substances and X-rays can all cause problems.

6 *Pregnancy and Childbirth*

From prehistoric times to the present day, women all over the world have used plants to enhance their health during pregnancy, to prepare for childbirth, and to help with various difficulties that may arise. Inspired by a greater confidence and self-reliance, women in recent years have increasingly taken much of the responsibility for their health during pregnancy, and for making decisions about their own labour and childbirth. They are advocating that optimum nutrition and healthcare, before and during pregnancy, combined with regular prenatal checks, is the best insurance for a straightforward, trouble-free birth. For it is now becoming increasingly clear that many kinds of medical intervention may carry some risk to health of mother and baby. As the self-help movement develops, many women are looking towards time-proved natural remedies to enhance their general health and to treat specific imbalances. Herbal medicines (with the exceptions noted on p.119) are safe alternative to drugs at all stages.

In the past, midwives had specific knowledge about which plants they should gather and prepare for an expectant mother. There were wild herbs which were taken several weeks prior to delivery in preparation for a safe and easy childbirth, and others to take for the various problems arising during gestation, such as nausea and heartburn. Herbs were taken to assist during the birth itself, and others used afterwards to aid recuperation, and for breastfeeding and babycare. More and more women today, including nurses and midwives, are interested in using herbs during pregnancy in preparation for childbirth and during the birth itself.

Many pregnant women are taking herbs at home and into hospital labour wards, taking more responsibility into their own hands with the support of their midwives. "Natural childbirth" is now a familiar phrase, describing the use of relaxation and breathing techniques, the avoidance of painkilling drugs, and the adoption of certain postures or positions during the birth to ease the birth process. Recently it has come also to include the use of natural therapeutics such as osteopathy, massage, homoeopathy and herbal medicine, to help ensure a straightforward delivery free from stress and medical interference.

Pregnancy can be a creative time, full of wonder and anticipation.

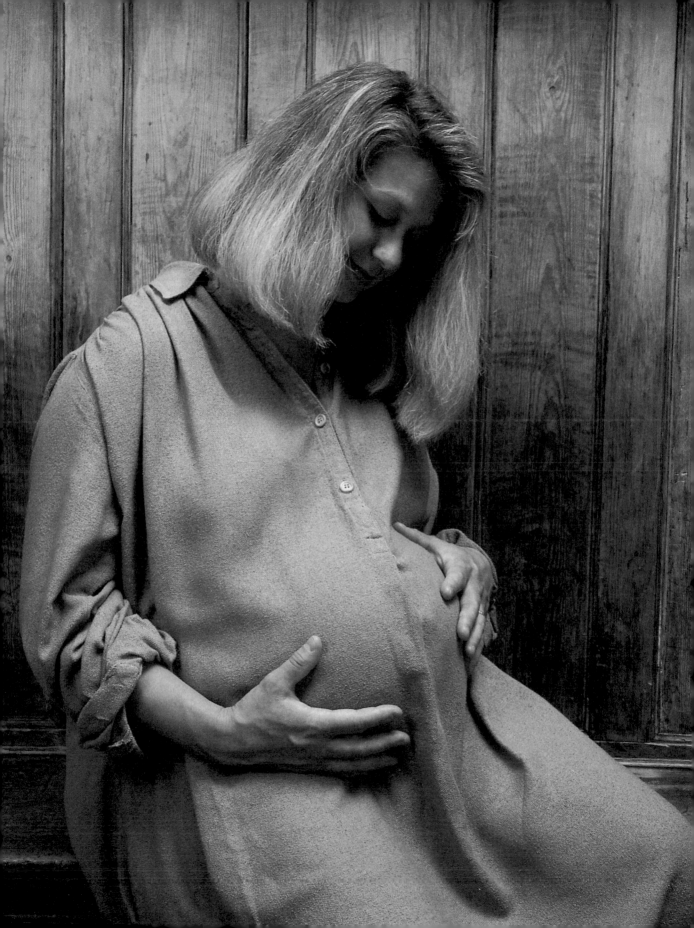

Healthcare during pregnancy

The good health of a mother-to-be during pregnancy prepares the way for a trouble-free nine month gestation period and a childbirth without complications. It also helps ensure that the baby will be born healthy and robust, with the head start in life that good health provides.

Pregnancy is a most special time for a woman, being the quintessence of her femininity. We celebrate the news that a friend or relative is pregnant, and share her joy as she prepares for the miraculous new arrival. The unborn child is totally dependent on the mother, and is profoundly affected by every aspect of her lifestyle. Her food and drink build the baby's physical body, her emotional reactions and the atmosphere around her have their effect on the baby's developing brain, senses and character. The more love and joy, peace and security, health and wholeness that a woman experiences in pregnancy, the richer the harvest for the whole family.

Diet during pregnancy

A good diet is vital to health during pregnancy, and to the normal development of the baby. The time to pay attention to diet, and if necessary change it for the better, is several months prior to conception and not when pregnancy is confirmed.

Most women who are pregnant do not realize it until they are six to eight weeks pregnant, by which time it is a little late to start changing the diet, since much of the crucial development of the baby occurs during the first eight weeks. During these critical weeks the normal, healthy development of the embryo depends on the mother's state of nutritional health and also her toxic state. Mineral and vitamin imbalances which would probably go unnoticed in a child or adult, can have a disastrous effect on the developing baby. This is because the cells in the embryo are growing at such a rapid rate, causing an exaggerated response to any harmful influences.

A natural wholefood diet is the only one which will adequately serve during pregnancy. Such a high quality diet is needed to maintain your own health and the best possible conditions for the baby to develop. It must also replace the nourishment and minerals which your body has provided the baby in preference to itself.

A well balanced diet is based on whole cereals and grains (brown bread, rice, pasta, buckwheat, rye and oats), nuts and seeds, pulses and beans, fresh fruit and vegetables, pure unrefined oils, with some fish and milk, eggs and meat if required. Fruit and vegetables are all excellent sources of vitamins, minerals and trace elements provided they are eaten in the right way. They should be fresh, either raw or quickly cooked, steamed or stir-fried, and preferably consumed immediately after they are harvested.

Salt is also essential, especially during pregnancy, except in cases of kidney and heart problems. It is needed to maintain the extra volume of blood, to supply enough placental blood, and to guard against dehydration and shock from blood-loss at birth. Most diets contain plenty of salt.

While you are pregnant there will be extra demands on your nutrition. You will require extra nutrients, especially protein, to provide for the baby's growth. Proteins form the basic building blocks of all our body tissues and cells, as well as many very important hormones and antibodies.. Food must also fuel the growth of the uterus, which can grow to 30 times its original size over the 9 months gestation period. Added to this, there is the extra work your body has to do to support the pregnancy: the development of the breasts and placenta, the expansion of blood and adequate blood flow through the placenta and the manufacture of breastmilk. All these demands as well as the development of the baby's body and brain are dependent largely on the protein we eat.

Proteins are divided into complete or first class proteins and incomplete or second class proteins. Complete proteins contain significant amounts of all the essential amino acids; you find them in meat, poultry, fish, eggs, milk and soya bean products. Vegetable proteins are incomplete proteins and contain only some of the essential amino acids. There are three types of second class proteins: nuts and seeds, beans and pulses, and grains. You can obtain the essential amino acids you need by combining two of the three types in the same meal. We often do this automatically – in beans on toast, for example – and those who eat no meat have no trouble in consuming enough protein, especially if they use soya products.

Plant proteins are easier for our bodies to digest and produce less toxic waste than animal proteins. The fibre in plants also has a very beneficial effect on the bowel; it ensures healthy bowel movements and the correct bacterial population in the gut, and prevents the build-up of putrefactive bacteria produced by excess animal proteins. Eating meat and meat products also carries the risk from chemical and hormonal residues found in intensively reared animals.

Essential Fatty Acids are vital to the normal development of the baby's nervous and immune systems. Fats are needed to build the cell walls in all our tissues, and so that trace elements and fat-soluble vitamins (A, E, D, and K) can be absorbed.   EFAs are needed to make adrenal and sex hormones, and to maintain a healthy population of bacteria in the gut. They are essential to normal development of the fetus's brain: 70 per cent of all EFAs go to the brain.

There are many different types of fatty acids which are broadly broken down into two different groups, saturated and polyunsaturated. The former are found mainly in hard fats such as in lard, meat and dairy produce. Polyunsaturated fats are liquid at room temperature and include vegetable, nut and seed oils.

Weight gain during pregnancy

The traditional view of eating during pregnancy is that a mother is eating for two, and so she is. Providing that the food she eats is healthy, the amount eaten is not crucial. A carrot or apple eaten as a snack will never have the same effect as a chocolate bar. Junk food will cause unwanted weight gain whether you are pregnant or not. Your weight is measured regularly at prenatal clinics, more to check water retention (because of its relationship to pre-eclampsia, see p.140), than as a monitor of your diet.

As they grow larger through pregnancy many women are afraid they will start to look less attractive and therefore want to limit their weight gain. However, it is true to say that most people, men and women alike, love the wonderful rounded shape of a pregnant woman and comment on how healthy and beautiful they look at this time of "blossoming". It is important not to restrict the intake of nutritious food, particularly towards the end of pregnancy, as this is the time when the stress on a woman's body is at its greatest. The

baby puts on a growth spurt at this time and the brain and central nervous system in particular are developing rapidly. It would even be a mistake to reduce intake of carbohydrates and increase proteins, fruits and vegetables, because if there are not enough calories consumed to meet the

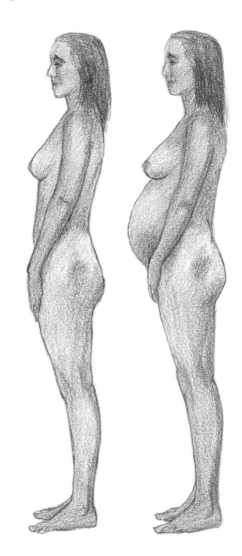

Much of the weight gained during pregnancy is made up of the placenta, amniotic fluid in the uterus, necessary extra uterus and breast tissues, and the increased amount of circulating blood. It is normal to put on 20-30 lb (13.5 kg), and although the baby will weigh only about 8-9 lb (3-4 kg) at birth, most of the rest of the weight gain is part of the pregnancy, and not unwanted fat.

increasing energy needs of a mother-to-be, her body will start to use protein instead, depleting the amount of protein available for her other needs and those of her baby. A good supply of protein to the baby is essential.

There is evidence to show that babies born to women who gained most weight in pregnancy were at least risk of developing problems both before birth and afterwards. They tended to be of more average weight and to develop normally, both mentally and physically.

Exercise during pregnancy

In pregnancy as at any other time, plenty of exercise, fresh air and sunlight are vital to health. Many pregnant women begin to doubt their robust nature and normal stamina, fearing that normal activities will carry unpredictable risks. This may be because other people view them as fragile or ill. However, exercise is always needed in order to bring the maximum amount of oxygen into tissues and organs, which is vital for their functioning. This is the case during pregnancy as at any other time.

There is no need to curtail a normal exercise routine in pregnancy unless you have a history of miscarriage, or your exercise is particularly vigorous or risky – such as skiing, horse riding or parachuting! Nor is there any need to take extra exercise unless yours is a very sedentary lifestyle or your exercise is infreqent. Yoga is particularly good in pregnancy, especially later on when specific practices are useful to prepare for the birth.

The best kind of exercise is natural and outdoor – walking (briskly rather than slowly), cycling, swimming, and dancing are all fine. Later on in pregnancy, when you are feeling very heavy, swimming can be wonderfully relieving, as the weight-bearing is done by the water instead of your back and legs. If you have backache or tired legs, simply floating on the water will lessen the discomfort. Swimming should be avoided after a large meal or in very cold water, which can cause cramp. High diving is to be avoided as it could result in a sudden change in blood pressure which could affect the circulation to the baby.

If yours is a largely sedentary lifestyle, it is important during pregnancy to introduce an exercise programme which builds up gradually. This will prepare your body for carrying the weight of the growing baby and lend strength for childbirth;

it will also help provide sufficient energy for the early weeks or months after the baby is born. Women who take plenty of exercise during pregnancy tend to have easier pregnancies and births than those who take little regular exercise, so this is another incentive to be active.

Rest during pregnancy

In the first few weeks of pregnancy, it is normal to feel tired and lethargic, and it is wise to follow the demands of your body by taking as much rest as you need. This is probably the most important time in pregnancy, when so much can influence the outcome of your pregnancy. After the fourteenth week most women feel considerably livelier. However, it is still sensible to take plenty of rest and relaxation – take heed of your body's needs and act accordingly. In the last few weeks of pregnancy most women go through a stage of feeling very tired again.

When you rest, put your feet up on the sofa or lie on a bed. Avoid sitting with one leg crossed over the other as this impedes the flow of venous blood from the leg and predisposes to varicose veins. As you rest, try to relax and let go of the day's anxieties. You may need to ignore your normal routine, cut down on your activities, and allow yourself some valuable time to treat yourself. Perhaps you unwind best listening to music; or you may like to read, go for a walk, sit in the garden, relax in the bath with your favourite aromatic oils, or have a soothing massage.

Time spent alone relaxing allows us to reflect on our own special needs. It is particularly useful for women who do not find it easy to relax and who feel stressed. The innate wisdom of the body, the vital force, is taking care of us if only we could heed its messages.

To be avoided during pregnancy

Caffeine The stimulant caffeine is an alkaloid found in tea, coffee, cocoa, chocolate and cola drinks. In pregnancy it passes from the mother's bloodstream via the placenta to the baby. Studies have shown that caffeine acts as a teratogen – a substance which can cause physical defects in the developing embryo – and as a result the USA's Food and Drug Administration (FDA) has suggested a limit of 500 mg of caffeine daily in pregnancy. Some studies in the USA have revealed that very high intake of caffeine (17-53 cups daily) is related to increased incidence of birth defects. It is also shown to increase the risk of miscarriages, stillbirths and premature delivery. Given the risks, it is sensible to avoid caffeine during pregnancy, as far as possible.

Smoking The dangers of smoking during pregnancy have been the subject over the last forty years of many studies. They leave very little doubt that smoking, especially smoking over ten cigarettes a day, is a major cause of problems during pregnancy, and contributes to defects and poor health in babies and children.

It causes thinning of the placenta, increasing the risk of placental hemorrhage, and narrowing of the arteries to the uterus, thereby diminishing both the oxygen in the blood and the blood supply to the developing baby. This can result in low birthweight babies, increased risk of miscarriage, premature delivery, mental and physical retardation, birth defects and increased susceptibility in the child to cancer, hypertension and heart disease. Many of these risks are increased if a woman also takes caffeine and alcohol regularly.

Alcohol The main risk of alcohol consumption during pregnancy is of the development of "fetal alcohol syndrome" (FAS). Alcohol passes through the placenta into the bloodstream of the baby, where it is found in the same concentration as in the mother. If a mother has one or two drinks daily, it may predispose to mild fetal dependence; if she drinks heavily it can result in birth defects, as large amounts of alcohol are teratogenic, affecting birth weight, physical and mental development and leading to joint and limb abnormalities as well as children's behavioural problems such as hyperactivity and nervousness.

Drugs As far as possible all orthodox drugs should be avoided during pregnancy, especially in the first three months. If you are taking prescribed drugs or buying them regularly from a pharmacist it is worth considering natural alternatives and visiting a medical herbalist, preferably prior to conception. Tell your practitioner that you are planning a baby so that any drug therapy can be altered if necessary.

All over-the-counter drugs such as painkillers and hay fever preparations should be used with great caution – check with your practitioner before taking them. Drugs cross the placenta and enter the baby's bloodstream. A therapeutic dose in an adult is a massive dose for a tiny embryo; most care should be taken during the early weeks of pregnancy when most potential damage could be caused.

Tranquillizers such as Librium and Valium can cause birth defects in some babies and could lead to fetal addictions. Analgesics can prolong pregnancy and childbirth and lead to bleeding in both baby and mother. Antacids like bicarbonate of soda could cause muscle problems in the baby and edema in the mother. Many antacids contain aluminium. Antibiotics may cause abnormalities, narcotics may cause fetal addiction, and sulphur drugs may cause jaundice.

Herbal remedies are for the most part quite safe to be taken during pregnancy; some are useful alternatives to drugs both in chronic illness and acute minor problems such as may arise during pregnancy. It is still preferable that no medication whatsoever is taken in the first three months, however, unless there is a specific problem that needs treatment.

There are certain herbs that should not be taken in pregnancy. Their emmonagogue or oxytocic properties may, in large amounts, cause contractions of the uterus and thereby risk miscarriage. They are as follows:

rue	*Ruta graveolens*
golden seal	*Hydrastis canadensis*
juniper	*Juniperus communis*
autumn crocus	*Colchicum autumnale*
mistletoe	*Viscum album*
bearberry	*Berberis vulgaris*
pennyroyal	*Mentha pulegium*
poke root	*Phytolacca decandra*
southernwood	*Artemisia abrotanum*
wormwood	*Artemis absinthium*
mugwort	*Artemisia vulgaris*
tansy	*Tanacetum vulgare*
nutmeg	*Myristica fragrans*
cotton root	*Gossipium herbaceum*
male fern	*Dryopteris felix-mas*
thuja	*Thuja occidentalis*
calendula	*Calendula officinalis*
beth root	*Trillium erectum*
feverfew	*Chrysanthemum parthenium*
sage	*Salvia officinalis*

Minor ailments of pregnancy

Herbs can be used throughout pregnancy for the various minor ailments which can arise, alongside the orthodox prenatal care that all pregnant women receive. Many herbs can be simply prepared at home, although many women find it reassuring to take herbs with the advice of a qualified medical herbalist. By caring for herself through the use of diet and herbs, used both to prevent and treat ailments, a woman can safely and effectively keep herself healthy throughout pregnancy and thereby increase her confidence in her ability to heal herself.

Anemia

Anemia is common in pregnancy because of the increase in the volume of blood in the body. Red blood cells contain hemoglobin, an iron and protein compound which carries oxygen from the lungs to every cell of the body, and in pregnancy to the placenta and the baby. The blood volume in pregnancy swells faster than our red blood cells are able to multiply, and the normal count of 10-15 grams per 100 cc of blood drops by 1-1.5 grams. Below the level of 11 grams, you have anemia. When the red blood cells are diluted, there is a relative drop in hemoglobin, which is why prevention of anemia during pregnancy is a very important part of prenatal care.

Those with anemia generally feel they are "making heavy weather" of a pregnancy, and there are often no actual symptoms.

However, anemia can give rise to:

headaches	lethargy
dizziness	indigestion
constant tiredness	
bad temper, irritability, depression	
breathlessness or palpitations on exertion	

If it occurs in pregnancy, it is known as iron-deficiency anemia. It is more likely to occur in the last two months of pregnancy, when a high proportion of the mother's iron is stored in the baby's liver, to supplement the low-iron milk diet.

Treatment of iron-deficiency anemia

It is best to build up iron stores prior to conception or in early pregnancy. During labour, a mother needs plenty of oxygen supplied by hemoglobin for energy and to supply her uterine muscles, and to continue free supply to the baby. If there is a history of heavy periods, bleeding piles or peptic ulcers, it is possible that iron supplies could be relatively low. In this case, the following suggestions will be particularly important to you.

Make sure there are plenty of iron-containing foods in the daily diet. The richest sources are:

> *organic meats*
> *egg yolk*
> *peas, beans and lentils*
> *molasses*
> *shellfish*
> *parsley*

The next best sources are:

> *meat*
> *fish*
> *nuts*
> *watercress*
> *beet and turnip tops*
> *other dark green leafy vegetables*
> *wholewheat bread, wheatgerm, brown rice*

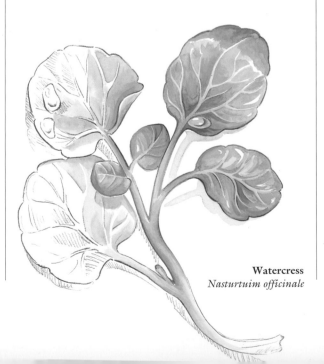

Watercress
Nasturtuim officinale

There are several herbs which contain iron. Use any of these in your cooking, in salads, or as teas:

dandelion leaves   chives
nettles   elderberries
chickweed   sorrel
purslane   coriander leaves
wood sage
hawthorn leaves and flowers
parsley (as a garnish – not in large amounts)

There are other medicinal herbs which contain iron, including:

burdock   vervain
yellow dock root   hops
rose hips   raspberry leaves
skullcap

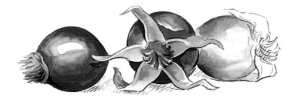

Rosehips
Rosa spp.

Help iron become absorbed

- Eat plenty of foods containing vitamin C which enhances absorption of iron.
- Avoid caffeinated drinks, especially tea.
- If you suffer from anxiety or tension this may impair digestion and absorption. Take vitamin B complex or brewer's yeast to help the nervous system and to prevent anemia caused by deficiency of vitamin B, B 12 and folic acid.
- For proper digestion and absorption there needs to be sufficient hydrochloric acid in the stomach. Sip a little cider vinegar in water half an hour before meals to increase acidity.
- Eat plenty of vitamin E-containing foods (for sources see diet chart on p. 70–73) to ensure iron absorption, and to prevent the destruction of red blood cells.

Folic acid deficiency anemia

Folic acid is one of the B complex vitamins and is vital for the formation of red blood cells. It is particularly necessary during pregnancy for the healthy development of the fetus and the supply of breastmilk. Deficiency of folic acid can be related to miscarriage and abnormalities, especially spina bifida.

As the name implies, folic acid is found in foliage – green leafy vegetables are a good source. It is also contained in brewer's yeast, beans and legumes, nuts and liver. It is found in the iron-containing leafy herbs.

Folic acid diminishes on storage and exposure to sunlight, which is another reason why vegetables should be eaten as fresh as possible. Folic acid is also destroyed by cooking, especially boiling, so ensure that you eat a fresh green salad daily and only lightly steam or stir-fry vegetables. Some drugs, such as aspirin, estrogens and sulphur drugs, destroy folic acid in the body, and alcohol slows down its absorption. High doses of vitamin C hasten its excretion.

Constipation

Constipation is a common complaint in pregnancy because of the hormone progesterone which dominates during pregnancy and which relaxes smooth muscle throughout the body. In the bowel, when the muscles relax under the influence of progesterone, they are less able to propel the bowel contents towards the rectum for defecation. As the baby and placenta grow larger and heavier, their weight puts pressure on the lower bowel and impedes circulation to it, aggravating any tendency to constipation.

Lack of fibre in the diet clearly contributes to constipation, as does any upset in the bacterial population of the bowel. A high proportion of harmful, putrefactive bacteria can slow down bowel movements. Such bacteria tend to thrive in the gut of those on a low-fibre, high meat and fat diet. They also produce toxins which, when absorbed into the bloodstream, slow down the transit time through the bowel of other harmful by-products from food digestion. This causes other toxins to be reabsorbed, producing a state of "auto intoxication" in the body which can contribute to symptoms such as headaches, aches and pains, malaise, irritability, lethargy and insomnia.

Treatment of constipation

A diet high in unrefined carbohydrates and plenty of fresh fruit and vegetables will ensure that beneficial bacteria predominate in the bowel. There is plenty of fibre in fruits and vegetables, beans and pulses, nuts and seeds, as well as whole grains. Prunes, dried figs and apricots can be eaten freely, as can rhubarb, apples, raisins, molasses, honey, sesame seeds and desiccated coconut, all of which are particularly laxative.

An old remedy for constipation is to drink lemon juice in a cup of warm water half an hour before breakfast with no sweetener added. Alternatively, a teaspoon of honey in a cup of hot water each morning before breakfast has also proved helpful. A daily (green) salad is recommended, for raw food is bulkier than cooked.

To ensure the right balance of bacteria in the gut, eat natural, live yoghurt or take a supplement of lacto-acidophilus. Garlic, onions and leeks are also helpful.

Tea and coffee are not recommended in pregnancy, and may aggravate constipation. Dandelion coffee acts as a tonic to the digestive tract and is slightly laxative, making this a useful alternative.

There is a large assortment of herbal remedies for constipation. Syrup of figs, linseeds, psyllium seeds, and slippery elm powder are traditional treatments which all work well. Health food stores supply these remedies.

There are other herbs which have a tonic, stimulating action in the bowels and a gentle action on the liver, increasing bile flow. They can be made into infusions, or bought as tinctures and taken as directed.

Such herbs include:

yellow dock root	*chamomile*
fennel	*raspberry leaves*
peppermint	*dandelion root*
burdock	*ginger*

If you have a particularly persistent problem, then senna pods may be your remedy. Tear up 5-10 pods and pour a cupful of boiling water over them. Add a pinch of ginger powder and let it stand overnight. Drink first thing in the morning before breakfast. Licorice may also prove effective.

Licorice water can be made by adding 1 oz (25 g) of peeled sticks to 1 pint (600 ml) of water. Bring to the boil and simmer for ten minutes. Drink a cupful three times daily or as required.

How to avoid constipation

Obey every urge to defecate, as you may only get the opportunity once in 24 hours. By passing a stool at least once a day, you will avoid the build-up of hard fecal matter which is so hard to pass. To ensure that the stools remain soft and easy to pass, it is important to drink plenty of liquid, approximately 4 pints (2.5 litres) daily.

Exercise – such as swimming, bicycling, walking or yoga – is essential to stimulate the bowels. Prenatal yoga exercises are pleasurable and highly recommended to help you maintain general health and good bowel function.

Relaxing herbal baths are ideal for women feeling particularly tense or stressed. Anxiety and tension can show itself in the bowel muscles, and make constipation worse.

To relax muscles and soothe the nerves, take these herbs as teas and add strong infusions to the bath water:

lavender	*lemon balm*
vervain	*skullcap*
chamomile	*rosemary*

Essential oils can be added to bath water or to massage oils. Choose from:

geranium	*ylang ylang*
rose	*marjoram*
fennel	*rosemary*
chamomile	*lavender*

Gentle massage to the lower back can also help the tension in the bowel.

Iron tablets can often cause constipation. If you require iron, look for natural sources (see p.120).

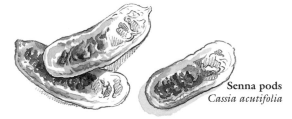

Senna pods
Cassia acutifolia

Cramp

Cramp during pregnancy probably occurs mainly because of low calcium levels, particularly in the last three months when the baby needs more calcium. Having enough calcium depends not only on the amount in your food, but also on hydrochloric acid levels in the stomach and having enough vitamin D and fats. Calcium deficiency may cause leg and foot cramps, twitchy muscles, restless legs, irritability, headaches and insomnia. Cramp may also be related to deficiencies of vitamins B and D, poor circulation, varicose veins and nervous tension. Cramps tend to occur at night, as the blood circulation is not as free as when you are active in the daytime.

When it happens, you can help relieve the pain if you:

try to relax as far as possible
try to pull your foot forwards with your hands
wiggle your feet up and down
massage your feet and legs vigorously

If you suffer from cramp frequently, help your circulation by raising the foot of the bed, and placing a pillow or two under the end of the mattress. Ensure that you keep your legs and feet as warm as possible, perhaps with bedsocks.

Treatment of cramp

Increase calcium in your diet (see food chart on p.70-75) especially from oats, sesame seeds, millet, figs, parsley and watercress. If you include herbs such as dandelion leaves, nettles, kelp and other seaweeds in soups, stews or salads, these will boost your intake.

Herbal teas rich in calcium can also be made from:

wild oats	*celery seeds*
meadowsweet	*nettles*
horsetail	

Drink a cupful two to three times daily.

There is a herb, suitably named cramp bark or guelder rose, which is specific for cramps. It can be taken as a hot decoction, singly or in conjunction with any of the above herbs three times daily.

If you consider that tension or stress could be causing your cramps, then add to the cramp bark herbs such as:

skullcap
passionflower
chamomile
vervain

Ginger, hawthorn or angelica can be taken regularly to aid circulation. Chamomile, marjoram, lavender or rosemary oils can be used to massage the legs, not only to relax over-tense muscles, but also to enhance the circulation through them. Hot foot baths can be taken at night before bed using the same oils. Take care with varicose veins – do not massage over them. Alternate hot and cold bathing will stimulate the circulation.

Help avoid cramps

- Do not be too active immediately following a meal.
- Leave at least two hours between eating and going to bed.
- Take moderate exercise daily – both inadequate or excessive exercise can induce cramp.
- Eat foods rich in vitamins B, C and E, or take supplements

Nausea

Nausea or vomiting generally starts around the fourth to sixth week and lasts, in most women who suffer it, until around weeks 14 to 16. It can make you feel terrible, but is only a serious problem when prolonged nausea causes an inability to eat properly or frequent vomiting carries a risk of dehydration – in which case you should consult your practitioner.

There is no clear cause of nausea or vomiting, but here are some of the theories about it. One or more of them may have a bearing on your nausea.

- The vital energy of the body is directed toward the uterus and away from the digestive tract, bringing to light any underlying digestive weakness. There may be associated tiredness and lethargy.

• A liver imbalance may occur in early pregnancy brought about by the circulatory change as more blood is directed towards the uterus.

• Rapid change of hormone levels in early pregnancy may irritate the brain's vomit centre.

• Relaxation of smooth muscle throughout the body, including the blood vessels, caused by high progesterone levels, produces a drop in blood pressure. This may cause a relative drop in blood supply to the brain, particularly on rising, which causes nausea.

• Low blood sugar; eating before getting up in the morning may help this, as can eating small meals frequently through the day.

• Food allergies can be to blame. Women often feel better when cutting out milk and wheat.

• Poor diet, junk foods and the toxic system produced by them may give rise to nausea and vomiting as the body attempts to cleanse itself in preparation for a healthy pregnancy. Food combinations may also be to blame. Many women feel better when taking a food combining diet, such as the Hay diet (see p.281).

• Stress may play its part. Fear, anxiety or apprehension about pregnancy or any other emotional problems can upset the digestion.

During the first 12-14 weeks of pregnancy, the hormones are mostly produced in the corpus luteum of the ovaries. After this time the placenta largely takes over, which may explain why most women feel better after this stage. Some researchers believe nausea or vomiting to be a positive sign that the body contains levels of hormones higher than are necessary to maintain the pregnancy. Women who vomit during pregnancy have been shown to have a lower rate of miscarriages, stillbirths and premature delivery than those who do not.

Treatment of nausea

The herbal remedies for nausea and vomiting are as wide and varied as the different theories associated with the symptoms. It is useful to assess which theory is most applicable to you, but if that is not clear, you can find your remedy through trial and error of those on offer. What helps one woman to relieve her sickness may not always work for another, and you may want to chop and change your remedies.

It is probably most simple to prepare teas of the suggested herbs, either singly or blended together to create pleasing tastes (for directions see p.18). You may want to drink the tea by the cupful three to six times daily, or it may suit you better to take sips every few minutes when the nausea arises. Lemon balm, lemon verbena, peppermint and lavender make delicious-tasting teas and can be blended with those herbs with less pleasant tastes. Tinctures of the herbs can also be used, especially for bitter herbs, as only small amounts need to be taken at a time. You can take up to about 15 ml through the day, as drops on or under the tongue as required. Use three to five drops at a time. Many of the herbs which aid digestion and relieve nausea are also relaxing or mildly sedative.

These herbs are useful for nausea which may be accompanied by anxiety and tension:

lemon balm	chamomile
lavender	raspberry leaves
wild yam	

Some herbs contain a strong component of volatile oil (see p.16). These include:

peppermint	chamomile
rosemary	lemon balm
lavender	ginger
cinnamon	fennel

Others contain bitters:

rosemary	meadowsweet
thyme	peppermint
lemon balm	verbena

All of these act to stimulate and enhance the function of the digestive tract and liver; they are useful where nausea is related to weak digestion or a liver imbalance.

Many are familiar with the strong aromatic taste and flavour the volatile oils lend to ginger and cinnamon – these can be ground to a powder or chopped finely and taken as teas, or added to cooking. You can also chew cinnamon sticks or pieces of crystallized ginger. Ginger beer is a most effective and refreshing drink, and ginger in various forms is recommended by midwives and health visitors for the relief it offers in nausea of all kinds – including motion sickness.

Slippery elm

Ulmus fulva

ALSO KNOWN AS: Indian elm, moose elm, sweet elm

PART USED: Inner bark

CONTAINS: Mucilage, tannin, starch

KEY USES: Demulcent, emollient, astringent, nutrient.

The powdered inner bark of the slippery elm is a wonderfully soothing remedy for the mucous membranes throughout the body. It will soothe irritation and inflammation in the stomach, bowels, kidneys and urinary tract, the reproductive system and the whole of the respiratory system. It makes a good remedy for gastritis, acidity, peptic ulcers, colitis, enteritis and for diarrhea. It will relieve cystitis, irritable bladder, nasal and bronchial catarrh, and soothe a dry irritating cough.

The powder can be mixed with warm water or milk to make a nourishing gruel, which will not only soothe indigestion and heartburn, but also provide an easily digested and assimilated meal, ideal for adults and children during convalescence or when debilitated. Honey or powdered cinnamon or ginger can be added to it to improve the flavour.

Slippery elm powder can be mixed with water or glycerine to form a paste to apply as a healing and soothing poultice for cuts and wounds, burns and scalds, inflammatory skin problems and ulcers. It makes a good drawing remedy for boils and abscesses.

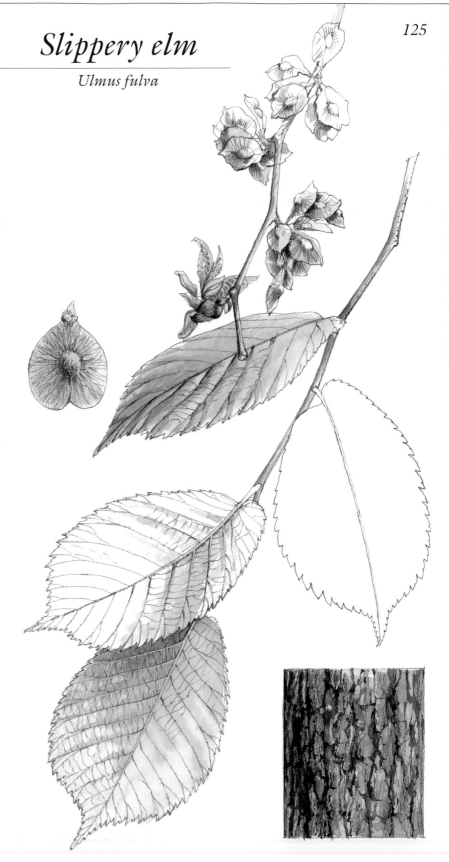

Slippery elm and Iceland moss both contain plenty of demulcent mucilage which acts to soothe the whole of the digestive tract. They are also highly nutritious and contain many minerals and trace elements. They are easily digested and make excellent food, as well as remedies for conditions associated with a weak digestion, including nausea of pregnancy.

False unicorn root and chaste tree are famous hormone-balancing herbs used to prevent or treat a wide range of problems in pregnancy. They can both be used to treat nausea.

During my own pregnancies, I have used a variety of remedies to relieve my nausea. I would suck slippery elm tablets on and off through the day when necessary, or chew pieces of cinnamon bark or peppermint leaves. I took a few drops of either chamomile or ginger tincture on or under the tongue, or I drank ginger tea. Each remedy worked for a while, and I would change my prescription whenever I felt the need for a change in taste.

Dilute essential oils can allay sickness when massaged gently into the stomach or back, dropped into bath water, or used in inhalations or room sprays. Exquisitely scented oils of rose, lavender or chamomile can be particularly effective, either used singly or together. For massage, add two drops of oil to each teaspoonful of base oil and they will pass through the skin to the bloodstream. Through inhalation they are carried through the nose both to affect the vomit centre in the brain, and also into the lungs and thus into general circulation.

Supplements of vitamins B6 (25 mg) with zinc (15 mg), and magnesium (500 mg) have helped some women.

Avoid greasy foods and caffeine. Make sure your diet is not highly acid, as this may aggravate your nausea.

Note If your nausea is frequent or severe, it may indicate a more serious problem, and you should consult your practitioner.

In the meantime, drink an infusion of a mixture of:

> *hops*
> *skullcap*

This remedy may prove effective, especially if the severe vomiting is accompanied by stomach pain.

Varicose veins

Varicose veins occur commonly during pregnancy. This is because high progesterone levels in pregnancy cause relaxation of muscles in the veins, making them dilate and enlarge. Blood then tends to pool in the veins, slowing the return of venous blood to the heart. This leads to further dilation and pressure on the valves in the veins, whose job is to keep the blood moving. If a valve becomes incompetent, the veins become swollen, engorged and tortuous. The result of this is that the legs often feel full and heavy. They may ache after you have been standing for long periods, and at the end of the day.

As the uterus enlarges, it puts pressure on the pelvic veins which further impedes blood flow from the legs. This puts more back pressure on the veins. Fluid retention, weight gain and constipation further aggravate the problem.

Varicose veins are often associated with swollen ankles and feet caused by accumulation of fluid in the legs leaked from over-full veins. The poor venous circulation in the legs can also cause cramp. Some women develop varicose veins, for the same reasons, in the vulva, which cause aching in the area particularly on walking and when standing.

Treatment of varicose veins

External treatments Bathe the site of the problem (legs or vulva) with herbal lotions such as those mentioned below. Used two to three times daily, more if necessary, this will improve the tone of the veins. Apply these to the affected part with cotton wool or a cloth.

A simple lotion can be made with:

> *1 part distilled witch hazel*
> *1 part glycerol*
> *1 part rose water*

Another easy recipe is made by steeping a handful of calendula flowers, if you have some available, in a cupful of distilled witch hazel for about one hour. Strain the liquid and discard the flowers before use.

Meadowsweet

Filipendula ulmaria

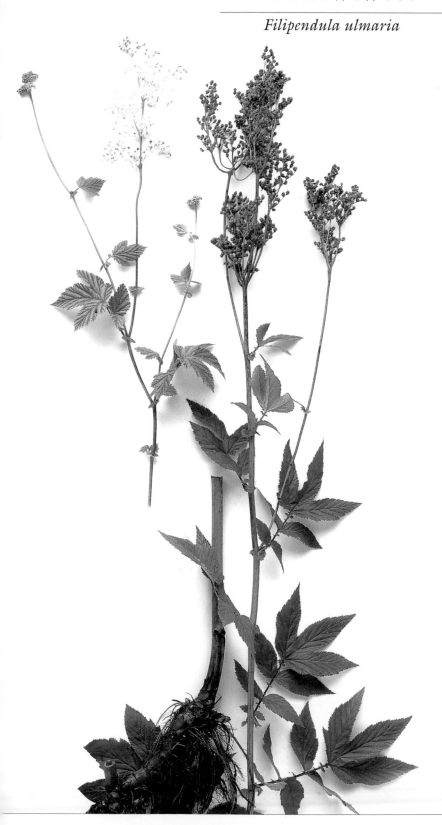

ALSO KNOWN AS: Queen of the meadow, bridewort

PART USED: Aerial parts

CONTAINS: Essential oil, salicylates, mucilage, sugar, tannin, citric acid

KEY USES: Antacid, astringent, relaxant, anti-inflammatory, antiseptic, diuretic, antirheumatic, diaphoretic, analgesic

Meadowsweet is one of the best antacid remedies for acid indigestion, heartburn, gastritis, peptic ulcers, and hiatus hernia. It relieves wind and distension and should be thought of in any inflammatory condition of the stomach or bowels. The tannins have an astringent action in the bowels, protecting and healing the mucous membranes and relieving enteritis and diarrhea; its mild antiseptic action combats infection and its relaxant properties soothe griping and colic.

The medicinal virtues of meadowsweet are very similar to those of aspirin, but without the side effectsg. Its additional tannins and mucilage protect the gastric lining, making it valuable for healing gastritis and gastric ulceration.

For aches and pains, rheumatism, arthritis and gout, meadowsweet has an anti-inflammatory action which relieves swollen joints, and diuretic properties which help eliminate toxic wastes and uric acid from the system. It also has an analgesic effect, helping to soothe pain, as well as relieve headaches and neuralgia. Its relaxant properties release spasm and induce restful sleep. Its diaphoretic action helps reduce fevers and eruptive infections such as measles and chickenpox.

The cleansing diuretic effect has given meadowsweet a reputation for clearing the skin and resolving rashes. Given its mild antiseptic action it makes a good remedy for cystitis and urethritis, fluid retention and kidney problems. The salicylate salts are said to soften deposits in the body such as kidney stones and gravel, as well as atherosclerosis in the arteries.

Wormwood

Artemisia absinthium

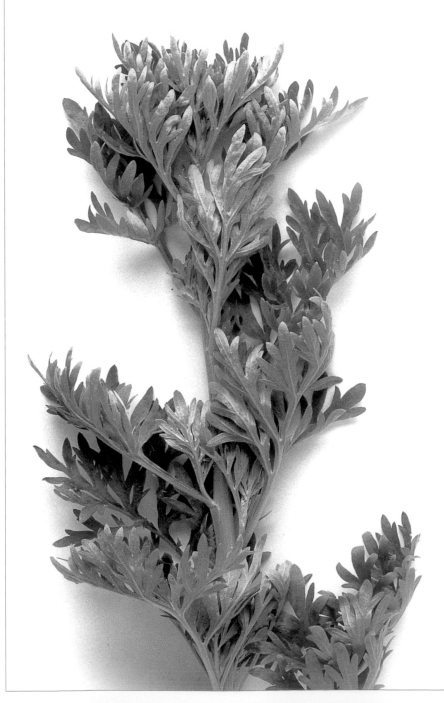

ALSO KNOWN AS: Green ginger

PART USED: Aerial parts

CONTAINS: Volatile oil (including thujone and chamazulene), bitters, tannins, carotene, vitamin C

KEY USES: Bitter tonic, anthelmintic, anti-inflammatory, diaphoretic, carminative, emmenagogue

Wormwood is a wonderful bitter tonic – in fact it is one of the most bitter herbs used in herbal medicine. It stimulates the appetite, and enhances digestion by increasing the secretion of digestive enzymes and bile from the liver and gallbladder and stimulating peristalsis. It can be used to expel worms, as its name suggests. It is an excellent remedy for those with weak, sluggish digestion, toxins and congestion in the gut, liver problems, those feeling run down and debilitated and during convalescence. The chamazulene in the volatile oil has an anti-inflammatory effect in the digestive tract.

Wormwood is a useful herb for treating fevers and infections. It boosts the immune system, detoxifies the body and clears heat and congestion. It can be taken in hot infusion (best mixed with mint to make it more palatable) for colds and flu, chronic fevers, food poisoning, catarrh, skin problems and arthritis.

Throughout history wormwood has been a favourite herb used by women to stimulate uterine contractions during childbirth. It is particularly beneficial when the birth is slow in getting going and contractions are weak and ineffectual. It can also be used to bring on delayed or suppressed menstruation due to stagnation in the uterus, and for painful periods. Its diuretic action is useful for any fluid retention around period time.

Note Avoid during pregnancy.

There is a wide variety of herbs from which astringent lotions can be made, including:

calendula	marjoram
oak bark	comfrey
elderflower	plantain

These can be used singly or in combination and made into infusions or decoctions in the standard way, cooled and applied frequently with cloths. They can also be used in tincture form, applied diluted or neat or added to an aqueous cream base to make application easier.

Some women find neat lemon juice applied to the area very relieving.

There are many essential oils that can be used to tone and strengthen the veins, and increase circulation.

Add to the bath water a couple of drops of oils of either:

peppermint	thyme
rosemary	lavender
lemon	cypress

You can also use warm hand and foot baths using ten drops of essential oils in a bowl of water. Here is a good recipe which has worked well for many women to relieve aching and heaviness in the legs from varicose veins.

Use the essential oils in these quantities:

4 drops cypress
4 drops lavender
2 drops lemon
2 drops marjoram

These oils can also be added to lotions made with herbal tinctures, or to a base oil or cream. They can be applied as such and massaged gently around or above the area of the affected veins, but never over the vein itself. The pressure of the massaging movement should always be towards the heart, using long sweeping upward strokes.

If your legs or vulva are aching severely you can spray the area with cold water, or apply crushed ice or a packet of frozen peas or sweetcorn for a few seconds until the cold feels uncomfortable. An arnica compress can also be very soothing. Mix one tablespoonful of arnica tincture into a litre of cold water, wring out a flannel in the mixture and apply to the area, repeating until the aching diminishes.

Internal treatments Several herbs will improve your circulation and encourage the return of blood from the lower part of the body.

Use these herbs in decoctions or infusions, or as tinctures:

St. John's wort	peppermint
hawthorn	cleavers
rosemary	burdock
linden blossom	

How to avoid varicose veins

• Avoid constipation.
• Avoid too much standing and sitting, especially with legs crossed.
• Avoid tight clothing.
• Get plenty of exercise, especially walking, swimming, yoga and deep breathing exercises.
• Rest as much as possible every day, with the legs higher than the head, and do this for 10 minutes at any time that your legs begin to ache badly to relieve the discomfort. Try lying on the floor with your legs against the wall. Alternatively you could use a slant board. Aid blood flow through the legs by pointing your toes away from and then towards your head 5-10 times.
• Raise the foot of your bed by putting a pillow or two under (your side of) the mattress.
• In severe cases wear elastic support stockings to promote better circulation through the veins by supporting them and the surrounding muscles, and preventing pooling of blood.
• Hot and cold bathing, or treading up and down in a cold bath reaching the knees, may help.
• If you have to stand for any length of time, try to keep your legs moving. Rock from side to side, flex your ankles or move your feet and toes, and you will resist the force of gravity pooling the blood in your legs.
• Eat plenty of foods containing vitamins E, C and bioflavonoids to help the circulation and strengthen the blood vessels. Zinc in brewer's yeast, buckwheat, grains and seeds speeds the healing of damaged blood vessels. Remember that garlic helps the circulation, and eat plenty of it.

Hemorrhoids (Piles)

When varicose veins occur in and around the rectum and anal canal they are called hemorrhoids. The cause is largely restricted blood circulation to the area, and they are common in pregnancy for these reasons:

● Progesterone relaxes veins in the rectal area, as elsewhere, and blood pools in the veins.

● The discomfort that hemorrhoids cause encourages constipation as passing a motion may prove quite painful and the whole area can tighten up as a result. Constipation and straining at stool aggravate the pressure on the veins.

● If there is a past history of constipation and straining at stool, the blood vessels in the rectal area may be weak, predisposing to hemorrhoids in pregnancy.

● As pregnancy progresses, hemorrhoids tend to become worse because pressure from the uterus impedes the return of venous blood from the pelvis to the heart.

● Obesity, hypertension and emotional tension will all help predispose to hemorrhoids.

● There is a strong hereditary factor in the incidence of hemorrhoids, and the more pregnancies a woman has, the more likely she is to develop them.

It is important to treat hemorrhoids, not only because their discomfort may encourage constipation, but also because if they bleed, regular blood loss may lead to anemia.

Treatment of hemorrhoids

Follow the guidelines for treatment of varicose veins (see p.126).

Avoid constipation and try to ensure that the stool does not become hard as this will worsen the hemorrhoids, and could cause pain and bleeding when passing a motion.

Take plenty of regular exercise and try not to sit for long periods as this will cause stagnation and pooling of blood in the rectal area.

External treatments Cold compresses applied to the area will increase local circulation and help reduce pain and swelling. Prepare strong infusions or decoctions of herbs, leave them to cool, then soak a flannel or cloth and wring it out a little and apply as a compress.

These are the most useful herbs to use:

catmint	witch hazel
calendula	oak bark
beth root	lady's mantle
horsetail	comfrey
plantain	

Alternatively you can apply ice cold distilled witch hazel on a compress to the area for as long as possible.

Comfrey leaves can be applied as a poultice (see p.20). They are very soothing and healing.

Tinctures of witch hazel, comfrey and calendula can be mixed into aqueous cream and applied regularly. Papaya juice has been used successfully both externally and internally.

Another remedy, which also works well, can be prepared simply at home. Cover elderflowers with olive oil in an airtight glass jar. Leave it on a windowsill in a sunny position for about two weeks, strain through muslin, and pour the oil into an airtight jar and keep in the fridge. Apply the oil two or three times daily.

Essential oils can also be used to relieve pain and discomfort. Add a few drops of any of these to your bath:

cypress	geranium
frankincense	chamomile
thyme	melissa

Alternatively, dilute a few drops in a base oil and apply to the hemorrhoids.

Internal treatments
Teas of the following herbs are particularly suitable and can be mixed into cocktails to suit your taste, and taken at least three times daily:

chamomile	St. John's wort
dandelion root	yellow dock root
cleavers	licorice
nettle	

To avoid constipation, follow advice on p.122. Eat plenty of fresh fruit and vegetables, and avoid refined carbohydrates, especially flour and sugar. Drink plenty of vegetable juices, pure water and flax tea. Foods rich in magnesium (fresh vegetables, whole grains, yeast extract, beans,

Feverfew

Chrysanthemum parthenium
Tanacetum parthenium

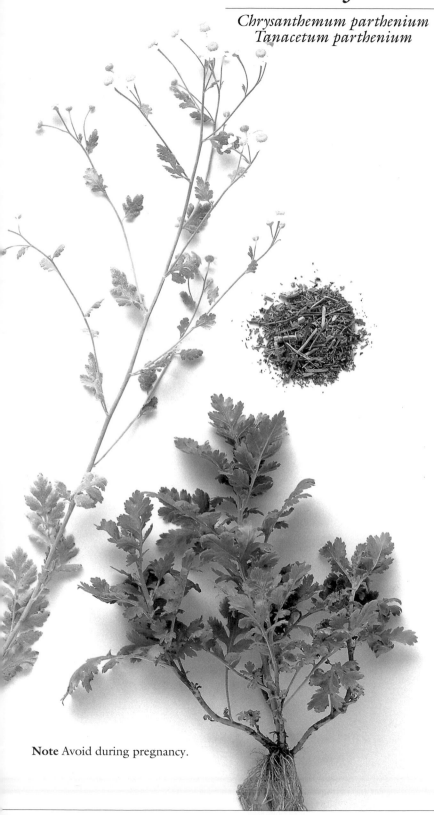

Note Avoid during pregnancy.

PART USED: Aerial parts

CONTAINS: Sesquiterpene lactones, volatile oils, tannins, bitter resin, pyrethrin

KEY USES: Diaphoretic, relaxant, uterine stimulant, anti-inflammatory, antihistamine, digestive bitter

Feverfew has a stimulant effect in the uterus but it also has relaxant properties. It can be used to bring on delayed or suppressed periods, to relieve period pains and reduce symptoms associated with PMS, such as headaches, irritability and tension. It has also been used traditionally for hot flashes during the menopause. Taken during childbirth it will equalize the circulation, make the pains and contractions more regular and contractions firmer if the birth is slow in getting going. It will also relieve tension in a rigid cervix.

More recently, feverfew has gained fame as an excellent remedy for headaches and migraine. In clinical trials, 70 per cent of people with intractable migraines improved when taking feverfew, while 33 per cent had no further attacks. The leaves can be eaten fresh every day between slices of bread (taken alone they cause mouth ulcers in some people).

Feverfew has a bitter taste, and has a beneficial action on the liver, enhancing the appetite and digestion, allaying nausea and vomiting and helping to clear heat and toxins from the system. It will help relieve the pain and inflammation of arthritis and reduce symptoms associated with a sluggish liver, such as lethargy, irritability and headaches. It acts as a tonic to the nervous system, relaxing tension and lifting depression and promoting sleep. It has also been used to relieve nerve pain, as in trigeminal neuralgia and sciatica.

A hot infusion of feverfew will increase perspiration and reduce fevers. It will also act as a decongestant, clearing phlegm, chronic catarrh and sinusitis. It has also been used for asthma, hay fever, dizziness and tinnitus.

dried fruit) and vitamin B6 (taken in B complex) may also prove effective in relieving symptoms. Raw garlic or garlic capsules taken daily will help improve circulation.

Insomnia

This is a common feature of late pregnancy, and usually caused by being uncomfortable for one reason or another and being disturbed in the night by the need to pass water.

Treatment of insomnia

You can feel safe about taking herbs for insomnia during pregnancy. Their gentle relaxant and sedative action is very different from that of powerful sleeping drugs with their habit forming and other often serious side effects.

These herbs can be taken, singly or in mixtures, as teas or tinctures:

chamomile	skullcap
lemon balm	catmint
vervain	passionflower
linden blossom	

Up to two or three cups of tea or teaspoonfuls of tincture can be taken before sleep, or during the night. Some find that a mixture of two teaspoonsful each of honey and cider vinegar in a glass of warm water just before bed is a great aid to sleep. Others take a nightcap of elderberry juice or celery juice.

A healthy wholefood diet is essential to maintain normal relaxation of the muscles and nerves, and to ensure sleep. B vitamins (especially B6) are particularly helpful, and are found in brewer's yeast, blackstrap molasses and wheatgerm. Dried figs, sesame seeds, molasses, parsley, watercress and dairy produce are rich in calcium, deficiency of which can reduce your ability to relax. Make sure you avoid stimulants such as tea, coffee, cocoa or chocolate. Take plenty of exercise in the fresh air and avoid eating a heavy meal too late in the evening.

A few drops of essential oils, or strong infusions of lavender, chamomile or lemon balm can be added to a bath before bed. A massage with the same oils would be wonderfully relaxing. A hot foot bath or a firm foot massage can also help induce sleep; as anyone who has ever had reflexology will know, these can be deeply relaxing.

Relaxation exercises can also be helpful. Just before bed, lie flat on the floor or bed, and have a good stretch. Start with your toes and focus your attention on each part of the body, consciously trying to let go of any tensions you may discover, and relax. To increase awareness of each part, you may find it easier to tense up or squeeze each part of the body for a few seconds, and then let it go. Breathe deeply and slowly to enhance relaxation. Once you have relaxed each part of you, just concentrate on the rise and fall of your abdomen while you breathe, or if you wish fill your mind with pleasing images, which will give you a great sense of wellbeing.

Thrush

Thrush (*Candida albicans*) is a fungus which thrives in moist, sweet, warm areas. During menstruation, normal blood estrogen levels which supply the vagina support the habitat of Doderlein's bacilli, bacteria which live there. They are responsible for maintaining the acid conditions which discourage the development of vaginal infections. During pregnancy, when the hormone balance changes, Doderlein's bacilli do not operate as effectively. In addition, there is a higher glycogen content in the cells lining the vagina at this time, on which the thrush fungus thrives.

Diabetics with higher blood sugar levels have an increased susceptibility to thrush. Taking antibiotics can upset the balance of acids and alkalis in the vagina by altering its bacterial population, predisposing to thrush by undermining normal immune responses.

For more about thrush, see Gynecological ailments, (p. 226).

Treatment of thrush

It is vital that vaginal thrush is treated vigorously, as it is possible for the baby to become infected as it passes through the vagina at birth. There are several ways of doing this using herbs.

The following herbs have antifungal properties:

calendula	fennel seed
rosemary	thyme
chamomile	

Take them as teas, three times daily, and hold herb-soaked pads to the vulva to soothe itching and burning for anything from five minutes to several hours, depending on the severity of the symptoms. Alternatively, you can use a sitz-bath of herbal tea, which is wonderfully soothing.

Tincture of calendula, with a few drops of any of these essential oils can be added to water to bathe the area:

tea tree	*oregano*
thyme	*cinnamon*
chamomile	*hyssop*
lavender	

Echinacea, cleavers, chamomile and thyme can be taken as teas or tinctures to enhance immune function and can also be used externally.

Use any of the above remedies to mix into an aqueous cream; apply it just inside and around the opening of the vagina.

Salt baths can also bring relief, as can a tablespoonful of lemon juice added to half a pint (300 ml) of water and applied to the area two to three times daily.

Avoid tight underwear and nylon tights which prevent circulation of air around the vagina, and encourage the conditions in which thrush thrives. Eat plenty of garlic, nature's best antifungal remedy, either raw in salads and sandwiches, or as garlic perles.

Japanese researchers have found that oleic acid, a fatty acid found in pure, unrefined olive oil, can prevent growth of a yeast infection. Add cold-pressed, unrefined olive oil to salad dressings, and try to take about one dessertspoonful daily. Heating the oil during cooking reduces its medicinal value (as in the case of garlic), so it's best taken raw.

Live, unsweetened yoghurt will help relieve and prevent thrush. Eat a little daily and add nothing except ripe bananas. If you apply yoghurt locally to the vaginal area, it will help restore the natural acidity of the vagina and so help to control the infection.

It is important to raise the strength of the immune system, so eat plenty of foods containing vitamins A, B, and C, zinc, iron, calcium and magnesium or take a multivitamin and mineral supplement (yeast free) daily.

Stretch marks

Stretch marks can develop overnight and commonly appear on the breasts, abdomen, and thighs – the areas which expand quickly when your weight increases during pregnancy. They are initially bright purple or red and, although they fade gradually over years they never go away, and remain as silvery white streaks on the skin. Lack of elasticity in the skin has been related to deficiencies of vitamins E and C, zinc, silica and pantothenic acid (B5). For foods containing these substances, see the Diet chart on p. 70.

As soon as you begin to put on weight, you can massage oils into the abdomen, breasts and thighs, at least once a day, to improve skin function and maintain elasticity.

Choose from these oils:

coconut	*wheatgerm*
almond	*olive*
vitamin E	

Essential oils of lavender and neroli have a particular affinity with the skin, and are healing and nourishing. Use a mixture of 20 drops lavender oil and 5 drops of neroli in 50 ml wheatgerm oil for massage. This is a simple remedy which also smells lovely.

Calendula flowers also have a beneficial effect on the skin. If you have some, steep them in wheatgerm oil for two to three weeks, and then use in the same way. Aloe vera gel may help.

As the birth approaches use any of these oils to massage around the vagina and perineum, which will help to improve the circulation and elasticity of the skin, and allow the area to resist tearing during childbirth.

Aloe vera

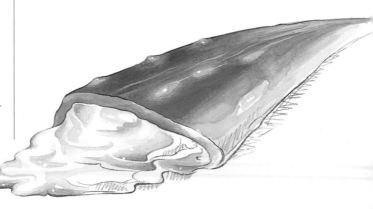

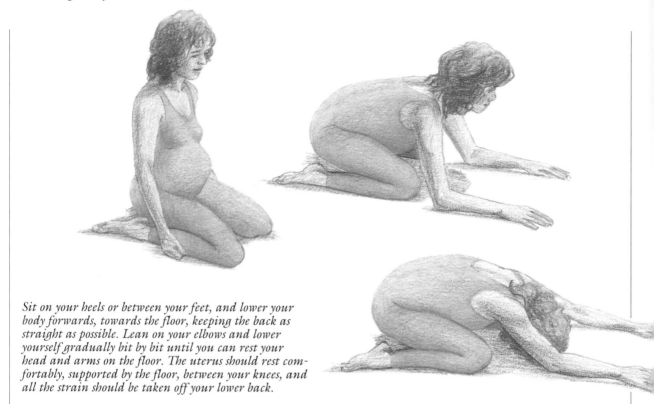

Sit on your heels or between your feet, and lower your body forwards, towards the floor, keeping the back as straight as possible. Lean on your elbows and lower yourself gradually bit by bit until you can rest your head and arms on the floor. The uterus should rest comfortably, supported by the floor, between your knees, and all the strain should be taken off your lower back.

Backache

Backache in pregnancy is related to high levels of progesterone, which have a softening effect on tendons and ligaments throughout the body, allowing them to expand where necessary to make room in the pelvis for the growing baby. This softening particularly affects the spine, where relaxation of the ligaments supporting the back, coupled with the increasing weight of the abdomen pulling on it, often produces low backache. As the abdomen enlarges later on in pregnancy, the characteristic posture adopted by many heavily pregnant women, leaning backwards, puts even more strain on the lower joints of the spine. Rapid weight gain during pregnancy may bring to light underlying back problems, as increasing strain is put on it. You may need to consult a chiropractor or osteopath to correct this.

Avoid standing for long periods, as this will aggravate any discomfort, and take plenty of rest. Sitting badly, or bending over as if to pick something up without bending the knees, can cause problems.

Yoga can be particularly helpful in relieving the strain on the back. A yoga therapist could devise a specific practice of asanas (yoga positions) for your individual problem. If this is not possible, try doing some at home. The frog posture (see diagram) may relieve backache considerably.

Back pain can frequently arise from or be aggravated by stress. The back is one of the areas most often affected by tense muscles causing neck and shoulder pain as well as lower back ache. Practise deep breathing and relaxation exercises if you feel your backache is stress-related (see p.163–4).

Massage is one of the best remedies for backache. Use dilute essential oils of either lavender, chamomile, geranium or rosemary, all of which have pain relieving and relaxant effects. Ginger or cinnamon oils are particularly useful for back pains if you tend to feel cold. (These oils can also be added to a hot bath.) Ask your partner or a friend to give you a firm massage to the painful area – if you feel the need for a more practised hand, have aromatherapy or a remedial massage.

If these measures do not bring relief, you may need to consult a chiropractor or osteopath, or you may have a kidney infection (see p.223) – take a urine sample to your practitioner to check.

Cayenne pepper

Capsicum minimum
Capsicum frutescans

PART USED: Pods

CONTAINS: Vitamins A and C, flavonoids, essential oil, carotenoids, alkaloid (capsaicin)

KEY USES: Stimulant, rubefacient, antiseptic, tonic, carminative, analgesic, diaphoretic, decongestant, expectorant, digestive, detoxifying

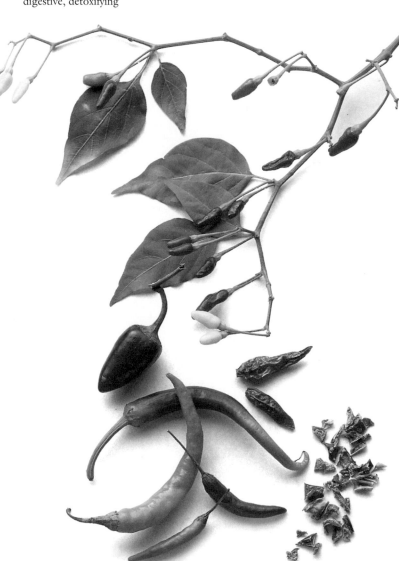

Cayenne is a powerful stimulant. It is a major stimulant to the heart and circulation, excellent for warming those prone to feeling cold and poor circulation, and for warding off winter blues, lethargy and chills. It reduces a tendency to blood clots and lowers cholesterol.

Taken hot at the onset of a cold or fever, it causes sweating and enhances the body's fight against infection. It has bactericidal properties and is also rich in vitamin C. Cayenne makes an excellent remedy for the lungs. Its pungency increases the secretion of fluid in the bronchial tubes, thinning phlegm and easing its expulsion. It relieves stuffiness and catarrh, and helps to keep the airways clear, thus preventing as well as treating coughs, colds and bronchitis.

In the digestive tract cayenne enhances the appetite, promotes the secretion of digestive juices and improves digestion and absorption. It can be added to cooking to relieve sluggish digestion that causes wind, nausea, and indigestion, and symptoms such as diarrhea, abdominal pain and dysentery. By warming the digestive tract, toxins are cleared from the gut, stagnant food wastes are removed and the work of the immune system reinforced.

In the reproductive system the warming effect relieves spasm and pain due to poor circulation. It has been used for infertility and is a rejuvenating tonic.

The burning sensation on the tongue that cayenne causes sends messages to the brain to secrete endorphins, natural opiates, which block pain and induce a feeling of wellbeing, sometimes even euphoria. A couple of drops of tincture can be applied to a sore tooth as an instant remedy for toothache.

Note Avoid cayenne if you are prone to over-heating or acidity of the stomach.

Thyme

Thymus vulgaris

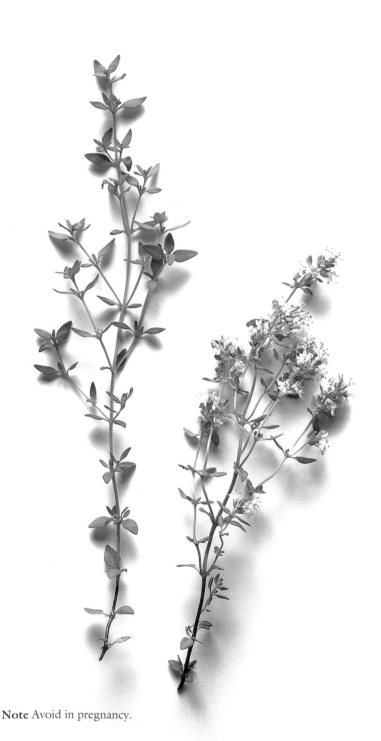

ALSO: *Thymus serpyllum, T. pulegiodes*

PARTS USED: Leaves and flowering tops

CONTAINS: Volatile oil, monoterpene hydrocarbons, alcohols, tannins, flavonoids, saponins

KEY USES: Antiseptic, diuretic, relaxant, expectorant, digestive, astringent, tonic, antioxidant, stimulant, decongestant, carminative

Thyme is a powerful antiseptic for both internal and external use. It enhances the immune system's fight against bacterial, viral and fungal infections especially in the respiratory, digestive and genito-urinary system, such as colds, coughs, flu, gastroenteritis, candi-da, cystitis and salpingitis. Its relax-ant effect on the bronchial tubes helps asthma and whooping cough, while its expectorant action increas-es the production of fluid mucous and helps shift phlegm. The relax-ing benefits of thyme can also be seen in the digestive tract, and used to good effect for wind and colic, irritable bowel syndrome and spas-tic colon. Its astringent action combined with its antiseptic prop-erties help curb diarrhea and its causes, and will re-establish normal bacterial population in the gut, especially helpful in candidiasis. Thyme also acts as a cleansing liver tonic, stimulating the digestive sys-tem and liver function, making it useful for indigestion, poor appetite, anemia, skin complaints, lethargy, and gallbladder complaints.

Thyme has a pungent taste and warming properties. It stimulates the circulation and helps to throw off chills and lethargy and acts as an exhilirating tonic to the whole sys-tem. Its tonic action on the nervous system makes it excellent for physical and mental exhaustion, relieving tension, anxiety and insomnia and to lift the spirits in depression. As a diuretic, thyme reduces water retention, infections of the urinary tract, rheumatism and gout. It also regulates the menstrual cycle and clears infections of the reproductive tract.

Note Avoid in pregnancy.

Bladder and kidney problems

Women in early pregnancy are particularly prone to urinary tract infections – in fact around 20 per cent of all pregnant women have them – related mainly to the relaxation of smooth muscle throughout the body, including the urinary system, caused by raised progesterone levels. The bladder and urinary tubules then have a tendency to dilate and kink, slowing down the flow of urine through them. The relatively stagnant urine encourages bacterial growth and infection.

Some women do not actually experience pain or discomfort, while others say they feel as though they were "passing broken glass". In some cases there has been a low grade infection which pregnancy has brought out. These bladder infections are best treated as soon as possible, to avoid complications.

A kidney infection is characterized by:

pain in the lower back, either side of the spine just below the ribs
fever and shivering
malaise
pain on passing water

Like other urinary infections, the onset may be insidious, or there may be an unnoticed chronic low grade infection, which only comes to light on routine urine analysis. Untreated kidney infections can have serious complications during pregnancy – possibly increasing the likelihood of high blood pressure, anemia and premature labour. So never ignore the first twinges, or even chronic headaches or malaise – consult your practitioner.

How to avoid kidney and bladder problems

Drink at least four pints (2 l) of liquid daily to help prevent stasis of urine. Apple juice, mineral water, herbal teas, cider vinegar and honey in warm water and barley water are all suitable.

It is important to eat healthily to support the immune system and maintain the correct acid-alkali balance in the body. Eat plenty of whole grains, pulses, nuts, fresh fruit and vegetables, and stay away from junk foods, refined carbohydrates, sugar, alcohol, excess meat and animal fats, tea, coffee and chocolate.

Over-consumption of certain other foods may irritate the urinary tubules. These include:

tomatoes	spinach
oranges	malt vinegar
rhubarb	sorrel

Other foods are therapeutic, including:

turnips	barley
leeks	onions
garlic	papaya
pineapple	

When washing around the urethra, vagina and anus, avoid using soaps, detergents or perfumed toiletries which may irritate. Wear only cotton underwear and avoid tight clothes. The distance between the bladder and the urethra is relatively short in women as compared to men, making women more prone to urinary infections. Because of this it is important, when wiping yourself after passing urine or stools, to wipe from front to back and never the reverse, otherwise germs may be carried towards the urethra, thence to the bladder.

Treatment of bladder and kidney problems

For an acute attack of either a bladder or kidney infection, first of all drink a pint of mineral water to flush out the system. Then add a teaspoon of bicarbonate of soda to a small glass of apple juice (unless you suffer from heart problems), which helps make the urine more alkaline.

Then take one cupful of herbal tea, prepared as any other infusion and left to cool a little. Drink it either lukewarm or cool.
Make your herbal tea using at least one herb from each of the following lists. Choose a mixture to suit your taste.

Recipe for barley water

Take 1.5 oz (40 g) of whole barley. Boil in 2 pints (1,200 ml) water. Simmer covered for 30 minutes. Add a slice of lemon for the last 10 minutes. Strain.

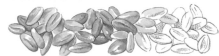

Urinary disinfectants for the infection:

echinacea	calendula
chamomile	thyme
meadowsweet	horsetail
plantain	rosemary

Anti-inflammatories and soothing demulcents:

corn silk	meadowsweet
chamomile	borage
plantain	

Diuretics to flush out the system:

raspberry leaves	corn silk
dandelion leaves	horsetail
meadowsweet	cleavers

Relaxants and painkillers to soothe the discomfort or burning pain:

pulsatilla	passionflower
lemon balm	vervain
skullcap	lavender
chamomile	

Follow each cup of herb tea with another half pint (300 ml) of water. Continue every 20 minutes through the day, and rest as much as possible.

You can also place a hot water bottle on your back, or wrap it in a towel and place it between your legs and over your bladder. Cranberry and bilberry juice can be very helpful as they have powerful antibiotic effects on the bacteria (*E. coli*) causing cystitis.

Whenever you pass water, wash afterwards very gently in warm water with a drop of lavender or thyme oil. Dab the area dry, don't rub.

You may also be greatly relieved by sitting in a bowl or shallow bath of chamomile tea, or by using warm compresses of chamomile tea over the back, abdomen or bladder area. Dilute essential oils can also be added to the water for these treatments.

Choose from:

frankincense	lavender
cypress	rosemary
bergamot	thyme
fennel	coriander
marjoram	pine

Heartburn

This is an unpleasant burning sensation in the esophagus, the food tube above the stomach, and is related to the relaxing effects of progesterone in pregnancy. The progesterone affects the cardiac sphincter – the valve at the upper end of the stomach, closing off the esophpagus above it – and can make it become incompetent. If this happens, and it fails to close as tightly as it should, it can allow regurgitation of the acid contents of the stomach into the esophagus. This is what causes the heartburn.

The condition is aggravated by bending over, sitting hunched up, and lying in bed, where you may feel better using several pillows to prop you up. It can be worse in late pregnancy when the enlarged uterus pushes up against the stomach, causing some degree of hiatus hernia. It also tends to occur more in women with a tendency to suffer from digestive problems.

Treatment of heartburn

It is best to eat slowly and take small amounts frequently. Avoid acidic, fatty and spicy foods, and also tea, coffee, alcohol, sugar and refined carbohydrates such as white rice, bread and pasta.

Take teas of any of the following herbs, singly or in mixtures, sipping them slowly and frequently to prevent and treat heartburn:

chamomile	peppermint
licorice	lemon balm
fennel	ginger
dandelion root	meadowsweet

Slippery elm food or tablets made into a gruel by adding water and a pinch of ginger or cinnamon powder is very soothing. Take as frequently as necessary. Sipping a little cider vinegar in warm water may also help.

Massage dilute essential oils gently into the upper abdomen. Choose from:

chamomile	rose
fennel	sandalwood
lemon balm	

Avoid buying tablets for heartburn from the pharmacist as many of them contain aluminium.

Horsetail

Equisetum arvense

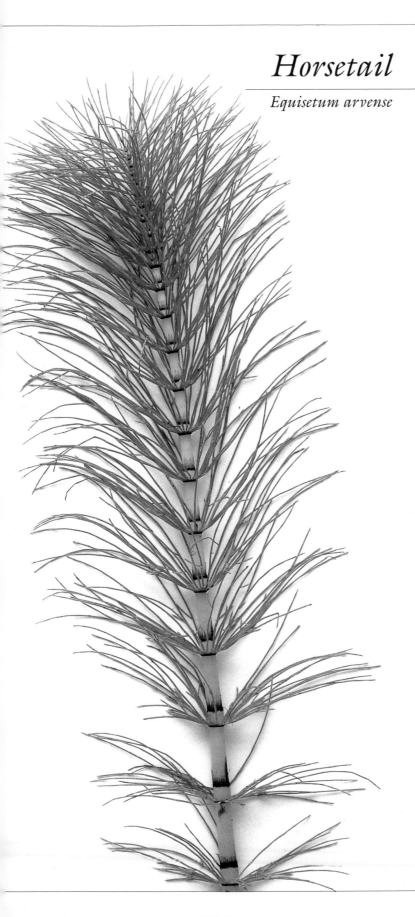

ALSO KNOWN AS: Mare's tail, shave grass, bottlebrush, pewterwort

PART USED: Aerial parts

CONTAINS: Alkaloids (including nicotine), silica, saponins, tannins, flavonoids, phytosterols, minerals (including potassium, magnesium, manganese), bitters

KEY USES: Diuretic, astringent, styptic, vulnerary

Horsetail is a descendant of prehistoric plants which grew as high as trees, and is a rich source of silica and other minerals, making it a valuable remedy for healing and a nutritious tonic. It has an affinity for the urinary system where it acts as a mild diuretic, soothing and healing irritation and infection of the urinary tract. Its toning and astringent properties make it a very useful herb for frequency of urination, incontinence and bed-wetting in children.

Horsetail is frequently used to treat inflammation or benign enlargement of the prostate gland. It acts as a tonic to the kidneys and urinary system. It also acts on the reproductive system, reducing hemorrhage and heavy bleeding, which it also does in the digestive tract, healing inflammation and ulcers, and in the respiratory tract where it was a traditional remedy for TB and coughing of blood. It can be used for brittle nails and lustreless hair, for debility and anemia. The silica helps absorption of calcium so it may help guard against osteoporosis and cramp, and has been shown to help prevent atherosclerosis.

A lotion of horsetail can be used for irritated skin conditions such as eczema, to heal cuts and wounds, sores and ulcers, and to apply to chilblains. A mouthwash and gargle can be used for mouth ulcers, bleeding gums and sore throats.

Edema

Edema is the swelling caused by fluid retention in the tissues, and some degree of edema is normal in pregnancy. Most pregnant women retain between three and six litres of fluid. It tends to appear to a minor extent in the ankles and calves.

The cause of this edema, also called gravitational edema, is the reduced level of the protein albumen in the blood. It is diluted by the increased volume of blood during pregnancy. Albumen normally holds water in the blood vessels by the process of osmosis, but when it is reduced some of this holding capacity is lost, and water seeps from the blood vessels into the surrounding tissues, which become puffy.

Because of gravity, most of this fluid gathers in the lower part of the body – mostly the ankles and calves – which swell. Edema can also affect the hands, fingers and face. Some edema in the legs is related to poor circulation and varicose veins.

Normally this gravitational edema in calves and ankles increases as the day wears on and is made worse by standing for long periods and hot weather. It is relieved by rest, putting up the feet, and reversed by sleep at night when the feet are raised.

Severe edema

The condition can worsen, until there is "pitting" edema, which pits or produces a hollow that remains after pressure is applied with the fingertips. This kind of edema usually goes with excessive weight gain, and is caused by further over-retention of fluid. This pitting edema may be a symptom of a more serious condition called pre-eclampsia.

Pitting edema normally appears in the calves and ankles. Unlike normal gravitational edema, some is evident in the morning on waking and is not much relieved by rest. It also tends to be more pronounced and causes stiffness and pressure on surrounding tissues. If you have pitting edema, contact your doctor immediately.

The cause for concern is that when it starts suddenly, and is linked with protein in the urine and high blood pressure, toxemia of pregnancy may be suspected. This is a very serious condition. If you have any of these symptoms, contact your practitioner immediately, go to bed and sleep as much as possible.

Treatment of edema

There are many herbs which have a mild diuretic effect and which may prove useful for edema. These include:

raspberry leaves	*dandelion leaves*
corn silk	*plantain*
meadowsweet	*horsetail*
cleavers	

Any of these can be prepared as a standard infusion and drunk cool three to six times daily. Add a few drops of essential oils of fennel, geranium, rose or orange to the bath, or use them diluted to massage swollen ankles and legs, always in the direction of the heart.

Adding apples, grapes, raw onions, garlic and asparagus to your diet may also prove useful as they all stimulate the kidneys. Lack of vitamin B6 has been related to fluid retention so it may be helpful to take brewer's yeast and other foods containing B6 (see p.71), such as blackstrap molasses and wheatgerm.

When edema is coupled with protein in the urine, false unicorn root is traditionally indicated. You can take lukewarm to cool infusions every two hours through the day. Plantain, horsetail and dandelion root may also be helpful.

Pre-eclampsia

This worrying condition is also called toxemia of pregnancy. Pre-eclampsia is caused by spasm in the tiny arteries in the body. The usual symptoms are rapid development of pitting edema (see above) together with protein in the urine and high blood pressure. This is another reason why regular prenatal checks are important, especially in later pregnancy.

Pre-eclampsia is something to watch for because, as its name suggests, it precedes eclampsia, a very dangerous condition which can occur in the second half of pregnancy, during labour or in the first few days after birth. Eclampsia involves mainly the sudden onset of fits or convulsions which can seriously threaten the life of both mother and baby. Other symptoms may include abdominal pain, vomiting, headaches and blurred vision. If these occur, they may not necessarily be related to eclampsia, but it is always safer to consult your practitioner immediately.

About one in ten pregnant women experience some degree of pre-eclampsia. During its development, a woman can have no apparent symptoms, and feel perfectly well. Some warning signs can be detected in routine blood tests, but generally it is picked up by taking the blood pressure, for high blood pressure tends to be the first sign of pre-eclampsia. Later in the development of pre-eclampsia, the kidneys begin to leak protein into the urine, by which time the condition may have been developing over weeks or even months. This is the reason for frequent routine blood and urine analysis, and measurement of blood pressure – these tests are vital to prevent the silent threat of eclampsia.

Causes of pre-eclampsia

Pre-eclampsia is not fully understood, though it seems that it is partly inherited, and it certainly occurs more often in first pregnancies. It may well be that the problem lies with the placenta and the supply of blood to it from the mother. Much depends on how well the placenta implants itself in the womb lining during the first four months of pregnancy. If it is not well implanted, then at some time in the second half of pregnancy it starts to outgrow its blood supply, and, starved of oxygen and nutrients, it starts to malfunction, producing pre-eclampsia. By the time it is diagnosed, scans are needed to monitor the health of the baby and the placenta, and early delivery may be necessary.

Another possibility is that pre-eclampsia occurs because of a failure on the part of the immune system. Dr. Tom Brewer and the Pre-Eclamptic Toxemia (PET) Society relate pre-eclampsia to liver problems caused by poor diet. He says that high blood pressure is caused by decreased blood volume and poor liver function, and that edema occurs when the blood is low in protein. Many doctors now relate pre-eclampsia to poor diet, particularly one deficient in protein.

Pre-eclampsia may also be related to general low health, long use of drugs, and other factors which deplete vitality and cause general toxicity in the body. While salt is conventionally restricted in edema and high blood pressure sufferers, in pregnancy this is not advisable as salt restriction has been associated with both pre-eclampsia and miscarriage.

To prevent the onset of pre-eclampsia, make sure your diet is sound, that you eat no refined foods, but plenty of foods rich in protein, calcium, vitamin B6, magnesium, potassium and natural salicylates (which are found in most fruits and vegetables, potatoes, nuts and seeds). Fatty fish such as mackerel, herring and salmon are also good.

Make sure you take plenty of exercise to ensure healthy circulation to the placenta, and rest for part of the day as well.

High blood pressure
High blood pressure can cause a restriction in the blood supply, and therefore the oxygen supply, to the uterus, the placenta and baby. This lack of oxygen and nutrients could cause growth retardation in the baby, or even stillbirth.

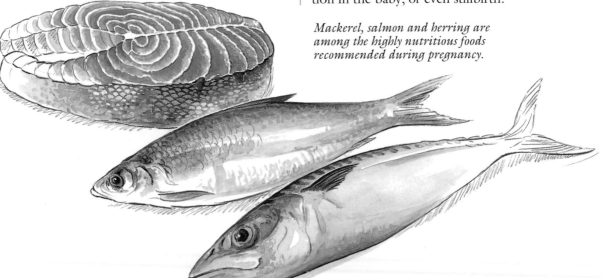

Mackerel, salmon and herring are among the highly nutritious foods recommended during pregnancy.

If you have a tendency to high blood pressure, your diet should include plenty of fresh fruit and vegetables, beans and pulses, nuts and seeds, whole grains and pure vegetable oils. Some fish, organic meat, eggs and dairy produce can be eaten to ensure you have plenty of protein. If you are vegetarian, be sure to combine your vegetable proteins to provide all the essential amino acids for your needs. The vegetable proteins are found in three groups – nuts and seeds, beans and pulses, and grains.

Eat plenty of foods rich in vitamin C every day, to help normalize the circulation and strengthen the blood vessels. Brewer's yeast is a valuable food supplement as B vitamins help to reduce blood pressure, as will raw garlic and onions. Do not restrict your salt intake. Tea, coffee, alcohol and cigarettes are best avoided.

Stress and tension frequently play a part in high blood pressure. They can cause the walls of blood vessels to tighten and narrow, thus raising the pressure within them. Rest and relaxation, quiet times alone, relaxation exercises, massage or baths in essential oils will all help to counteract the effects of stress throughout the body.

If you feel particularly anxious, or your blood pressure is worryingly high, then bed rest may be the best remedy for you. Plenty of calcium in your diet will help the muscles to relax. Frequent and gentle exercise can also prove helpful.

Treatment of high blood pressure

Hawthorn flowers, leaves and berries are nature's best remedies for normalizing blood pressure. linden blossom, passionflower, lemon balm, skullcap and cramp bark are also useful for relaxing the arteries and soothing away tension. These can be taken as teas, singly or in mixtures, three to six times daily.

There are also foods which will help. Eat oats, leeks, olive oil, garlic, onions, carrots and barley, all of which regulate blood pressure. Nettles and raspberry leaves are also helpful. Take dandelion root and leaves to regulate the action of the liver and kidneys.

High blood pressure may also be related to imbalances in the kidneys, such as chronic infection. It is sensible to have your urine analysed for infection and treat the problem accordingly (see Bladder and kidney problems p.221).

Tension and anxiety

There are several relaxing herbs you can take regularly at any stage of pregnancy, as teas or dilute tinctures. Chamomile, lavender, passionflower, linden blossom, lemon balm, skullcap and vervain will all relax both mind and body, reducing tension and anxiety, slowing respiration (useful during labour), lowering blood pressure if necessary and relaxing tight muscles. Add strong infusions to bath water, and hand and foot baths.

Raspberry leaf tea and partridge berry help to strengthen the nerves; vervain, skullcap and wild oats act as tonics to the nervous system and are very supportive during emotional upheavals, reducing tension and providing energy to help you cope with your feelings.

Cramp bark and wild yam will help relieve cramping pains, tension, uneasiness, nervousness or restlessness during pregnancy which result from stress and tension. Wild oats, false unicorn root and partridge berry are particularly useful when you feel weak, tired and low. If you feel really depressed take either St. John's wort, wild oats, vervain, chamomile, lavender or lemon balm singly or in combinations made to taste – add a little licorice to any of these remedies to sweeten them and support the adrenal glands. In later pregnancy if you feel very tired and heavy, then rosemary, vervain or wild oats will give you strength and help you feel better.

Oils of jasmine, frankincense, clary sage and lavender can help boost morale, especially towards the end of pregnancy when each day can seem like an eternity. Sandalwood is a plant native to India, where it is used for women in pregnancy who feel agitated, very nervous or fearful and panicky. In India they say that a particular kind of wind, called anant vayu, can enter a pregnant woman through the soles of her feet and cause great fear and anxiety. Sandalwood, applied in Ayurvedic medicine as a paste between the toes, helps to earth and balance you and calm the wind and fear. Try it – it smells delicious. You can also burn sandalwood incense and use essential oil of sandalwood.

Bach Flower Remedies are also excellent for easing emotional problems, and easing transition from one phase of life to another. Take mimulus for fear and anxiety; rock rose for panic; mustard for depression; olive for exhaustion; walnut for easing transitions. You may find others which are more specific to your needs.

Peppermint

Mentha piperita

PART USED: Flowering herb

CONTAINS: Volatile oil, carotenoids, betaine, choline, flavonoids, phytol, tocopherols, azulenes, rosmarinic acid, tannin

KEY USES: Carminative, antispasmodic, diaphoretic, anti-emetic, nervine, anti-septic, analgesic, astringent, deconges-tant, tonic, bitter

Peppermint is both cooling and warming. When taken internally it induces heat and improves the cir-culation and by dispersing blood to the surface of the body it causes sweating. This can be put to good use for chills and fevers, colds and flu. Its astringent and decongestant action helps relieve stuffiness and catarrh.

Peppermint makes a good gener-al tonic, to recharge vital energy and dispel lethargy. The refreshing taste of mint is followed by a cool-ing and numbing effect which extends to the respiratory tract, also apparent on the skin. It has an analgesic effect and makes an excel-lent local application when the fresh leaf or lotions are applied to relieve the pain of inflamed joints in arthritis and gout, for headaches, neuralgia, sciatica and general aches and pains.

Internally, it has a relaxing effect, calming anxiety and tension and relieving pain and spasm. It can be used for menstrual pain, asthma and insomnia. In the digestive tract it relaxes smooth muscleand reduces inflammation, relieving pain and spasm in stomach aches, colic, flatulence, heartburn, indigestion, hiccoughs, nausea, vomiting and travel sickness. The tannins help protect the gut lining from irritation and infection and make it useful for griping in diar-rhoea, spastic constipation, Crohn's disease and ulcerative colitis. The bitters stimulate and cleanse the liver and gallbladder, helping to prevent gallstones.

The volatile oils have an antisep-tic action, and are now confirmed as antibacterial, antiparasitic, anti-fungal and antiviral, useful for treating skin problems such as cold sores and ringworm.

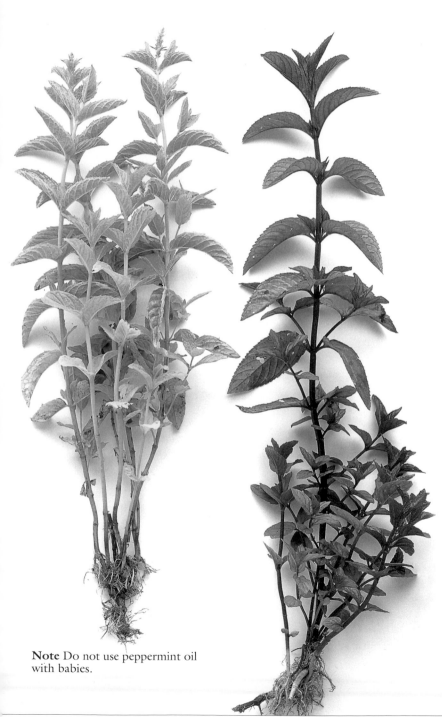

Note Do not use peppermint oil with babies.

Preparation for childbirth

In the last few weeks of pregnancy as the birth approaches, many women want to start actively preparing themselves for giving birth and being a mother. The LaLeche League, International Childbirth Education Association, Active Birth Centre and National Childbirth Trust have information and run classes which are wonderfully helpful, enhancing the ability of women to prepare themselves both emotionally and physically for the birth. They help women learn how to draw on their inner resources, enabling them to be more responsible for their own health and inner harmony, and that of their baby.

If you have not tried them before, now is the time to take up regular practice of yoga, meditation, and of massage and breathing techniques. It is better to start yoga earlier in pregnancy rather than later. These practices can go hand in hand with the use of herbs and will help to bring you positive health in both body and mind as the birth approaches and during the birth itself. This will help to increase your confidence in the inherent feminine wisdom you will need during childbirth, reducing the need for medical intervention.

There are herbs you can use in the last few weeks of pregnancy which prepare your body physically for childbirth. Several herbs have the ability to ease and shorten labour by their influence on uterine muscles and contractions, and reduce the risk of complications. Raspberry leaves (see p. 25) are the most well known of these herbs and should be taken as an infusion, made up in the normal way, once daily from the third month onwards and three times daily from the sixth month. You can add aromatic herbs such peppermint, fennel, lemon balm or rosemary if you wish. In the last week or so before the birth, add a little ginger to each cup of tea, and at the first signs of contractions add 1 tsp. Composition Essence to each cup and take it every hour or so while you can. Partridge berry (see p. 24) is another famous herb with a long history and excellent reputation for preparing women for childbirth. It can, like raspberry leaves, be taken quite safely through pregnancy.

Prepare an excellent pelvic tonic for the last three months of pregnancy using equal parts of:

partridge berry	*cramp bark*
false unicorn root	*blue cohosh*

I have recommended this to many women approaching childbirth and it has always, in my experience, worked well, making for a safe, easy and short labour, generally of no more than four to six hours.

This alternative recipe can be taken in the last six to seven weeks of pregnancy.

Mix equal parts of:

raspberry leaves	*motherwort*
blue cohosh	*false unicorn root*

This will help keep the muscles in your pelvis elastic and relaxed. It strengthens them for normal effective contractions, and will support the action of the heart, helping to ensure a good flow of blood to the uterine area.

I have often recommended equal parts of black cohosh (see p.27) and blue cohosh (see p.26) to be taken three times daily in the last six to eight weeks of pregnancy, in decoction or tincture form, as well as raspberry leaf tea.

If you are feeling particularly tired or stressed, it is a good idea to add to your chosen prescription herbs to support the nervous system and adrenal glands. These will also help give you the extra strength and stamina needed for the birth, and to speed recovery.

Choose from:

ginseng*	*wild yam*
vervain	*licorice**
ginger	*skullcap*
borage	

* but not if your blood pressure is high. Use motherwort and cinnamon instead.

If you tend to get powerful Braxton-Hicks contractions – a tightening of the uterus, and hardening of the abdomen – take herbs which are particularly relaxing to the uterine area, such as cramp bark and wild yam.

Essential oils

When preparing for the birth you can dilute essential oils and massage the abdomen and lower back, add them to the bath, or hand and foot baths, or use them as perfumes. One of the loveliest oils to use is rose, especially if you are feeling tense and anxious about the birth, and lacking confidence in your ability to cope when the time comes. Rose oil will help you to relax, and it will also relax the uterus and the whole pelvic region. It has a slight analgesic effect so it can help control pain.

Lavender oil is a wonderful balancer, helping to calm and soothe if you feel tense, volatile or vulnerable. Clary sage relaxes the uterine muscles and helps prepare them for childbirth. Geranium is a useful circulatory stimulant and has a particular affinity for the uterus, where it helps prepare the muscles for contractions. It has antidepressant effects which can be very helpful in the last few days or weeks of pregnancy, when you may feel heavy or clumsy, or feeling as if the day will never come. Some women feel quite low just before the birth because of a drop in progesterone levels.

Herbal baths and oils to massage the perineum are certainly worth recommending. You can add essential oils of rose, lavender, geranium, clary sage, clove, nutmeg and chamomile to bath water, and to a base of linseed or wheatgerm oil (2 drops of oil per 5 ml of oil) to massage the abdomen and perineum to help soften and prepare the tissues for contraction and dilation. You can also add strong infusions or decoctions of motherwort, raspberry leaves, partridge berry, chamomile, or black or blue cohosh to warm baths and soak luxuriously in these as a pleasant way to help prepare your body for childbirth.

Geranium
Pelargonium graveolens

Culinary herbs

Herbs can also be added to cooking to prepare you for childbirth. Nutmeg has long been used in this way in Malaysia; women add it frequently in small amounts to their cooking during the last few weeks of pregnancy to strengthen and tone the uterine muscles and prime them for contraction.

Note large amounts of nutmeg are dangerous, being hallucinogenic and oxytocic and should never be used in early pregnancy.

Cloves act as a tonic and antispasmodic to uterine muscles, preparing them for childbirth. You can add them to your diet in the last few weeks – only use one clove per dish as they taste very strong.

Over the last week of pregnancy you can drink clove tea two or three times a day, made by decocting one coffeecupful of cloves in a litre of water. Clove oil is highly antiseptic; dilute 2 drops in 5 ml of base oil and massage the abdomen up to two weeks before the baby is due.

Sage can also be used as a prenatal tonic; you can add it to cooked dishes, or drink an infusion two or three times a day for the last two weeks.

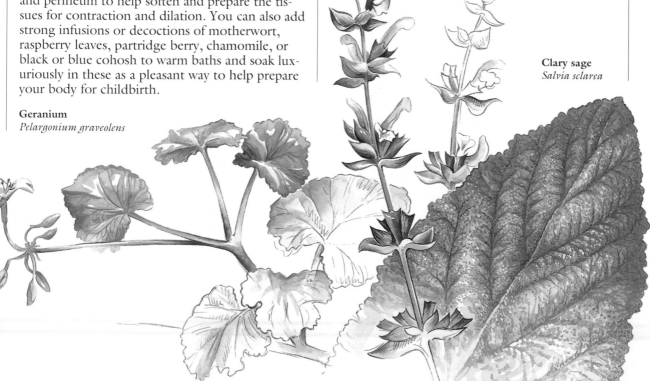

Clary sage
Salvia sclarea

Herbs for childbirth

In the last few weeks before the birth, you may notice changes in your body that indicate that the birth is imminent. Among these will be frequent Braxton-Hicks contractions (see p.144) as the uterine muscles practice for the real thing, increased vaginal discharge, a spurt of energy, pelvic pressure as the baby's head drops into the pelvis and slight weight loss a few days before the onset of the birth. At this time, decide what remedies you would like to use during the birth and gather together your birth kit.

Childbirth

Once contractions have started or the waters have broken, you can continue to use herbs to relax or tone, depending on what you need. In the first and second stages of delivery the birth can be delayed, mainly because of inadequate uterine contractions ("uterine inertia") and here herbs have a great part to play.

Sometimes the uterus takes a long time to get going – contractions may occur at irregular intervals, about every 10-30 minutes, and are weak and ineffectual. As a result, the cervix dilates only slowly and labour can become very prolonged and tiring. Poor contractions at the second stage may be the result of a long and tiring first stage, or be caused by sedation with drugs, or over-distension of the uterus because of a multiple pregnancy.

On the other hand, "uterine inertia" can also occur when the uterus contracts strongly and fiercely, but only for a few seconds at a time. Sometimes this is because of the way the baby is lying and this can cause quite severe backache. Frequent short, sharp uterine contractions are not as efficient as normal contractions. Again, the cervix can take a long time to dilate and the birth is prolonged. This kind of inertia may be part of a "fear-pain-tension" syndrome, where fear and anxiety about the birth can cause tense muscles, and increased pain, and thus can further increase tension and anxiety.

Many women feel anxious, especially with a first baby, as they do not really know what to expect. Some fear they will not be able to cope with the pain of childbirth. Many worry about performing what is essentially a private act in a

The herbal birth kit

This should consist of herbs and essential oils that you may need, dried herbs for infusions, a thermos flask in which to keep them warm, and tinctures in dropper bottles. You can make herbal ice cubes from frozen tea and suck them during the birth. Include essential oils for inhalation, baths and massage. Choose remedies from each category – you never know exactly what you are going to need – and label them well. If you are having a hospital delivery, it is also worth packing remedies for after the birth as well.

For weak, irregular contractions:

> blue cohosh
> black cohosh
> beth root
> feverfew
> raspberry leaves
> wormwood
> sage
> calendula
> golden seal
>
> tincture of myrrh and capsicum

For overstrong, painful contractions:

> blue cohosh
> black cohosh
> wild yam
> cramp bark
> raspberry leaves
>
> *And essential oils of:*
> clary sage
> lavender
> rose
> geranium
> ylang ylang
> frankincense
> rosemary
> chamomile

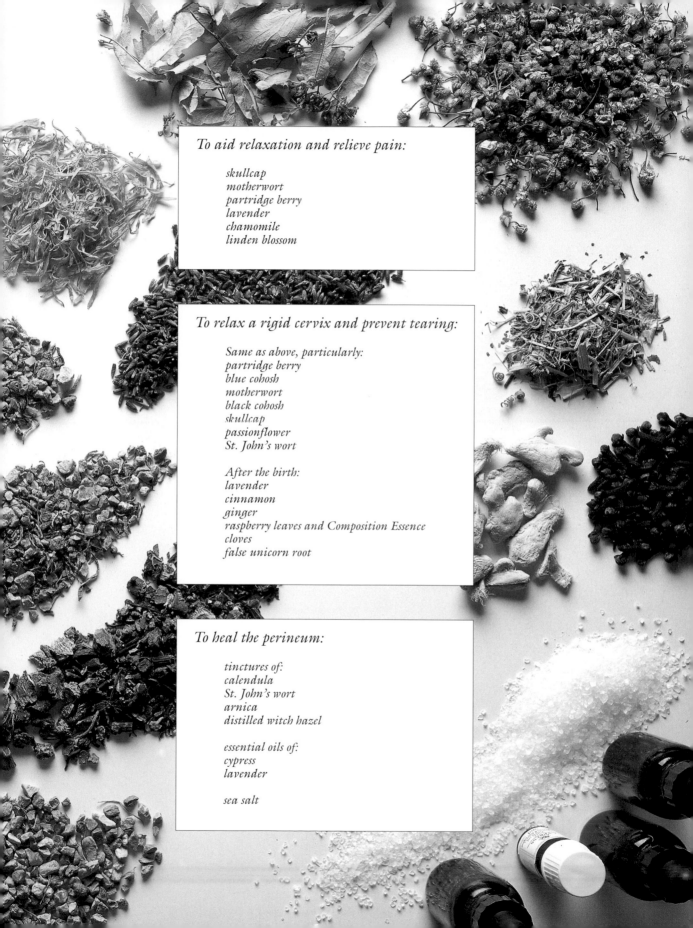

To aid relaxation and relieve pain:

  skullcap
  motherwort
  partridge berry
  lavender
  chamomile
  linden blossom

To relax a rigid cervix and prevent tearing:

  Same as above, particularly:
  partridge berry
  blue cohosh
  motherwort
  black cohosh
  skullcap
  passionflower
  St. John's wort

  After the birth:
  lavender
  cinnamon
  ginger
  raspberry leaves and Composition Essence
  cloves
  false unicorn root

To heal the perineum:

  tinctures of:
  calendula
  St. John's wort
  arnica
  distilled witch hazel

  essential oils of:
  cypress
  lavender

  sea salt

Corn silk

Zea mays

ALSO KNOWN AS: Indian corn, maize

PART USED: Stigmas (fine soft threads from the female flower), called silks

CONTAINS: Fixed oil, gums, fats, resin, glycosides, saponins, alkaloids, albuminoids, sterols, plant acids, potassium, calcium, allantoin and tannin

KEY USES: Diuretic, demulcent, tonic, lithotriptic, alterative

Corn silk is a soothing, relaxing diuretic and a wonderful remedy for acute inflammation and irritation of the genito-urinary system, such as cystitis, urethritis and prostatitis. It is particularly useful for calming bladder irritation and infection in children. It clears toxins, catarrh, deposits and irritants out of the kidneys and bladder, and has a gentle antiseptic and healing action. It makes a good remedy for frequency of urination and bedwetting due to irritation or weakness of the urinary system, and has been used for urinary stones and gravel.

By reducing fluid retention in the body, corn silk may help reduce blood pressure, and by aiding elimination of toxins and wastes from the body it may relieve gout and arthritis, and act as a gentle detoxifying remedy.

Corn silk's healing and soothing properties are helpful for relieving skin irritation and inflammation and for healing wounds and ulcers.

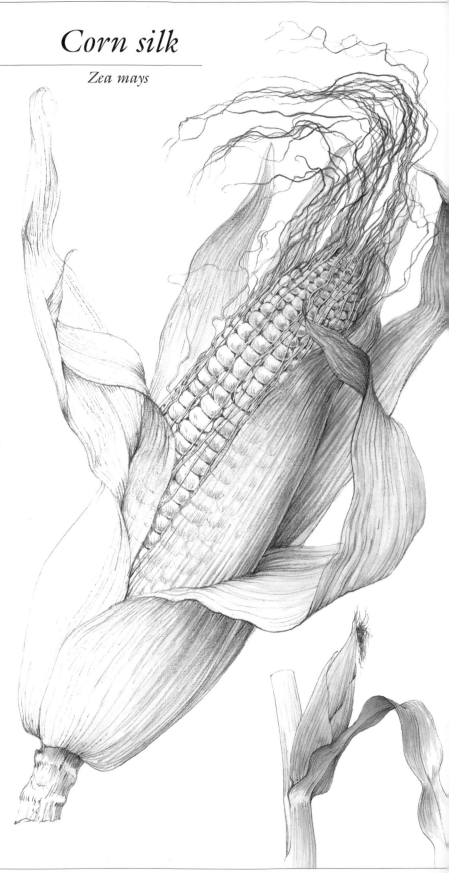

public place, exhibiting themselves to strangers. Preparation for birth using yoga, relaxation and breathing, and implementation of these and massage during the birth, can go a long way to help let go of much of this fear and anxiety. If it does cause delay in the birth, then look to support from your partner, and to massage, rhythmic breathing and herbs.

To help the actual birth you can drink herbal infusions throughout labour every half hour or every few minutes, as required, until strong contractions prevent any more liquid from being taken into the stomach. After that, take sips of tea or drops of teas or tinctures under your tongue which will bypass the digestive system. Oils can be massaged into the skin, hand and foot baths can be taken and compresses applied wherever you feel they would bring relief.

Firm massage to the lower back during the first stage can be very relaxing, reassuring and pain-relieving. Your partner, a friend, or the midwife can do this with the heel of their hand between contractions. Dilute essential oils can be used for relaxation and pain relief.

A beautifully smelling blend can be made, using the following in 2 tablespoons of base oil:

> *15 drops clary sage*
> *10 drops geranium*
> *5 drops rose*
> *5 drops ylang ylang*

This combination has a particular affinity for the uterus.

Hot compresses using a drop or two of any of these oils, or strong infusions of calendula, chamomile, lavender, or verbena, can be applied just above the pelvic bone when you are lying down, to give pain relief and help you to relax. Once the compress cools, replace it with another hot one.

For weak, irregular contractions

Black and blue cohosh help to establish a normal birth with regular and strong contractions. Sip teas or dilute tinctures (ten drops in a little water) or place a few drops under the tongue every 15-30 minutes as necessary. You can also use compresses and hand and foot baths.

Other herbs which can be taken similarly to enhance the birth and promote contractions include:

> *raspberry leaves and Composition Essence**
> *feverfew   cloves*
> *golden seal   nutmeg*
> *beth root*

> **Composition Essence is a stimulating mixture of herbs and tinctures.*

These remedies should not be taken early in pregnancy, but are excellent for the birth:

> *sage*
> *myrrh*

One drop each of tinctures of myrrh and capsicum taken in a little water, and repeated as necessary, helps to promote regular and effective contractions, increases circulation, and helps prevent post-partum hemorrhage.

Dilute oils of clove, jasmine, nutmeg, cinnamon, juniper or myrrh can also be used in the room, in vaporizers or for steam inhalations or massaged into the lower back. These stimulate contractions and promote the birth, and can help to lift the spirits if you are feeling tired or low and your strength is waning.

For over-strong, painful contractions, fear and tension

Blue cohosh can be very effective to relax the uterine muscles, soothe the nerves and relieve restlessness or irritability. At the same time its tonic action increases tone and vigour to help with the birth effort.

Black cohosh promotes relaxation and helps to regulate contractions, making them less painful and yet more productive. Black cohosh is very helpful to calm pain and relax you if you get very tense, overexcited or panicky.

Raspberry leaves relax the uterus, calm and strengthen the nerves, normalize contractions and reduce pain.

Wild yam is specific for those who are tense and nervous, cramp bark is a general relaxant and also reduces uterine tension.

Skullcap is an excellent relaxant and tonic to the nervous system. It is useful to combine it with

Myrrh

Commiphora molmol

ALSO: *Balsamodendron myrrha,*
Commiphora myrrha

PART USED: Gum resin

CONTAINS: Volatile oil (about 8%), resin
(up to 40%), gums (about 50%)

KEY USES: Stimulating, detoxifying,
astringent, anticatarrhal, carminative,
vulnerary, expectorant, rejuvenating
tonic, antiseptic

Myrrh has been valued since antiquity for its antiseptic and detoxifying properties. Myrrh is bitter, astringent and pungent and its predominant effect is warming and stimulating. It makes a wonderful rejuvenating tonic for those feeling tired and run down. It increases the circulation, dispels cold and any resultant weakness. It pushes out eruptions as it brings blood to the surface of the body, helping to resolve rashes and eruptive infections and to bring down fevers. Myrrh increases circulation to the reproductive system, relaxing spasm and regulating periods. At childbirth, it helps promote efficient contractions and relieves pain.

Myrrh acts as a stimulating expectorant and decongestant in the respiratory system, useful for bronchitis, asthma, colds and catarrh. The additional benefit of its powerful antiseptic action, active against viral and bacterial infection, helps fight off disease and it stimulates the body's immune response. Its astringent action helps arrest discharges, phlegm and chronic catarrh.

In the digestive tract its warming effect stimulates the appetite and the flow of digestive juices, improving digestion and absorption. It both relaxes and invigorates the stomach, dispelling colic and spasm, wind and distension, and fatigue associated with weak digestion. By improving digestion it clears toxins from the digestive tract and acts as a general detoxifying and anti-inflammatory remedy, useful in arthritis, rheumatism and gout. Its antibacterial and antifungal action helps restrain infection and candidiasis in the gut and clears intestinal parasites.

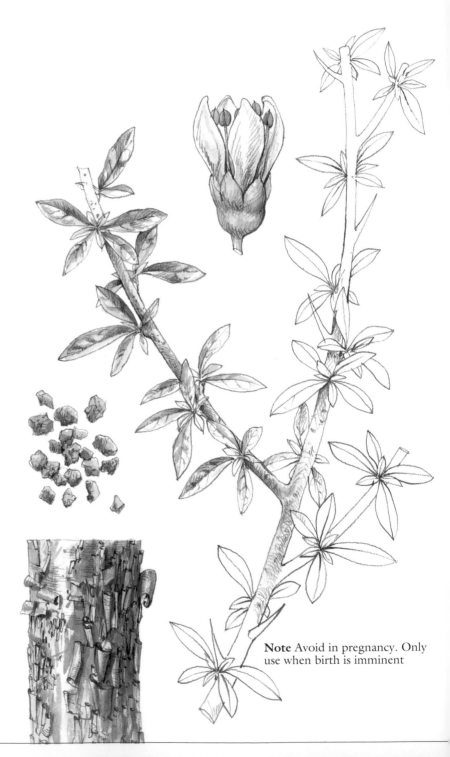

Note Avoid in pregnancy. Only
use when birth is imminent

blue cohosh. Motherwort and partridge berry both help to relax and relieve pain and distress.

Essential oils can be used to imbue the atmosphere in the room. Choose which ones you would like around you in the delivery room – their fragrance will be uplifting and reassuring, especially if you have used them previously at home in a relaxed atmosphere. A few drops can be put on lights (before they are switched on), radiators, in vaporizers, or bowls of hot water. You can also use them for massage and compresses.

Lavender helps balance the emotions and restores energy when you are feeling tired or fed up. Chamomile is particularly recommended if you get irritable or cross, or are sensitive and cannot stand any pain. Try a foot massage of these oils together when your energies are waning and you feel your ability to cope is diminishing.

If you are in great pain, especially when approaching transition (or the swearing stage as some call it) firm massage to the lower back can bring relief.

For this massage use dilute oils of:

clary sage	*ylang ylang*
geranium	*rose*
lavender	

Chamomile, rosemary, nutmeg or geranium can be used for intense back pain.

Frankincense, neroli and clary sage are calming to the nerves, relaxant to the muscles and help to slow down and deepen breathing. This in turn enhances relaxation and helps you to keep your deep rhythmic breathing going and reduces pain. They increase oxygen supply to the brain and help prevent hyperventilation. Clary sage helps make the birth easier by its specifically relaxing effect on the uterine muscles. Cold or hot compresses using any of these can be applied to the back, temples, wrists, or anywhere that feels soothing.

Strong infusions of rosemary, chamomile, mint, sage, lavender or linden blossom used in this way can relieve pain and soothe nerves. Take sips of these teas, especially when your mouth becomes dry from breathing or panting.

The relaxing effects of the herbs and essential oils described so far will all help relieve an overtense or rigid cervix, allowing it to stretch enough to let the baby pass down it without tearing.

Particularly useful at this stage are motherwort, blue cohosh, black cohosh and wild yam.

One herb worthy of note during the second stage, when you are trying to push the baby out, is ginseng. If you are feeling stressed, tired or even so exhausted you can't find the energy or enthusiasm to push any more, try chewing good quality ginseng (panax ginseng) root. It can have quite miraculous healing effects, imparting a new burst of energy just when you need it to complete the birth successfully. I have recommended it many times and tried it myself with amazing results.

For the afterbirth

The placenta usually separates from the uterine wall within five minutes of the baby's birth, and the contractions of the uterus push it out through the cervix in about half an hour. One more push from you should finish the job. It is important to ensure it all comes away, as heavy bleeding can be caused by retained placenta. Your midwife should check for this.

Once you put the baby to the breast or simply have skin contact, a hormone called oxytocin is released into the bloodstream which stimulates the uterus to contract and expel the placenta. Sometimes the uterus fails to contract properly at this time (the third stage of the birth) either because the muscles are overtired from a long birth or because they are overstretched from distension caused by multiple pregnancy. Sedatives and painkillers given during childbirth can also cause over-relaxation of uterine muscles.

There are certain herbs which can be taken to prevent retained placenta, or taken at the time should the placenta not come out whole.

These will help contract the uterus, and prevent any over-relaxation:

partridge berry	*black cohosh*
black haw	*raspberry leaves*
beth root	

A tea of raspberry leaves and beth root helps expel the placenta and can be taken through the birth to ensure proper contraction at the third stage. Feverfew and all the other oxytocic herbs can now be used. Calendula, golden seal, wormwood, bayberry, dang gui and ginger are also useful.

7 *Postnatal Care and Motherhood*

Immediately after childbirth, a new mother may feel overwhelmed by a whole range of feelings – joy over the birth of a new baby, exhilaration, excitement, and a wonderful feeling of accomplishment and fulfilment, as well as a deep love for the new baby. If the birth did not go as expected, or medical intervention was needed, this can be tinged with disappointment or sadness, or maybe just relief. During the first hours after the birth, mother and baby may experience a new energy and alertness. Both are entering distinct new stages of life; the baby in the world outside the womb, and you as a new mother. Both need comfort and reassurance. Holding your baby in your arms against your skin, and letting the baby suck on the breast will be therapeutic for you both. You will now be going through the third stage of the birth, during which the uterus contracts. After the birth comes a time of great excitement and change, when you may feel intense and uplifting emotions. You may also feel exhausted, physically and emotionally, from the birth. The hormonal system is still active but in new ways, for example controlling milk production.

Both mother and baby need comfort and reassurance after the birth.

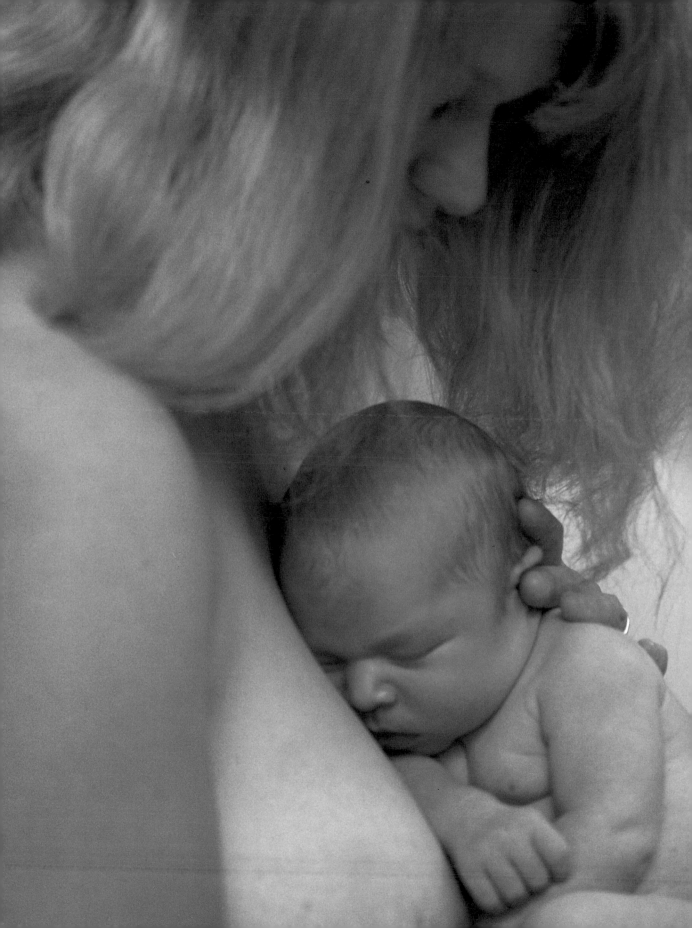

Recovery from childbirth

The Bach Flower Remedies, particularly Rescue Remedy and Star of Bethlehem, will help both parents and baby to recover from the birth, soothing the "shock" of so many new, intense experiences coming so closely together. They are especially helpful after physical shocks to the system such as Caesarean section, the use of forceps or an episiotomy. Dab a drop or two on the baby's head or wrists, and take a few drops in water yourself.

Treatments for the mother

To help restore energy after the birth you can make a tasty brew with equal parts of cloves, ginger and cinnamon. Pound the spices and mix a teaspoonful in a pint of sweet wine. Drink warm or cold. These are particularly fortifying herbs, and have long been used for weakness and tiredness after childbirth. These spices can be added to food over the next few weeks. Raspberry leaves can also be used in this mixture to speed recovery, contract the uterus and enhance the flow of breastmilk.

Another restorative herb is lavender; drink an infusion or rub the essential oil into your wrists and temples, or simply crush fragrant lavender flowers in your hands to release their beautifully uplifting aroma. You can also drink a glass of water with six drops of tincture added, to restore strength and vitality. Oils of rose, frankincense, neroli, geranium and fennel can also be used, in baths, for compresses or hand and foot baths, or in the atmosphere of the room. They are emotionally uplifting, relaxing and yet energizing and have the added benefit of being cleansing and antiseptic.

Ask your partner, midwife or friend who supported you through the birth to give you a relaxing massage using any of the oils mentioned, paying special attention to the abdomen, the back and the soles of the feet. This will help you to feel refreshed and revitalized. If you feel like it, hot and cold bathing will help revive you and tone you up generally.

There are a variety of famous herbs used as tonics for women after childbirth. Dang gui has an ancient and honourable reputation for this, and actually tastes delicious. Take dang gui in decoction or tincture three times daily over the next few weeks.

Alternatively, false unicorn root is a celebrated Native American remedy which can be taken three times daily to restore vitality when feeling tired from childbirth, or fatigued through the following weeks from breastfeeding and disturbed nights. It is a nutritious and reviving tonic, with a particular affinity for the reproductive system, where it has a special toning effect.

You can also take raspberry leaves with a little Composition Essence; a cupful of the tea three times daily after the birth will tone and strengthen the pelvic tissues.

If you have had a Caesarean, a forceps delivery, an episiotomy or tearing from the birth, and are feeling very sore and bruised, homeopathic arnica will help. Or take one drop of arnica tincture stirred into a glass of water every two hours or so. This can be enormously helpful in easing the shock and bruising of a difficult birth and speeding recovery.

If you are in a lot of pain, take the following sedative and anodyne (pain-relieving) herbs regularly throughout the day until you feel better:

> pulsatilla   lavender
> black cohosh   wild yam

Mix them with the following to aid healing:

> St. John's wort
> calendula

Treatments for the baby

Your baby is now having to adapt to all the new conditions of the world outside the womb. He too needs soothing and restoring. Use herb scented water to bathe your baby; use herbs which will help calm and reassure him.

Lavender flowers, chamomile, lemon balm, rose petals, meadowsweet or rosemary are all suitably gentle and can be made up as infusions and added to the warm water. One teaspoon of calendula, lavender or chamomile tea can be added to a cup of distilled water and used to clean the baby's face and eyes.

Cinnamon

Cinnamomum zeylanicum

ALSO: *Cinnamomom cassia*

PART USED: Bark

CONTAINS: Volatile oils, including eugenol, tannins, mucilage, gums, sugars, resin, calcium-oxylate, coumarins

KEY USES: Circulatory-stimulant, relaxant, tonic, nerve tonic, antispasmodic, astringent, digestive, antiseptic

This delicious aromatic spice is a wonderfully warming and strengthening remedy to dispel cold, winter chills and a variety of conditions associated with cold, congestion and deficiency of vital energy. It acts as a tonic to the whole system. A hot drink of cinnamon will stimulate circulation and cause sweating, preventing and resolving flu, colds, catarrh and other infections. It helps to reduce fevers. Oil of cinnamon can be inhaled for head colds and chest infections. Its general warming and stimulating properties can give direction in the body by other remedies – such as thyme for bronchial congestion and infections, or blue cohosh as a uterine remedy to treat irregular and painful periods, heavy bleeding, uterine infections and vaginal discharge.

Cinnamon acts as a relaxant, reducing anxiety and stress, relieving cramp and colic. Eugenol in the volatile oil relieves pain, for example when used as a liniment for arthritis, to deaden the nerve in toothache and for such conditions as headaches, muscle pain and neuralgia.

Cinnamon warms and stimulates the digestive system, useful in weak digestion, colic, griping, diarrhea, nausea and vomiting, wind and distension. The tannins have an astringent action, stemming bleeding in nosebleeds, heavy periods and resolving diarrhea and catarrhal congestion. When taken cold, cinnamon has been used to stop sweating.

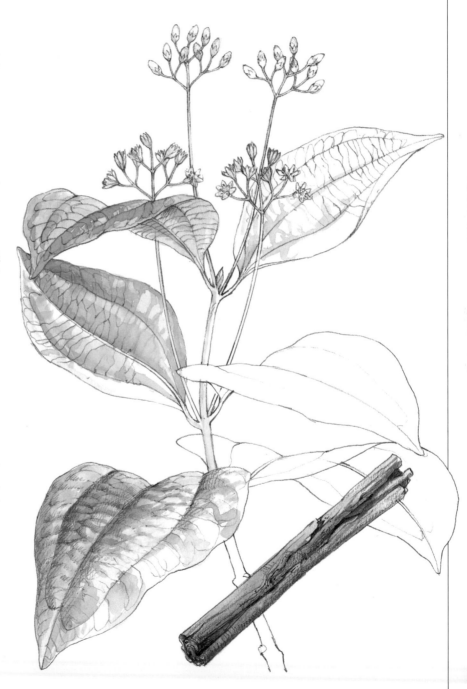

Massaging your baby with aromatic oils can be delightful. Use dilute oils, (1 drop of oil to 5 ml of base oil – preferably almond oil) of either lavender, chamomile, rose, geranium or rosewood. Your baby will probably love it! St. John's wort oil is also beneficial. There is an Arab tradition of sprinkling dried, powdered rosemary leaves on the umbilicus of the newborn baby. Rosemary has astringent and antiseptic properties and is good for nursing mothers.

Postnatal herbal treatments

Healing the perineum

The area between the anus and vagina, called the perineum, is often bruised or torn in childbirth, or may have been cut (in an episiotomy) during delivery. It can feel extremely sore and tender, and makes moving about, passing water and having a bowel movement very uncomfortable and often painful. The sooner it heals the sooner you will be able to move about again, and tend to your baby and other children you may have, without discomfort. Bathe the area frequently, either in a sitz-bath or in the bath.

Add to the water any of the following remedies which are wonderfully soothing and aid speedy healing:

Calendula add a strong infusion or a teaspoon of tincture to the water in the bath.
Arnica take 1-2 drops of tincture stirred into a glass of water 2-3 times daily, and add few drops to water in the bath. This is particularly useful for bruising but should not be used where the skin is broken, or has been cut and stitched.
St. John's wort add a strong infusion or a teaspoon of tincture to the water, and take internally 2-3 times a day.
Witch hazel add a teaspoon of tincture to the water or apply distilled witch hazel gently to the area on some cotton wool.
Comfrey add a strong infusion or a teaspoon of tincture to the bath water. A poultice of fresh comfrey root or leaves can be applied directly to the perineum to speed healing.

Essential oils can be added to bath or applied to the area as compresses. Try two drops of cypress oil, which has an astringent action, with three drops of lavender oil, which is healing and encourages growth of new skin, while protecting raw areas. Chamomile tea or oil can be added to bathing water, as can a teaspoon of myrrh, which can be an excellent healer, and has antiseptic properties. You can also add to the bath a dessert-spoonful or handful of sea salt which is greatly soothing and antiseptic, and speeds healing.

Contracting the uterus and avoiding post-partum hemorrhage

Once the baby and the placenta have been delivered, the uterus starts to contract immediately, beginning the process of involution, the return of the uterus to its normal, non-pregnant state. The whole process takes about two months to complete, but most of it occurs during the first two weeks after the birth. It is remarkable how relatively flat the abdomen becomes so soon after the baby is born.

It is important that the uterus contracts immediately after the third stage of delivery to prevent excessive bleeding from the area where the placenta was attached in the uterus and any infection which might follow. In hospitals it tends to be routine procedure to give an intramuscular injection of ergometrine or syntometrine, to ensure proper contraction of the uterus and prevent post-partum hemorrhage.

Breastfeeding is a natural trigger to uterine contraction. When your baby starts to feed, the hormone oxytocin is released into the bloodstream, causing tiny muscles around each milk-producing cell to contract and squeeze milk down the ducts to the nipple. It also contracts the uterus. You can enhance the process using herbs, once your perineum has healed.

Black cohosh, partridge berry, black haw and raspberry leaves all promote normal uterine involution and help draw the pelvis back into its normal, non-pregnant state. They also help speed general recovery after the birth.

Essential oils of geranium, rose and clary sage act as uterine tonics, and help the pelvic tissues to regain their elasticity after the birth. Geranium has a particularly contractive effect, pulling the dilated pelvic tissues back together.

Oak bark

Quercus robur

PART USED: Bark

CONTAINS: 20% tannin, gallic acid, ellagitannin

KEY USES: Astringent, anti-inflammatory, antiseptic

Oak bark contains a high percentage of tannins which give it powerful astringent properties, toning mucous membranes throughout the body and protecting them from irritation and infection. Oak bark makes a good remedy for diarrhea, catarrh, and sinus congestion. It reduces excessive menstrual bleeding and can be used to tone pelvic and abdominal muscles, very useful for treating prolapse. By clearing catarrh and toning mucous membranes in the digestive tract it aids digestion and absorption. By toning muscles throughout the circulatory system it is useful for varicose veins and hemorrhoids.

A decoction of oak bark can be used as a gargle for tonsilitis, pharyngitis and laryngitis. As a mouthwash it is good for bleeding gums and mouth ulcers. As a lotion it can be used for varicose veins and hemorrhoids, burns and cuts and as a douche or lotion for vaginal discharges and infections. It was used as a snuff when powdered for stopping nosebleeds.

Borage

Borago officinalis

ALSO KNOWN AS: Bugloss, burage

PARTS USED: Leaves, flowers, seeds

CONTAINS: Saponins, mucilage, tannins, essential oil, potassium, calcium, pyrrolizidine alkaloids

KEY USES: Diaphoretic, diuretic, antidepressant, nervine, expectorant, tonic, anti-inflammatory, galactagogue, detoxifying, decongestant, demulcent

Borage is a cooling, cleansing herb used for detoxifying the system and for any condition associated with heat and congestion. It increases sweat production, and has a diuretic action, hastening excretion of toxins via the skin and the urinary system. Borage tea can be taken to clear skin problems, such as boils and rashes, for arthritis and rheumatism, during infections and to bring down a fever. It is also good for clearing children's eruptive diseases such as measles and chickenpox, and for feverish colds, coughs and flu. It has a decongestant and expectorant action in the respiratory system and makes an excellent remedy for catarrh, sore throats and chest infections. The mucilage in borage soothes any sore, irritated condition of the throat and chest. It has the same action in the urinary system and the digestive system, making it useful for gastritis and irritable bowel syndrome. The leaves and seeds increase milk supply in nursing mothers.

Borage has an ancient reputation as a heart tonic; it calms palpitations and revitalizes the system during convalescence and exhaustion. It has a relaxing effect and is said to give courage and help relieve grief and sadness. It stimulates the adrenal glands which can prove valuable in countering the effects of steroids and helpful when weaning off steroid therapy to encourage the adrenal glands to produce their own steroid hormones. It is also useful during the menopause when the adrenal glands take over estrogen production. These properties are also present in the seeds which contain gamma linoleic acid.

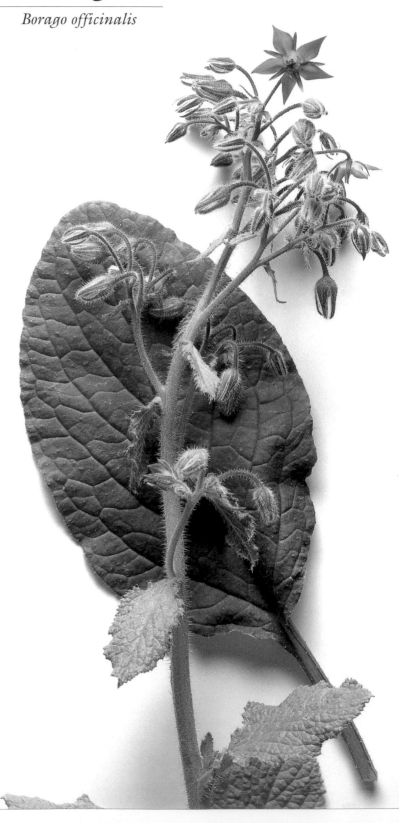

Post-partum hemorrhage

Should you bleed excessively after the birth there are several herbs which may prove beneficial.

Use any of:

golden seal	beth root
false unicorn root	wild yam
black haw	

In China, huang qi and dang gui are famous herbs used for post-partum hemorrhage as well as any weakness after childbirth, including that arising from anemia after heavy blood loss. They also promote healing of the pelvic tissues.

Uterine infections

After the birth of a child it is quite normal to bleed lightly for anything up to three weeks. During this time it is possible for an infection to develop, although it tends to occur more in women who bleed heavily or whose uterus is not contracting down as efficiently as it should be, perhaps due to retained placenta. If the lochia (vaginal discharge following delivery) starts to smell strongly, you may well have an infection. To confirm this, check with your midwife.

If you have an infection, take echinacea tea or ten drops of tincture in a glass of water every two hours.

Add to this astringent tonics for the uterus which are also antiseptic, such as:

golden seal	myrrh
wormwood	thyme
beth root	

Cramp bark taken in decoction is also specific for uterine infections.

Add dilute tinctures, strong infusions or decoctions of the above to water in the bath and sit in it for 10-20 minutes twice a day. Sea salt added to the water is also helpful.

After-pains

As the uterus rapidly contracts to its normal size, uterine contractions can be so powerful that they feel like cramp or the pains of childbirth all over again. These are known as after-pains. They tend to occur more in women having a second or third child, and can occur immediately after the birth and continue for a few days afterwards. Apart from the discomfort or pain, there is no real cause for concern, as they are quite normal. It may well be that the powerful contractions reflect a general level of muscular tension in the body, so it is important to try and relax as much as you can.

Many women only feel after-pains when their baby starts to suckle. This is because oxytocin is immediately released as the baby feeds, causing the uterus to contract. Try to be aware of any tension in your body, or anxiety you may feel as you feed, and let it go. Some soothing music, or a relaxing herbal tea, or the use of relaxing essential oils before or during feeding may help you to release some of the tension, and relieve the after-pains considerably.

To help reduce uterine contractions, try this very effective and pleasant herbal tea:

> 3 parts skullcap or passionflower
> 1 part sliced fresh ginger
> 2 parts wild yam

Mix 1 oz (25 g) of herb to a pint (600 ml) of boiling water. Infuse for 20 minutes. Take a cupful 3 times daily.

Other herbs can be equally effective as teas or dilute tinctures:

black haw	cramp bark
blue cohosh	black cohosh

These all relax the uterus and the whole pelvic area and reduce or relieve after-pains. They are all excellent remedies and recommended for over-powerful contractions of the uterus both during pregnancy and after the birth.

Another useful tea is made by mixing together equal parts of:

> wild yam
> blue cohosh
> black cohosh
> 1 tsp Composition Essence per cup

Take a cupful every two to three hours as necessary.

Postnatal depression

After the birth, that wonderful hormone progesterone – responsible for many of the physiological changes during pregnancy and that feeling of well-being and relaxation experienced by many pregnant women after about the third month – starts to decrease back to the levels in a non-pregnant woman. On the third or fourth day after the birth when this shift in hormone levels begins, and the milk supply starts to come through, many women feel a little low and depressed with the "baby blues" (or the "third day blues"). You might feel vulnerable and weepy, perhaps made worse by the fact that your friends and family around you are radiantly happy for you and your new baby and you feel concerned by your inability to feel the same. You may have mood swings, maybe from happiness and elation about your beautiful baby, to feelings such as guilt, anger or resentment about the shortcomings of your birth experience.

Once the hormones settle down, most mothers feel better again and those breastfeeding can often feel in a state of heightened sensitivity for many months. However, there are some mothers whose "baby blues" settle into chronic postnatal depression or who start to feel very depressed months later once they stop breastfeeding.

The enormous changes in every aspect of a new mother's life present new challenges which can serve to increase your vulnerability or inability to cope. There are the unrelenting demands of the baby, who might have colic and feeding problems, which you have to interpret; there is your partner, who is not only a lover now, but also a father; there is tiredness from breastfeeding, broken nights and apparently endless washing and cleaning; seeing single friends with their freedom and exciting activities – all these can contribute to your feelings of depression.

It is often helpful to understand why women can feel so low and vulnerable after the birth of a child – after all, it is the biggest change physiologically, hormonally, emotionally and socially a woman will experience and not something to be brushed off lightly. It is something that many women experience and it is certainly not anything you should feel ashamed of. Talking about your feelings, whether they are about the birth, the hospital attendants, your family, the baby or your inability to cope, can be an enormous relief. It may be very important for you to find a listening ear, either from your partner, a fellow mother, a friend or relative, or a professional counsellor.

You will need all the loving, understanding, help and support from your partner and family that you can get. Try and support yourself as well; you can pamper yourself without feeling guilty. Relax as much as you can, leave the ironing, forget about the housework, and spend time just getting to know your baby and reflecting on your new way of being. If you have plenty of rest, and eat and drink properly, you may find that you soon regain your strength and are better able to cope. A little time to yourself may show you that within you is an innate feminine wisdom which understands and knows the needs of your child, perhaps even before he asks, without worrying about him every time he starts crying or sleeps longer than normal. You may find that this crisis, painful though it is, brings old problems to light, and helps heal emotional problems from a long way back – but support during this process is essential. Your partner may turn out to be the last person who is able to help you, and may experience a very difficult time himself. There are organizations and professionals who you can consult – the organizations mentioned on p.280, your health visitor or maybe a counsellor or psychotherapist.

Diet and herbs can also be very supportive during this difficult time. Your diet is as important now as it was during pregnancy, and you may need to take supplements of B vitamins, in B complex or brewer's yeast, vitamin C, calcium, magnesium and zinc.

Take teas or tinctures of the following to help your nervous system and help lift depression:

rosemary	vervain
wild oats	borage
St. John's wort	skullcap
lemon balm	pulsatilla

Hormone-balancing herbs such as chaste tree or false unicorn root can be added to your prescription.

Dilute oils of jasmine, clary sage, ylang ylang, bergamot, neroli, and rose are all lovely aromas to help lift the spirits and are specific to postnatal depression. Choose two or three and mix them together as perfumes, for massage, hand and foot baths, and add them to long, luxurious warm baths. Drop a little on the pillow before you go to sleep, or on your clothes in the day, so that the healing aromas are about you for the best part of the day and night.

Bach Flower Remedies can be very helpful during such difficult times. Cherry plum, olive, mustard, or willow are particularly indicated.

Bladder problems

Stretching of the pelvic floor muscles, and trauma to them from pregnancy and the birth, can cause them to slacken. The result of this can be a degree of uterine prolapse and leaking urine when you exert yourself (stress incontinence). Postnatal exercises will help put your muscles back in shape, and many of them are designed to tighten the pelvic floor muscles specifically.

Sit well back on a hard chair, and lean forward with your elbows on your knees, or lie on your back with your knees bent up and your feet flat on the floor.

1 Pull the area between your legs, which is the pelvic floor, up as tight as you can, try to hold it there for up to 5 seconds, and then gently let go.

2 Tighten different groups of muscles, one at a time. Imagine you want to pass water but have to wait, and tighten the muscles around the urethra. Then tighten the anus and then vagina and pull them up as far as you can. Hold them all for a count of 5 then gently let go.

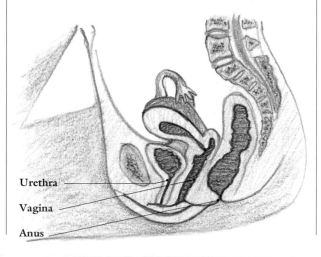

Urethra

Vagina

Anus

Repeat these as frequently as you can for a few days and then try them standing up.

Associate certain activities with your pelvic floor exercises so that you never forget to do them – for example, every time you stand at the basin to clean your teeth, or when you put the kettle on, stand at a bus stop, scrub the potatoes or do the dishes.

If you need to cough or sneeze, tighten your pelvic floor before you do, to stop any leaking of urine. But remember that to prevent it from happening every time you run or jump, you need to practise these exercises regularly every day. When you are actually taking physical exercise, you will need to consciously tighten up your pelvic floor muscles, until they regain their elasticity. Practise strengthening them under exertion – empty your bladder first and then run or jump on the spot while tightening your muscles, for as long as you can. You will soon see an improvement.

If you have put on a lot of weight during pregnancy, it is important to try to reduce it slowly if you are having bladder problems, but make sure that you do not compromise your nutrition. The Hay diet (see p.281) would be particularly helpful at this time, when you may not benefit from a calorie-reducing diet, and your baby may suffer nutritionally if you are breastfeeding. Avoid constipation as this puts pressure on the pelvic floor muscles (see constipation p.121)

Alternating cold and hot sitz-baths every morning and evening will help tone up your pelvic floor muscles. If you cannot bear those, add strong herbal infusions or tinctures to your baths.

Use any of:

beth root	*horsetail*
golden seal	

Also add uva ursi to your chosen prescription. These should also be taken internally three or four times daily to help tone the bladder muscles.

Other postnatal problems you may experience include backache, piles and constipation and anemia. These are ailments also common during pregnancy and are dealt with in an earlier chapter. Turn to the relevant section discussed in Chapter 6 (p.108-136) for herbal and nutritional help for these problems.

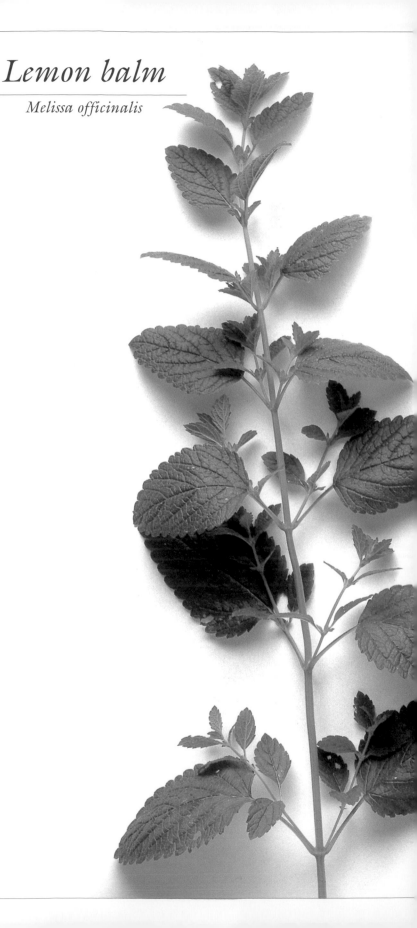

Lemon balm

Melissa officinalis

ALSO KNOWN AS: Bee balm, melissa, sweet balm

PART USED: Aerial parts

CONTAINS: Volatile oil, polyphenols, tannin, flavonoids, rosmarinic acid, triterpenoids

KEY USES: Antiviral, decongestant, antihistamine, antiseptic, carminative, antispasmodic, antidepressant, nervine, diaphoretic, hypotensive, bitter tonic

Lemon balm is an excellent remedy for soothing the nerves and lifting the spirits. It has a particular affinity with the digestive system, where it calms and soothes nausea, vomiting, poor appetite, colic, dysentery, colitis and any stress-related digestive problems. The bitters gently stimulate the liver and gallbladder and enhance digestion and absorption. Lemon balm makes a useful remedy where nervousness or depression affect the action of the heart, causing heart pains, palpitations or an irregular heartbeat.

In the reproductive system, lemon balm relaxes spasm causing period pain, and relieves irritability and depression associated with PMS. It also helps regulate periods and has been used traditionally to relax and strengthen women during childbirth and to bring on the afterbirth. Both postnatally and during menopause lemon balm can help relieve depression.

The relaxant effects of lemon balm help relieve pain and spasm in the kidneys and urinary system. It makes a good remedy for headaches, migraine, vertigo and buzzing in the ears, and when combined with linden blossom it can help reduce blood pressure.

In hot infusion it causes sweating, reducing fevers and making a good remedy for childhood infections, colds and flu, coughs and catarrh. Its relaxant and mucous-reducing properties are helpful during acute and chronic bronchitis, as well as harsh irritating coughs and asthma. It makes a good remedy for allergies and its antiviral action makes it excellent for cold sores.

Herbs for early motherhood

If you feel tired or stressed from the huge demands imposed upon you, then you need some help and support. You need to compensate for the amount of energy that life is taking from you at this time, while you are breastfeeding, having broken nights, attending your baby's and other children's needs as well as the housework. Take naps in the day when you can, and go to bed as early as possible. Reduce the number of your visitors unless you feel they will be supportive, and try to find at least one hour a day to be on your own to relax, or do whatever is pleasurable or energizing for you. You may have to ask your partner, family or friends to support you for a while until you recuperate your energy.

Make sure that your diet is as nutritious as it was when you were pregnant; it is just as important now. However, if you don't have enough energy to cook, you can manage on raw meals and snacks, which can be just as nutritious as cooked foods. Supplements of vitamin B complex, vitamin C and a multi-mineral and vitamin tablet will boost your nutrition.

Add nutritious herbs to your salads and cooking, and your herbal teas. These will increase your iron:

nettles	burdock
dandelion leaves	chickweed
watercress	coriander
basil	parsley

These will help increase calcium:

horsetail	chamomile
oats	borage
plantain	nettle
skullcap	

Kelp and other sea herbs are also very nutritious. They can usually be found in health food shops. For tiredness and exhaustion there are tonic herbs which will revitalize you and feed the nervous system. Try drinking the tea made from the following recipe over the next few weeks.

1 cup of tea or 1 tsp. of tincture 3-6 times a day made of equal parts of:

wild oats	vervain
skullcap	dang gui
ginger	

Add a little licorice to flavour it and to support the adrenals.

If you feel tense or anxious, try relaxing in a luxurious warm bath and add your favourite oils to make it smell good. Lavender, geranium, rose or clary sage are all soothing and relaxing and will help you release tension. Relaxation exercises, rhythmic breathing and meditation are all very beneficial when practised regularly.

Herbs will help alleviate the wearing effects of stress on the body and nervous system. Take any of the following, in combinations of your choice, to help you relax:

lavender	wild oats
rosemary	passionflower
wood betony	vervain
chamomile	valerian
linden blossom	skullcap
lemon balm	catmint

Add licorice and borage to support the adrenal glands in these stressful times. The Bach Flower Remedies can be enormously helpful – try olive for exhaustion, mustard for gloom and depression, mimulus for fear and anxiety, and rock rose for panic. A full list is on p.246–7.

If you find yourself becoming very tense, try to deal with it practically as soon as you become aware of your feelings. A crying baby can be a source of great distress and anxiety, as well as pure frustration. Sometimes your baby can seem to be asking for help but you have no idea what to do. If you have tried all the usual things – a feed, a drink, a winding, a diaper change, a walk round the room or just a cuddle – and the crying continues, it may be that your distress is being transferred to your baby. Put the baby down or give him to someone else for a while and get right away, to somewhere you cannot hear him.

Now is the time to take your Bach Flower Remedies and herbal mixtures. You can also try this relaxation exercise; either lying flat on the floor or sitting comfortably in a chair.

Concentrate on each part of your body in turn and let go of any tension that you find there. This will relax you, centre you in your body, and take the energy away from those disturbing emotions which can very often get out of proportion. This simple relaxation exercise helps put life back into perspective and in my own experience can be wonderfully helpful.

If your anxiety or fatigue is extreme or long lasting, you will need plenty of support from your family and friends. You may find it beneficial to talk out your fears and anxieties. There may be a local support group of new mothers which you may find comforting, and of great practical help. Refer to the list of helpful organizations on p.280. Try not to be afraid to ask for help when you really need it – you will find that most mothers know exactly how you feel and will be only too happy to lend a hand.

Exhaustion and stress

Making a new human being from your own tissues and giving birth to this little being are enormous feats in themselves. If the birth is prolonged or stressful, you may feel tired or exhausted before you even start feeding or caring for your baby through the day and night.

If you feel drained after the birth, take raspberry leaf tea with a teaspoon of Composition Essence frequently through the day.

Take 3-6 times a day a remedy made from equal parts of:

false unicorn root	*dang gui*
ginger	*nettles*

A short course of ginseng for a few days may prove beneficial if you feel very depleted. Essential oils of frankincense, rose and lemon are all restorative and energizing. Try these in baths, massage oils, vaporizers or just use them about you as perfumes.

Relaxation exercise

When you really need to relax, try this exercise which is often used to release muscle tension at the end of a yoga practice. It works just as well if you sit comfortably instead of lying down; the important thing is to be perfectly at ease and out of reach of disturbances and possible interruptions.

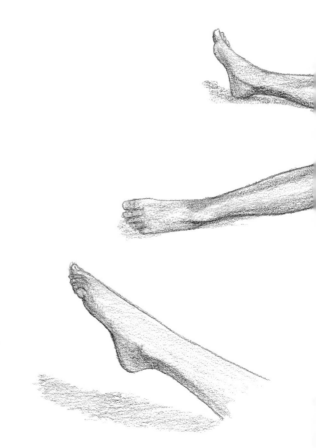

Feet and legs *Lift your right foot just off the floor. Tense the leg for a few seconds, then let it drop. Do this with the other leg.*

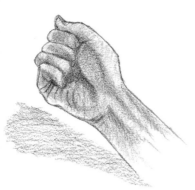

Hands and arms *Lift up your right hand slightly from the floor. Clench it, tense the arm, then let it drop. Repeat on the other side. Relax.*

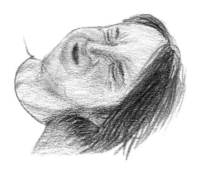

Face *Squeeze up your face so every muscle is tight, drawing the face into the nose. Now stretch the face wide.*

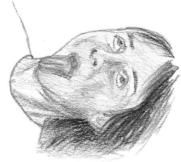

Open your eyes really wide, and stick your tongue out as far as it will go. Relax.

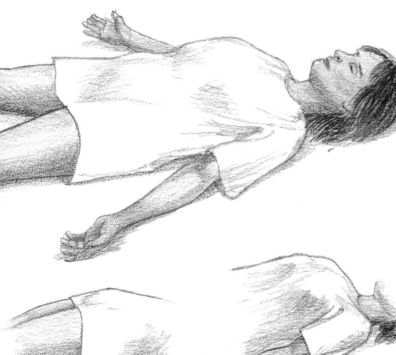

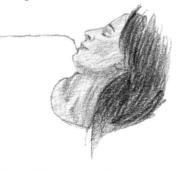

Head *Tuck your chin in a bit and move the head gently from side to side. Find a good central resting place for the head to lie, and then relax.*

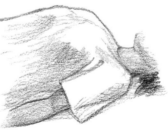

Chest *Keeping your hips and head on the floor, tense and lift up the back and chest. Relax and drop them down.*

Buttocks *Tighten up your buttocks, and lift the hips slightly off the floor for a few seconds. Drop them down and relax.*

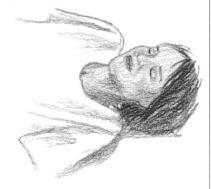

Shoulders *Lift your shoulders and hunch them tightly around your neck. Let them drop, relaxed. Now bring each arm, in turn, down beside the body, and relax.*

8 *Breastfeeding and Infant Care*

At birth, the new baby makes an enormous transition from one state of dependency, inside the womb, to another outside the womb. The baby still needs to be fed, nurtured, kept warm, secure and loved, just as he was in the womb. Breastfeeding is a wonderful way of providing nurture of all these kinds to ease the transition from one world to another.

To many, breastfeeding is a vital part of mothering. In fact there is much research to prove the beneficial effects of breastfeeding on the baby's emotional as well as physical development, particularly breastfeeding and skin contact immediately after the birth. Separation from the mother at birth, which can happen in hospital, prevents the signals of birth completion being given, so the adrenal glands of the baby stay in a state of alert. This can cause exhaustion and prolonged sleeping or prolonged crying.

Most women are eager to breastfeed their babies but find it is not as straightforward as they thought. There is quite an art to breastfeeding that in the past midwives would have been able to teach to new mothers. Many women start well enough and continue until they develop such sore nipples that they cannot go on. Others stop through lack of sufficient milk. Help is available, however, both to prevent and treat most breastfeeding problems. There is also practical advice available in books and from midwives and health visitors, so don't give up too easily!

The sooner after the birth you start to breastfeed, the easier it will be in the long term. So keep your baby with you, lie him on your abdomen and let him find the breast, or put him gently to the breast, and you will find that he will be much less stressed than if he is taken away to be washed and weighed. Less stress will mean easier breastfeeding, and will start your relationship off on the right foot. If you have had painkillers during the birth the baby may be very sleepy, and you may find it takes a while for him to suck strongly on the breast. Don't worry, it will happen in time. Let your baby determine how long and how often he will feed. This will make for a plentiful supply of milk, and prevent engorgement of the breasts, which can be very uncomfortable.

Breastfeeding is a healthy start to your baby's physical and emotional life.

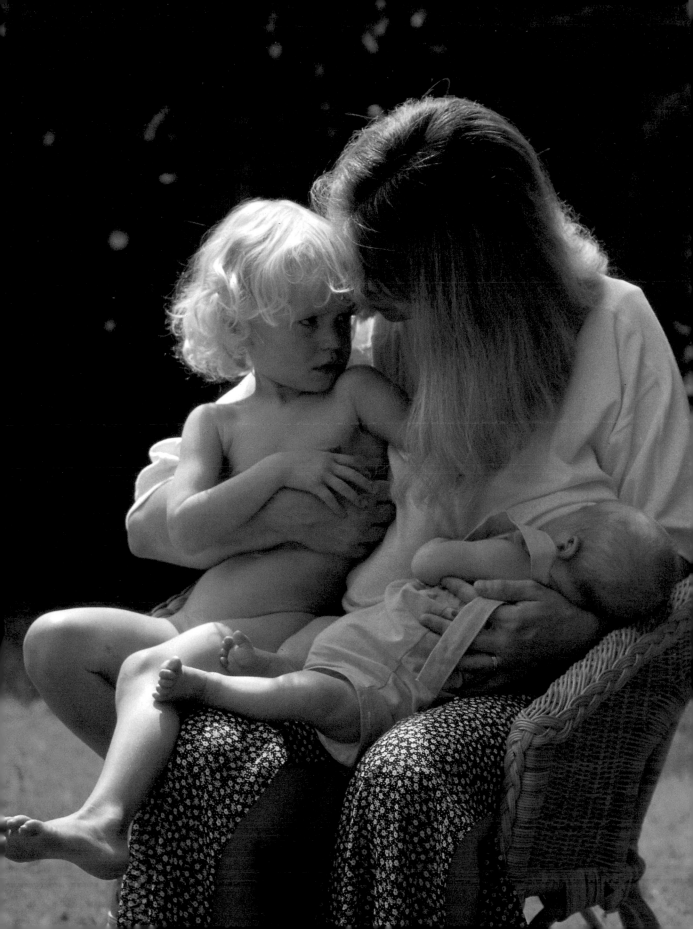

The advantages of breastfeeding

There are many advantages to breastfeeding as opposed to bottle feeding. Breastmilk helps to protect the baby against digestive infections, such as enteritis and diarrhea, respiratory and urinary infections. The first milk that comes into the breasts is colostrum, containing antibodies to many of the diseases the mother has had or has been immunised against. If you breastfeed for at least 13 weeks this will help protect your child from gastro-enteritis for the first two years of life. Lactose in breastmilk is a sugar which supports the growth of beneficial bacteria in the baby's gut, and discourages pathogenic ones, preventing the development of infection. Commercial baby milks contain glucose, maltose or dextrose which pathogenic bacteria thrive on. Infective diarrhea, chest infections, meningitis, and septicemia are more common in bottlefed babies all over the world. Breastmilk contains certain sugars which are carried from the baby's gut to the lining of the lungs, where they prevent pathogenic organisms from damaging the lungs.

Breastmilk boosts a baby's immunity to allergies as well as infections. So if there is a family history of allergy, it is best to breastfeed exclusively for as long as you can. A baby's immune system is immature for the first four to six months, during which time his food can affect the development of allergies as an older child or even as an adult. Symptoms of allergy in a baby may include colic, insomnia, constipation, diarrhea, crying, diaper rash, skin problems, catarrh and convulsions.

Breastmilk is the perfect food for babies, just as cow's milk is for calves. Cow's milk has to be radically altered to make it suitable for feeding babies, while the nutritional composition of breastmilk is just right for building the body of a human infant, especially during the first few weeks when it doubles its birth weight and develops its co-ordination. The high proportion of fat compared to protein and carbohydrate in breastmilk is particularly important for humans, as fat aids brain development and the human brain develops far more quickly than those of animals. Breastmilk contains plenty of essential fatty acids necessary for the nervous system while cow's milk contains much more protein, necessary for body building. As a result, bottlefed babies often put on more weight than breastfed ones, which may predispose them to infections, weight problems and arterial disease later on in life.

The physical relationship between a breastfeeding mother and her baby is a wonderful one. By sucking, a baby calls for food, and breastmilk is produced as a response. The more the baby sucks, the more milk is supplied, until the baby is replete. Your baby's needs are hard to gauge when bottle-feeding.

Because breastmilk is better digested and assimilated than formula milk, breastfed babies tend to have fewer digestive upsets such as colic and constipation. Added to this, the absorption of the other nutrients depends on the kind of milk a baby has. The lactose in breastmilk is broken down by bacteria to become lactic acid. Vitamin C and several B vitamins are easily destroyed unless they are held in acid until they reach the bloodstream and iron, phosphorus, calcium and other minerals can only dissolve in acid. So because of the greater proportion of lactic acid produced in a breastfed baby's intestines, he will absorb far more of these vitamins and minerals than one fed on formula milk.

Breastfeeding involves contact between mother and child for quite some time during the day and night. In this holding comes bonding, and nurture that far exceeds the nutritional value of the milk. For a mother too, breastfeeding can give a wonderful feeling of joy and fulfilment, along with the pleasure of knowing that your baby is having the best possible nourishment.

Breastmilk is readily available, requires no preparation, comes at the right temperature, germ-free and full of antibodies to protect the baby against illness and infection. Breastfeeding stimulates the contraction of the uterus to its normal size and uses up excess fat, helping you to regain your figure. Research shows that prolonged breastfeeding can also reduce the incidence of breast cancer.

Herbs to increase and enrich milk supply
There are many herbs which women have used for centuries to stimulate milk production and to enhance and enrich their milk supply while they are breastfeeding.

These herbs can be taken as tinctures, but are best taken as teas, frequently through the day:

borage	*nettles*
raspberry leaves	*fennel seeds*
blessed thistle	*goat's rue*
saw palmetto	*false unicorn root*
dill	*vervain*
chaste tree	*cinnamon*
garlic	

Caraway seeds and fenugreek can also be added to your diet at this time. Any of these herbs can be combined together to suit your taste, and you can alter the mixture when you feel the need for a change.

A delicious recipe for enhancing milk supply is raspberry leaf tea with honey and half a teaspoon of a mixture of powdered ginger, cinnamon and cloves; take this as soon as the baby is born to speed recovery and to revive you when you feel tired.

Many of these herbs are very nutritious, especially nettles, raspberry leaves, borage and garlic. Others have relaxant effects which soothe tension and anxiety while breastfeeding – these include cinnamon, vervain, borage, blessed thistle and raspberry leaves. Some are warming and antispasmodic, helping to relieve muscle tension, and include fennel, caraway, cinnamon and dill. Borage contains calcium and phosphorus, and has been used traditionally to "gladden the heart" and lift depression – particularly useful if you feel sad or depressed when the time comes to wean your baby.

Chaste tree seeds stimulate the pituitary gland to regulate secretion of the hormone prolactin which governs breastmilk production. Saw palmetto berries promote the normal function of the mammary glands in the breast. You can take three to five berries daily in the last month of pregnancy and while nursing.

While these nutritious and therapeutic herbs benefit the feeding mother, they also pass through the milk to the baby. Several of the herbs which enhance milk supply contain volatile oils, which are antiseptic, antibiotic and antispasmodic. These will boost the baby's immune system, aid digestion, and soothe tension or colic. Such herbs as lavender, thyme, rosemary, chamomile, peppermint, yarrow, lemon balm, elderflowers and garlic can all be taken to treat and prevent minor infections such as coughs or colds, or digestive problems (see Herbal babycare p.174–183). They can be taken as teas or added regularly to your cooking or used in salads.

You can also use essential oils to enhance milk supply. Choose either fennel, geranium or clary sage. Add about 10 drops to 30 ml of almond oil and massage it into each breast with gentle, circular movements once a day.

Your diet and milk supply

A healthy diet is important for maintaining your milk supply, and to provide nutrition for both you and your baby – you need about 2000 extra joules (500 cal) a day. You can also enhance and enrich your milk supply by the foods that you eat every day.

Maize, oats, barley, peas and beans and pulses have been used traditionally to produce plentiful and nutritious milk. Onions and leeks enrich the milk and have antiseptic properties, so try to include plenty in your diet.

Nuts, particularly walnuts and almonds, are good for milk production. The same reputation applies to seeds, including sunflower, sesame, linseed, celery and fenugreek seeds. Most fruits are beneficial, especially bananas, blackcurrants, rosehips, grapes, pears, peaches and apples.

Make sure you eat raw vegetables, particularly carrots, watercress, chicory, as well as dandelion leaves, and green herbs such as coriander, borage, land cress, alfalfa and spring onions. They will all help enhance your milk supply.

Treatments for breastfeeding problems

Poor milk supply

It may be hard for some women to get milk production properly established; others find they cannot maintain a plentiful supply to satisfy a hungry baby. There may be a variety of reasons for this. A poor diet, or reduction in food intake if you are trying to lose weight after the birth, may leave you tired and run down, and this could affect your milk supply. Exhaustion after a long labour may

Blessed thistle

Cnicus benedictus
Carduus benedictus

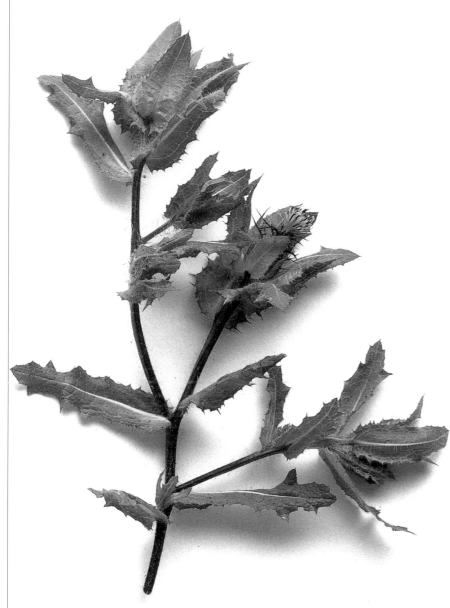

ALSO KNOWN AS: Holy thistle, St. Benedict thistle, spotted thistle

PARTS USED: Root, aerial parts and seeds

CONTAINS: Alkaloids, mucilage, tannin, bitter compound (cnicine), essential oil, flavonoids

KEY USES: Stimulant, tonic, digestive, diaphoretic, emmenagogue, expectorant, antibacterial, astringent

Blessed thistle is a very useful herb for women. It can be taken to relieve painful periods, and for menstrual headaches. As an emmenagogue it will help bring on suppressed periods (and so should be avoided during pregnancy). It is excellent for increasing milk production in nursing mothers and can be helpful during problems with the menopause, such as heavy bleeding.

The bitters in blessed thistle enhance the appetite and aid digestion, while stimulating the liver and the flow of bile. It is a good remedy for anorexia, indigestion, wind, colic and any condition associated with a sluggish liver such as headaches, lethargy and irritability. Its astringent action is useful for treating diarrhea.

The bitters have been shown to have an antimicrobial action, useful for enhancing the function of the immune system. Blessed thistle has also been shown to act as an antineoplastic, hindering the formation of abnormal cells, useful in cancer treatment. It also has diuretic properties and when taken in hot infusion is a useful diaphoretic for fevers and an expectorant for chest problems.

Blessed thistle can be used to staunch bleeding of cuts, and speed healing of wounds. It also acts as an antiseptic.

Note Do not use this herb internally in pregnancy. Strong infusions may be emetic and cause diarrhea.

stop breastfeeding being well established in the first week or two, and overtiredness from broken nights, stress, or trying to do too much may cause milk supply to dwindle once it has begun. Any anxiety or tension associated with feeding can inhibit the let-down reflex and stop the flow of milk.

The hormone prolactin is responsible for producing milk. When a baby sucks at the breast, the message is sent to produce more prolactin and so more milk is made. Since breastmilk is produced on demand, if your production is scanty, try letting the baby more frequently. Let it be your baby who decides how long and how often to feed, not you. Once the baby starts to suckle, the hormone oxytocin is released into the bloodstream, and on reaching the breasts it causes the tiny muscles around each milk-producing cell to contract and squeeze the milk down a system of ducts which lead to the nipple. This "let-down reflex" can easily be inhibited if you feel anxious or tense about breastfeeding. If you have problems with the let-down reflex, it is best to feed your baby quietly, on your own, so that you can relax properly. Put on some music you like, have a warm relaxing drink, or an aromatic bath – why not take him with you and feed in the bath?

Sore, cracked nipples

Your nipples may become very sensitive from so much sucking during the first week after the baby is born, but after that any soreness should subside. Some women, however, have particularly delicate nipples which may continue to feel tender and sore, or even become very dry and crack.

It is important to make sure your baby is feeding properly, as sore nipples are frequently caused by the baby not being latched on to the breast correctly. Before you start to feed, make sure that you are comfortable. Sit on pillows if your perineum is sore, or place one on your lap to raise the baby to the breast. Rest your feet on a stool if you need to. Try to relax and let go of any tension you feel. Breathe slowly and calmly. When you hold the baby tilt his head back and rest his chin against your breast, so when he sucks he can get the areola of the breast into his mouth. If he is latched on properly his ears will move as he feeds. If the cheeks go in and out as he feeds, then he is not on correctly. Take him gently off the breast and start again.

Once he is feeding properly, he will feed in spurts and then rest. When he has had enough he will stop feeding and may continue just to "comfort suck". If he starts chewing the nipple and the cheeks go in and out, take him off the breast, as this could make your nipples very sore. If he cries and wants to suck, but then only comfort sucks when he is offered the breast, you could give him a dummy, or let him suck your finger. As long he is able to feed sufficiently, he will feel satisfied and sleep for long stretches between feeds which will give your nipples a chance to recover. If he is taken off the breast too soon, he could wake again soon for another feed, and if this happens a few times he will suck harder to make sure he gets all he needs quickly before he is taken off the breast again. This also could make the nipple sore.

To prevent your nipples from becoming sore you can apply buttermilk, honey or comfrey ointment to keep the skin supple – you can massage the nipples with these before the birth to accustom them to being touched frequently. Calendula or chickweed ointment, thick honey, almond oil, wheatgerm oil or rose water can also be used to prevent and to heal sore nipples. One drop of rose oil in two teaspoons of almond oil is also very effective. Apply your chosen ointment frequently, particularly after feeding.

If your nipples become so sore that you find feeding difficult, it is important to express any excess milk, to avoid the breasts becoming engorged, as this would only add to your problems.

Care of the breasts

It is best not to wash your breasts more than once a day or with soap as this can wash the natural oils out of the nipple and make the skin more delicate. Let the nipples dry naturally after each feed. If you express a little milk, rub it in and allow it to dry on the nipple, this will help protect it. Keep your nipples dry between feeds by using breast pads and change the pads when they get damp. Expose your nipples to the air as often as you can, especially after feeds. Avoid wearing a bra and breast pads at night, even though you may get quite wet, to allow circulation of air around the breasts. Start each feed on a different breast, and change your position frequently so that the pressure is not all in the same part of the nipple.

Engorgement of the breasts

Engorged breasts feel very hot, swollen, hard and painful, and as the nipple becomes flattened it is hard for the baby to suck properly. This leads to further engorgement and discomfort, and makes for a hungry, unhappy and tired baby.

If your breasts become engorged, try to ease the extra fluid in the breast away from the nipple with your fingertips, so that the nipple stands out for the baby to latch on to. If you let the baby feed frequently and on demand when you start breastfeeding, you will probably find that the engorgement that normally occurs in the first few days is mild and soon goes. If not, try applying ice-cold flannels after feeding to constrict the blood vessels and reduce swelling. Swing your arms vigorously or wash your breasts with warm water just before feeding to get the milk flowing.

To help reduce congestion and discomfort in the breast take the following together as a tea frequently through the day:

> *lady's mantle*
> *cleavers*
> *calendula*
>
> *dandelion root decoction is also helpful*

Make a hot compress of decoction of poke root or infusion of cleavers, and apply it frequently to the breasts. Alternatively, you can use fresh rhubarb or cabbage leaves placed inside the bra for about three hours; this works very effectively and can reduce congestion and swelling very quickly.

You can also use essential oils of fennel, rose, lavender and geranium. Put a few drops of oil in a bowl of hot water, wring a cloth out in it, and apply frequently to the breast. A few drops of rose or peppermint oil in calendula tincture can be mixed into aqueous cream to rub into the breast.

Inflamed breasts and mastitis

The prevention and treatment of sore nipples is important so that feeding difficulties do not lead to breast engorgement. Try to reduce any engorgement that develops as quickly as possible so that the breast does not become inflamed through a blocked duct, making the breast even more painful and swollen. Flushing or redness of the skin on the breast may indicate a blocked duct which can lead to an infection (mastitis). This produces a sharp rise in temperature, flu-like symptoms, tenderness, usually on the outer part of the breast, and flushing of the skin. Keep feeding as often as you can, to help reduce the engorgement. Express any milk left in the breast after each feed.

To bring down a fever, and clear infection, drink plenty of fluid – teas of calendula, yarrow and elderflower mixed with cleavers are best.

For hot, red inflamed breasts and mastitis, dandelion root tea is an effective remedy. Alternatively, take equal parts of golden seal, ginger, echinacea and black cohosh as tea or tincture three to six times daily.

There are also good external treatments. Pound up lady's mantle and sweet violet leaves with a little hot water and honey; spread it on to a piece of gauze and apply it as a poultice to the inflamed breast. Warm cooked bran, linseed or slippery elm also make effective poultices. You can use linseed oil with a few drops of rose or geranium oil to rub into the breast or alternatively, distilled witch hazel, buttermilk, St. John's wort, poke root, comfrey or raspberry leaves.

Hand and foot baths can be a very effective treatment. A chamomile or eucalyptus foot bath every two hours will help bring down the fever; garlic, thyme, echinacea or lavender will help resolve the infection, and poke root, cleavers, calendula and dandelion root can be used as strong teas or dilute tinctures to reduce congestion and inflammation.

Weaning

When you stop breastfeeding, it is best to wean gradually. This way you will reduce discomfort through engorged breasts and flooding, for once you stop feeding it can take quite a while for the milk glands to stop working.

Should circumstances force you to stop feeding more abruptly, then seek out sources of red sage, herb robert and periwinkle which will reduce milk flow. They are, naturally, best avoided while you wish to continue breastfeeding.

You can also try eating plenty of garden mint, sorrel and sage with your meals. A glass of carrot juice first thing in the morning has also been said to help dry up milk.

Goat's rue

Galega officinalis

PART USED: Aerial parts

CONTAINS: Saponins, flavone glycosides, bitters, tannin, alkaloids

KEY USES: Galactagogue, diuretic, diaphoretic, hypoglycemic

Goat's rue is a wonderful galacto-gogue, increasing milk production in nursing mothers – often by up to 50 per cent. It is also said to stimulate the development of mammary glands.

In hot infusion goat's rue makes a useful remedy for increasing sweating and bringing down fevers – and for this reason it was an old remedy for the plague.

It is notable for its action on the pancreas and has the ability to reduce blood sugar, making it useful for diabetics.

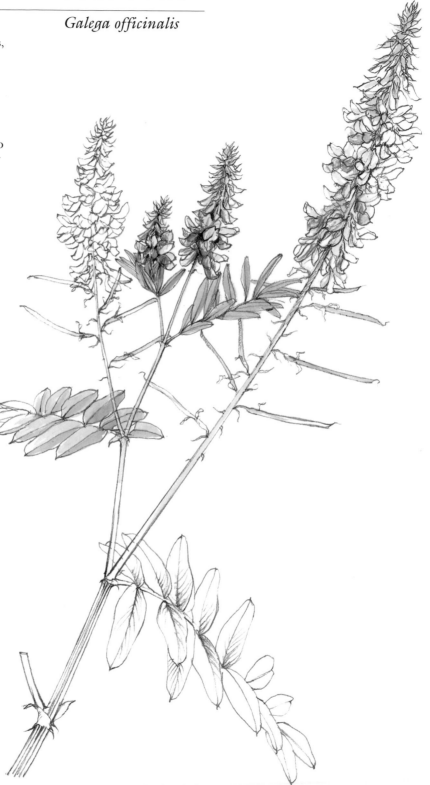

Herbal babycare

Herbs can be used in many helpful ways for babies. You can add aromatic infusions to the bath or use them to wash the eyes, face and diaper area, and use herbal oils to massage your baby's feet, tummy and back. You can give your baby weak infusions of herbs between feeds, using a quarter of a teaspoon of herb per cup of boiling water. To treat a specific problem, such as fever or colic, you can use any of these methods, hand and foot baths, sponging or applying compresses of herbal infusions. Essential oils can be used in vaporizers, in baths, or dropped on to radiators and light bulb burners where the baby can inhale them. If you take herbs yourself some of the constituents will pass through your milk to the baby.

When you bathe your baby, use infusions of rosemary, thyme, lemon balm, chamomile, lavender or linden blossom, mixed with tepid water. Clean the eyes, face and diaper area with antiseptic lavender, thyme or calendula infusion instead of soap. Once the baby is crawling, you can use coarse oatmeal in a muslin bag on dirty areas, and dilute essential oils or herbal oils of rosemary, chamomile, thyme or lavender in the bath. Rub any sore or dry skin with a couple of drops of chamomile or calendula oil in almond oil diluted with rose water.

Cleaning the umbilical cord

The umbilical cord which joins the baby to the placenta is clamped and cut after the birth, and over the following ten days it shrinks and finally drops off. Until it does it should be cleaned daily as it may be contaminated by urine. Use antiseptic herbs and oils, especially dilute oil of cloves, distilled witch hazel or rosemary tea.

For any redness or inflammation, use comfrey tea, alternated by infusion or tincture of calendula, applied on cotton wool. Dilute tincture of myrrh, thyme or echinacea could also be applied or added to the bath water.

Diaper rash

To avoid diaper rash, wash the baby's bottom regularly with dilute herbal infusions of lavender, thyme, chamomile or calendula, or with rose water. Dry the skin well and leave the baby with no diaper on for a while in a warm room or out-side in the sunshine. Try to prevent the delicate skin being enclosed in a wet, chafing diaper for too long and without enough air reaching it.

Use any of these to apply to the baby's bottom before replacing the diaper:

chamomile	calendula
comfrey	chickweed

Use infusions in aqueous cream or use fresh or dried herbs to make ointments. These herbs are healing and soothing and help protect the skin against the corrosive effect of the urine and stools.

Alternatively you can also use herbal oils such as comfrey or St. John's wort, while essential oil of lavender or chamomile in a base of almond oil are also good. It is best not to use talcum powder as it holds in the damp and encourages bacteria, and can cause or aggravate diaper rash.

Treatment of diaper rash

At the first sign of any rash on your baby's bottom, act straight away, otherwise a secondary infection may set in.

Make sure you change diapers frequently. At each change, wash the bottom with herbal infusions such as thyme, chamomile or lavender, or use distilled witch hazel. Let it dry then apply calendula, chamomile or comfrey cream to protect and heal it. Where you suspect an infection, use antiseptic herbs, calendula or chamomile cream.

If your baby has white patches inside the cheeks or on the tongue, this indicates oral thrush which can spread through the digestive tract as far as the anus, and cause diaper rash. (For treatment of thrush see p.226.) Use a couple of drops of calendula tincture and thyme or oregano oil (1 drop per 20 ml tincture) in the mouth two or three times daily, or rub a little plain live yoghurt round the mouth with your finger. You can apply yoghurt, calendula cream and powdered golden seal to the bottom, after washing it with either dilute cider vinegar, rosemary or thyme infusion.

Egg white and oxygen is an old and effective remedy for diaper rash. Apply egg white repeatedly to the affected area and between each application dry it with a hair dryer. This way, you build up a thick protective layer of albumen which protects the skin and allows it to heal rapidly.

Sometimes diaper rash can be severe, with spots, raised red patches which may develop into red raw areas, or even shallow ulcers. Your baby will be very unhappy when he passes urine or a stool. To comfort him give chamomile tea between feeds, and apply soothing and healing comfrey or plantain ointment alternated with more antiseptic calendula or chamomile cream. You can wash the bottom with infusions of calendula, lavender, rosemary or elderflowers or dilute tincture of myrrh or calendula.

Cradle cap

This is a thick yellow-brown encrustation on a baby's scalp, and is a condition caused by overactivity of the glands in the skin which secrete oily sebum. It can last until the child is about three.

Since it has nothing to do with cleanliness or hygiene, don't wash your baby's hair overfrequently, or with soap, as this aggravates it by increasing sebum secretion. It is best to leave it alone until the baby's sebum production settles down. If you do want to clear it, rub the scalp regularly with olive oil mixed with a few drops of essential oil of lavender, rosemary or lemon, and wash the loosened crusts off with shampoo the next day. Rinse the hair after shampooing with meadowsweet or burdock infusion or ordinary tea. Remove any loose flakes then with a brush or clean fingernail, but never pick off crusts that are not loose, as this may cause bleeding, inflammation or infection of the scalp.

Colic

Colic is a cramp-like abdominal pain that comes intermittently and is caused by spasm of the gut. Some babies have "three month colic" – the crying and discomfort occurring mostly in the first 12 weeks of life. Others tend to cry more in the evenings and are said to have "evening colic".

It is not easy to be sure when your baby has colic, but when you have tried every other remedy for his crying (feeding, changing, cuddling, walking him up and down) and he still cries, or when he cries so much that his face goes red and both legs are drawn up, then it may be colic. It tends to occur after a feed, or in the evening when the baby is tired and the digestion does not work so well. It is especially upsetting for mothers, because they feel they have tried everything and still the baby is distressed.

Colic can be related to tension in the digestive tract for a baby's digestion is closely connected to his general sense of wellbeing and security. This in turn relates very much to his mother and how she is feeling. The more anxious and tense you feel, the more your baby may cry. If you feel yourself becoming upset or tense, try passing the baby over to someone else for a little while, and try to relax a little on your own.

A baby's colic can also be related to feeding problems; check that the baby is latched on properly to the nipple and is not gulping too much air while feeding, as can happen if your milk comes out too quickly at the beginning of a feed. Express a little first by hand. If you are bottlefeeding, the hole in the teat may be the wrong size.

Many colicky babies have been found to react to cow's milk both in formula milks and breastmilk, particularly if from a family prone to allergies where problems such as eczema, asthma and hay fever occur. Other foods coming through breastmilk can also cause reactions; examples of these are wheat, corn (maize) and citrus fruits, especially when the mother eats them a good deal.

There are certain other foods which come through the breastmilk and tend to cause colic or other digestive upsets in babies:

too much fruit	*alcohol*
coffee	*onions, leeks, garlic*
green peppers	*eggplant*
beans	*lentils*
cucumbers	*zucchini*
chocolate	*tomatoes*
eggs	*sugar*

brassicas: cabbage, cauliflower, brussels sprouts curry or highly spiced foods

If you eat a lot of any of these foods, try omitting one at a time completely for up to a week to see if there is any change. Then reintroduce the food after a week and watch for any reaction. Through this method you should be able to determine if any foods are causing colic. Once you start him on solids, introduce foods you suspect last of all, and only in small amounts.

Be careful not to compromise your nutrition when you are breastfeeding. If you omit suspect foods from your diet, be sure to replace them with something of the same nutritional value.

Treatment of colic

Make sure you are breastfeeding in the correct way. Read the advice given on breastfeeding under Sore, cracked nipples on p.171.

Before each feed give the baby herbal tea to relax the digestive tract and ease the digestion. Choose from:

fennel	*cinnamon*
dill	*lemon balm*
chamomile	*angelica*
catmint	

Use a quarter to a half a teaspoon of herbs to 4 oz (100 ml) of boiling water. Give the baby 1 oz (30 ml) of the tea. After the feed, if he seems uncomfortable or fretful, give the tea again. Slippery elm powder mixed with warm water is often very soothing.

You can use a stronger infusion of the same herbs in the bath water, or in hand and foot baths. You can also drink stronger herbal teas yourself, as their volatile oils pass through the breastmilk to the baby.

If you feel anxious or your baby seems tense, add more relaxing herbs to the tea or bath for the baby, such as:

catmint	*linden blossom*
chamomile	*lemon balm*
hops	

Use any of these for yourself:

skullcap	*vervain*
passionflower	*wild oats*
lemon balm	*chamomile*

Essential oils can also be used; geranium, lavender, chamomile, rosemary, ginger or fennel can be diluted (2 drops per 5 ml base oil) and added to bath water, used for massage or as compresses to the abdomen. A warm bath with herbal infusions or essential oils will often relax your baby wonderfully before you feed, so that feeding goes more smoothly.

If none of these remedies help, and your baby is still crying hard and frequently, consult your practitioner.

Vomiting

First consider what kind of vomiting appears to be the problem. When your baby regurgitates a little milk (known as posseting) this is quite normal and harmless. If your baby is less than ten weeks old and vomits forcefully (projectile vomiting) during or immediately after a feed, it could possibly be more serious, and you should consult your practitioner. Also, if the baby is very distressed, in severe pain or passes stools containing blood and mucus, contact your doctor immediately as the baby may have a blocked bowel.

Between these extreme cases lie various kinds of vomiting that can be treated at home. If the baby is on solids and vomits during or after food, it may be that the food is upsetting him, or he is allergic to it, or the food is too lumpy for him to digest.

If your baby has a runny or blocked nose or a catarrhal cough, he may swallow mucus which is brought back up, often after coughing.

Vomiting may be just one symptom of an infection or mild gastro-enteritis; if so, the baby will seem unwell, be off his food, flushed and irritable, and may have watery stools.

Treatment of vomiting

Make sure you offer the baby water, dilute juice or herbal teas mixed with honey, frequently through the day to replace lost fluids. Reduce fever with tepid sponging and suitable herbs such as elderflowers (see Fever p.181).

If your baby does not want to feed, express your milk so that your milk supply does not dwindle nor your breasts become engorged.

Give weak herbal teas, sweetened with honey, to settle the stomach. Use herbs such as:

chamomile	*lavender*
meadowsweet	*dill*
catmint	*cinnamon*
fennel	*lemon balm*
ginger	

If there are signs of infection, use:

linden blossom	*rosemary*
lavender	*lemon balm*
elder flowers	*echinacea*
thyme	

Comfrey

Symphytum officinale

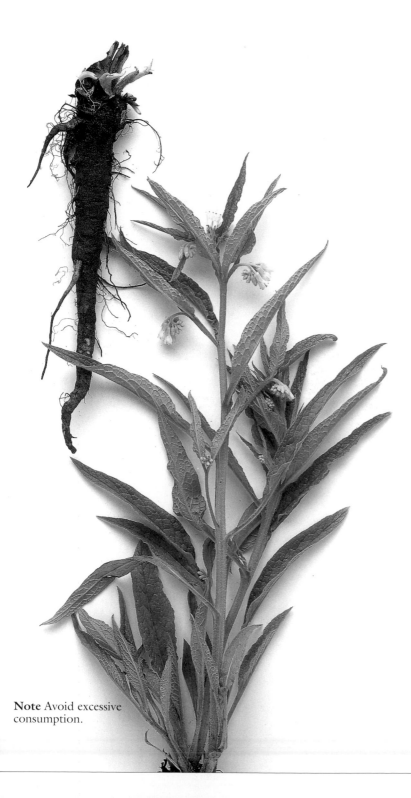

Note Avoid excessive consumption.

ALSO KNOWN AS: Knitbone, boneset, bruisewort, consormol, knitback

PARTS USED: Roots: external use only. Leaves: internal and external use

CONTAINS: Mucilage, allantoin, tannins, resin, essential oil, pyrrolizidine alkaloids, gum, carotene, glycosides, sugars, beta-sitosterol, steroidal saponins, triterpenoids, vitamin B12, protein, zinc

KEY USES: Demulcent, cell-proliferant, vulnerary, astringent, expectorant, anti-inflammatory, restorative

Comfrey is the prime first aid remedy. When applied to the skin allantoin diffuses easily into the underlying tissues so that when applied over a fractured bone it can accelerate healing and closure. Applied fresh to wounds, sores or ulcers, the mucilage in the roots or leaves seeps out onto the injured skin, dries and then thickens and contracts, drawing the sides of the wound together, inhibiting infection. Where the wound is fairly superficial it will heal the skin with little scarring.

A poultice or ointment can be used for bruises, sprains and strains, gout, arthritis, bleeding piles, varicose veins, phlebitis, and ulcers, swellings and burns. A decoction of the root or infusion of the leaves makes a good eyewash for sore, inflamed eyes and a wash for skin problems such as psoriasis, eczema, acne, and boils.

The leaves have healing properties and a particular affinity with the respiratory, digestive and urinary systems. Comfrey is used for sore throats and laryngitis, as a soothing expectorant for dry coughs, pleurisy and bronchitis. In the gut it soothes and heals gastritis, gastric and duodenal ulcers and can be used to reduce irritation causing diarrhea, dysentery and ulcerative colitis. In the urinary system it relaxes urinary spasm, soothes cystitis and clears irritation and infection. Comfrey is taken for gout and arthritis, as well as other painful or inflamed conditions such as tendinitis, sprains, and fractures.

If there is accompanying diarrhea, add elderflowers or meadowsweet. Drinks or gruel made with slippery elm powder, a pinch of powdered cinnamon or ginger, mixed with warm water or expressed milk will help soothe an upset stomach.

You can also massage the abdomen or feet with dilute oils of:

lemon balm	lavender
chamomile	geranium

Alternatively you can apply compresses of these oils or herb infusions to the abdomen. Add stronger infusions or dilute essential oils to the water when bathing the baby.

If your baby is eating solids, it is best to give no solid food, just plenty of fluids, until the stomach has settled down.

Diarrhea

Babies often have loose stools, resembling French mustard, but providing your baby is well and gaining weight, there is no cause for concern. It may be worse when the baby is teething.

Diarrhea can sometimes be related to food intolerance. Even when being entirely breastfed, babies may react to substances in foods coming through in breastmilk. Bottlefed babies can react to formula milks. Once on solid food, a baby's allergies can become more apparent, so if diarrhea occurs on introduction of a new food, stop giving it and see if the diarrhea improves.

Excessive fruit, such as citrus fruits, green apples, strawberries and plums can cause diarrhea. So can dried fruit and fruit juice.

If your baby seems unwell, irritable and flushed and has vomiting or frequent, watery stools, it may be an infection, gastro-enteritis. This is more common in bottlefed babies, as cow's milk formulas tend to encourage putrefactive bacteria in the bowel and, unlike breastmilk, do not protect a baby from infection. Give plenty of liquid, either water or herbal teas, to replace lost fluids and prevent dehydration. Don't give solid food until the bowels are back to normal, and then start with ground rice with a pinch of cinnamon, or mushy brown rice and yoghurt, or yoghurt with a little honey and banana.

If you give the baby water, add a little fresh lemon to help settle the bowels.

Give herbal teas frequently through the day, made from any of these, singly or mixed:

raspberry leaves	chamomile
fennel	cinnamon (a pinch)
lemon balm	meadowsweet
plantain	ginger

If your baby is weaned, try this drink.

1/2 cup live yoghurt
1/2 cup boiled water
1 teaspoon grated fresh ginger
a pinch of nutmeg

To soothe the gut use slippery elm powder with a pinch of ginger or cinnamon powder, made into a drink with a little warm water.

If you feel tense and anxious it may affect your baby, and upset the bowels, so try to stay calm while feeding, and use relaxing herbs – lavender, chamomile, linden blossom, catmint, lemon balm – for yourself and your baby.

If your baby has acute, frequent diarrhea for more than 24 hours, this may be a sign of something more serious and you should call your practitioner.

Constipation

Constipation tends to occur more in bottlefed babies, whose bowels breed more putrefactive bacteria. If a breastfed baby develops constipation it may be that certain foods are irritating your baby's gut and causing intolerance. Foods containing wheat and milk are the most common culprits. For a week or two remove any foods you suspect and watch for any improvement.

In babies on solid food, constipation can be caused by such factors as:

insufficient fluids
a low fibre diet with too much refined food and sugar
too much animal protein from meat and dairy produce
tension or spasm in the gut
poor diet with a deficiency of vitamins and minerals, particularly vitamin C and magnesium
anemia

To remedy constipation, between feeds offer drinks such as water, dilute fruit juices, water from cooked dried fruit, or herbal teas.

Poke root

Phytolacca decandra
Phytolacca americana

ALSO KNOWN AS: Coakum, pigeon berry, poke

PART USED: Dried root

CONTAINS: Triterpenoid saponins, resins, alkaloid, phytolaccid acid, formic and oleanolic acids, tannins, amino acids

KEY USES: Purgative, anti-inflammatory, decongestant, alterative, emetic

Poke root is a powerful herb, and one quarter of the normal dose is quite sufficient. It is an excellent remedy for the lymphatic system, relieving lymphatic congestion, swollen lymph glands and swollen, congested breasts. It is also recommended for breast lumps and cysts. By promoting lymphatic circulation and drainage, poke root has a cleansing action, clearing toxins, reducing inflammation and aiding the body's fight against infection. It is good for tonsilitis, laryngitis, swollen glands, glandular fever, mumps, catarrh, ear infections, and other respiratory infections. It is also recommended for arthritis and rheumatism.

Poke root will also help clear the skin of inflammatory problems such as acne, boils, psoriasis, eczema, and a tendency to skin infections such as athelete's foot. It enhances the liver's detoxifying action and also promotes digestion and absorption, making it useful for problems associated with a sluggish liver such as constipation, headaches, irritability, nausea, abdominal distension and lethargy. It has also been used for indigestion, gastritis, peptic ulcers and a sluggish digestion.

A decoction or dilute tincture can be used externally to promote repair, reduce inflammation and check infection on the skin – for boils, sores, ulcers, abscesses, psoriasis, fungal infections and breast congestion. A poultice can be applied in mastitis. A gargle is useful for tonsilitis and sore throats.

Note: Never use in pregnancy. Only use poke root dried and in small doses, as large doses cause diarrhea and vomiting.

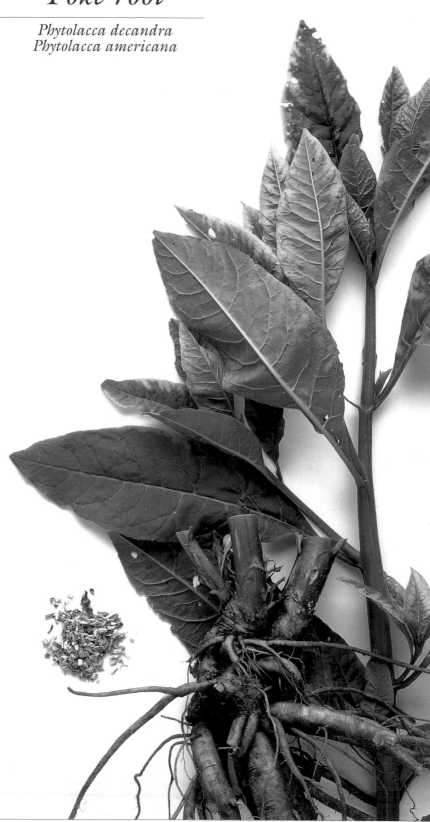

These herbs will all help release tension or spasm in the gut:

chamomile   linden blossom
cinnamon   catmint
rosemary   lavender
lemon balm   fennel
ginger

These will soothe an irritated gut lining:

plantain   slippery elm powder
borage   meadowsweet

If you add a little licorice water or a teaspoon of molasses to hot drinks it will have a more laxative effect. Honey also has a slightly laxative effect. Give mashed prunes and apricots to babies on solids. Give plain natural yoghurt with a little mashed banana, and add garlic and unrefined vegetable oils to their vegetables – both will help re-establish the right bacteria in the gut.

To encourage bowel movements, massage the baby's abdomen with dilute oil of cinnamon, chamomile or fennel, always in a clockwise direction (the same way as the bowel movements) or try hot compresses applied to the abdomen.

Allergies

If you have a family history of allergies, it is possible that your baby has inherited them. There are several symptoms to look out for which could indicate that your baby has an allergy.

These are the main symptoms of allergies:

crying a lot for no apparent reason
difficulty in feeding or digesting
frequent posseting
colic
constipation, vomiting, intermittent or frequent
    diarrhea
eczema, urticaria, diaper rash or other rashes
frequent infections such as colds, coughs, ear infections
    or chronic catarrh

If you are breastfeeding, the baby is probably reacting to a food you are eating, such as milk, wheat, eggs, chocolate or citrus fruits. Bottlefed babies may well be reacting to their formula feed. Try a soya based milk and, once your baby is on solids, try almond milk, goat's or sheep's milk.

Treatment of allergies

If you are breastfeeding, you can boost your baby's immune system via the breastmilk. Read the advice on p.169 and take recommended mineral and vitamin supplements, essential fatty acids and herbal remedies, as these will be passed through the milk to your baby.

You can take and give to your baby dilute herbal teas made from these herbs to aid digestion and soothe the allergic response:

chamomile   wild yam
yarrow   fennel

As long as your baby does not have diarrhea you can flavour the teas with a little licorice; otherwise use honey. Slippery elm gruel is also good.

Dilute essential oils can be used to reduce the allergic response. Chamomile is particularly useful for skin irritation.

Add two drops of any of the following oils to 5 ml base oil and use in the bath, as massage oil, or in a vaporizer in the bedroom:

chamomile
lavender
lemon balm

Try to avoid your baby being in contact with allergens or toxins which may make the allergy worse, such as cigarette smoke, pesticides or chemicals in tap water (use filtered or spring water). Check the effects of any drugs you may be taking, and try not to give your baby antibiotics, as candidiasis (see p.227) greatly aggravates allergic problems. Keep away from foods with artificial additives and buy organic produce where you can.

Sleeping problems

The amount of sleep that a baby needs varies, as does the pattern of that sleep. Your baby may sleep for several hours at a stretch and sleep through the night at just a few weeks old, or he may want feeding every hour or two, even through the night. He may sleep for long periods through the day and very little at night. Some babies will sleep through the night at six months, but others will wake at night for some years.

Babies feel most happy and secure when near their mother, so if you have a very wakeful baby, try carrying him in a sling across your front, and at night, if you have the baby in your bed, you will hardly have to stir when your baby wants to feed and he may well sleep longer.

When putting a young baby in a cot, if you wrap him snugly in a sheet or shawl and then tuck something firmly over him, he will feel more secure and may sleep longer. If he wakes it is usually for a feed and for reassurance. As the baby grows older he will probably not want to be so restricted and will have longer periods awake, interested in looking around and wanting to play or be amused. This is fine in the day, but better discouraged at night!

Babies spend about half their sleeping time in a light sleep, known as rapid eye movement sleep, when they are dreaming. Because of this, it is quite normal for a baby or toddler to wake up several times in the night, however difficult this is for the tired parents. If you have a particularly restless or sleepless baby, try some of the herbal remedies to be found under Crying baby on p.183.

If none of the remedies or suggestions work for your baby, it may be that there are other factors involved, such as teething, colic, an infection, an itchy skin, being too hot or not warm enough, a snuffly nose or a sore bottom. It may be that your baby has a food allergy or is hyperactive.

Teething

Babies normally produce teeth from about five to six months onwards, and very often do so with no trouble at all. Some dribble a lot when teething, develop rashes on the face, become irritable, clingy and restless, have a poor appetite, or have trouble sleeping. These troubles may predispose them to other symptoms which often accompany teething, such as fever, diarrhea, rashes, catarrh, colds and other infections, and rubbing their ears. However, these should always be checked out as they could indicate other problem altogether.

If you suspect teething, check the baby's gums. If they look red and swollen or there is a blister on the gum overlying an emerging tooth, give him something to chew on – either your finger, hopefully not your nipple, a marshmallow root or licorice stick, or a teething ring. Rub the gums with a little honey, or honey with a drop of clove or chamomile oil.

To reduce pain and soothe inflamed gums, give infusions frequently through the day made from any of these:

chamomile	*lemon balm*
linden blossom	*yarrow*
lavender	*catmint*

Fever

The temperature-regulating mechanisms of babies are less effective than those of adults, and so fevers can develop easily in babies and quickly swing up and down, though tending to be higher in the afternoon or evening.

If your baby is off his food, irritable and has a fever, it probably indicates the presence of an infection. A fever shows the body is fighting an infection, it is a healthy reaction and not something that needs to be suppressed unless it is high. If the baby feels very hot, and the temperature is over 100°F (38°C), remove the clothes and leave just an undershirt and diaper on, or cover with a sheet. Give plenty of liquids to prevent dehydration: either breastmilk, dilute juice, water or herbal teas.

These teas will increase perspiration and help to bring down the fever. Their volatile oils also have antiseptic properties to help fight off accompanying infection:

elderflower	*lemon balm*
thyme	*borage*
yarrow	*linden blossom*
chamomile	*catmint*

Use the same infusions for tepid sponging. Don't use cold water as this will reduce heat loss via the skin by closing up the pores. You can also use the herbs in a tepid bath.

Essential oils of chamomile, lavender, eucalyptus and thyme can be used in the bath and for tepid sponging; just a few drops in plenty of water. Use them also in vaporizers in the room. You could also apply compresses to the baby's head, abdomen or feet using these infusions and essential oils.

If your baby seems particularly restless and cannot settle, use predominantly linden blossom and chamomile tea, and essential oils of chamomile or lavender. See if you can get the baby to sleep.

Lavender

Lavendula officinalis

PART USED: Flowers

CONTAINS: Volatile oil, tannins, coumarins, flavonoids, triterpenoids

KEY USES: Relaxant, antispasmodic, anti-depressant, nerve tonic, antiseptic, decongestant, expectorant, diaphoretic, detoxifying, analgesic, rubefacient

Lavender has been one of the best loved scented herbs for thousands of years. An infusion or tincture of lavender or inhalation of the essential oil has a wonderfully relaxing effect on mind and body. It makes a good remedy for anxiety, nervousness, and physical symptoms caused by stress such as tension headaches, migraine, palpitations and insomnia. Lavender oil is considered a balancer to the emotions, lifting the spirits, relieving depression and balancing inner disharmony. Lavender also has a stimulating edge to it, acting as a tonic to the nervous system, restoring vitality to people suffering from nervous exhaustion.

Lavender's relaxing effect can be felt in the digestive tract, where it soothes spasm and colic related to tension and anxiety and relieves distension, flatulence, nausea, indigestion, and enhances the appetite. Its powerful antiseptic volatile oils have been shown to be active against bacteria including diphtheria, typhoid, streptococcus and pneumococcus. As tea, oil inhalation, or vapour rub, lavender is effective for colds, coughs, asthma, bronchitis, pneumonia, flu, tonsilitis and laryngitis. The tea or tincture can also be taken for stomach and bowel infections causing vomiting or diarrhea.

Taken as hot tea, lavender causes sweating and reduces fevers. It helps to detoxify the body by increasing elimination of toxins via the skin and, with its mild diuretic action, through the urine.

Lavender is a useful external disinfectant for cuts and wounds, sores and ulcers. It stimulates tissue repair and minimizes scar formation when the oil is applied neat to burns and diluted in cases of eczema, acne and varicose ulcers.

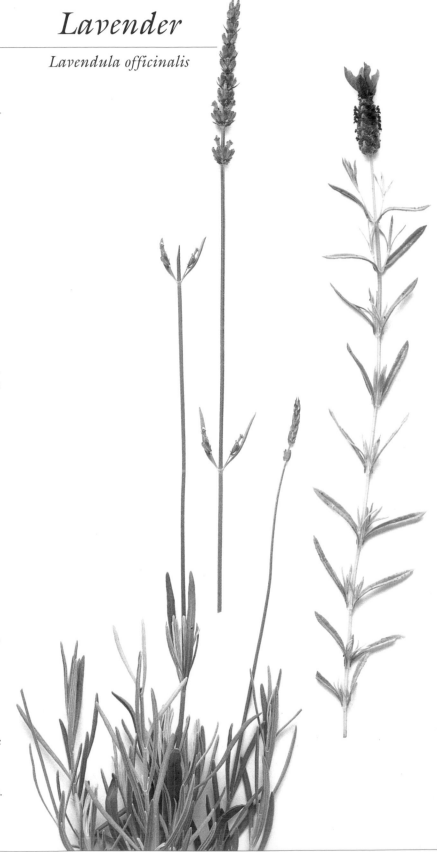

If a fever persists for over 24 hours or you are worried about any accompanying symptoms, consult your practitioner.

Crying baby

Crying is perfectly normal; it is a baby's way of telling you he is uncomfortable, hungry or bored. If your baby is breastfed he may cry from hunger more than a bottlefed baby as breastmilk tends to pass through the stomach quite quickly. Your baby may cry often in the evenings if your milk supply is dwindling, or perhaps if he has 'evening colic'.

It will not be long before you understand what your baby means when he cries: whether he is bored or hungry or wants to be picked up, whether he feels hot, cold or uncomfortable, or whether he is feeling insecure or irritable because he is tired. If he has colic his cry will be more distressed, or if he doesn't feel well his cry will vary from the normal pattern and could continue on and off through the day. This could indicate teething, so check his gums and see if he dribbles a lot (see p.181) or it could mean an infection is developing.

Once you have attended to all the possible needs of a crying baby, you can use herbs to calm him and encourage a restful sleep for you both.

Bathe the baby at night in warm water, to which add strong infusions of relaxing herbs. Choose from:

linden blossom	*lavender*
catmint	*chamomile*
lemon balm	*hops*

Give the baby dilute teas of these herbs before bed, on a spoon or in a bottle and again if he wakes and does not go back to sleep quickly.

Alternatively, dilute essential oils can be added to bath water. Chamomile, lavender, geranium, neroli and rose are all very helpful. The warmth of the bath is relaxing in itself, and the addition of herbs will help induce calm and sleep, releasing tension in muscles and in the gut, and soothing discomfort related to colic, fever or skin problems. If your baby seems to wake distressed from sleep, lavender or catmint are particularly recommended.

When you put your baby to bed, massage his feet or abdomen, or stroke his head with some dilute essential oils until he drops off. Alternatively, rock the cradle and use the oils in a vaporizer near the bed.

The Bach Flower Remedies often work well with a crying baby or one with sleeping problems, especially when they are related to insecurity, fear, or not wanting to be left alone (see p.246–7).

It is not easy to comfort a crying baby when he cries and nothing you do seems to make any difference. A baby often responds better to rhythmic, noisy and fast motion as in a car or carriage, rather than quiet and gentle rocking as in a cot. Your baby may stop crying if you talk to him and show him things to catch his attention, instead of trying to relax him into sleep. He may just be bored.

It may be hard for you to find your own way through the wealth of often conflicting advice from others, but you will probably find that if you give your baby what he needs, once you understand what that is, and respond to every cry for help, that he'll be generally more contented and secure, even if he does have crying times. A baby is helpless and totally dependent on you for nurture on every level of existence – you need to be there for him now more than at any other time, to lay the foundations for his sense of security, wellbeing, self worth and identity.

Naturally, a crying baby can have a disturbing effect on a mother's feelings: from anxiety, panic, and pure frustration to relief once the crying stops. It is important that you regularly take a break, get your partner, family or friends to look after your baby for a while. This may even stop him crying, if he has been picking up on your anxiety or frustration. If you feel very tired and drained, or tense and anxious, see p.163.

The Bach Flower Remedies are very useful (see p.246–7) at times like these.

It is perfectly normal for a mother to feel concerned or distressed if her baby cries – nature has made this powerful connection between mother and child to ensure that the baby is nurtured until it is more able to look after itself – and a signal such as crying cannot be ignored. It may be that sometimes you have to give up other activities or plans just to be with your baby. Let go of ideas about how you want things to be or how they should be, and be there for him, until he settles.

If you feel that your baby's crying may indicate an underlying medical condition, consult your practitioner.

9 *Adult Life and Menopause*

The middle years of a woman's life have both their joys and their sorrows. With children growing older and more physically independent, we may begin to have more time to ourselves, to look forward and make plans for our own pleasures rather than for the family as a whole. The middle years can also be a time of great change, both at home and at work. Changes are taking place in family relationships, which may bring conflict with teenagers as they struggle to establish their identity. Elderly parents may begin to need extra care and attention; children may be leaving home or marrying. We may be returning to work, taking a new job – maybe a low-paid job with low status – and suffer the economic insecurity many working men and women over the age of forty feel in a society which discriminates against them. These changes sometimes feel stimulating and challenging, but they can also be very stressful, and may contribute to a sense of great vulnerability at this time. Added to all this, sooner or later we also have physical changes in the shape of the menopause.

Hops

Humulus lupulus

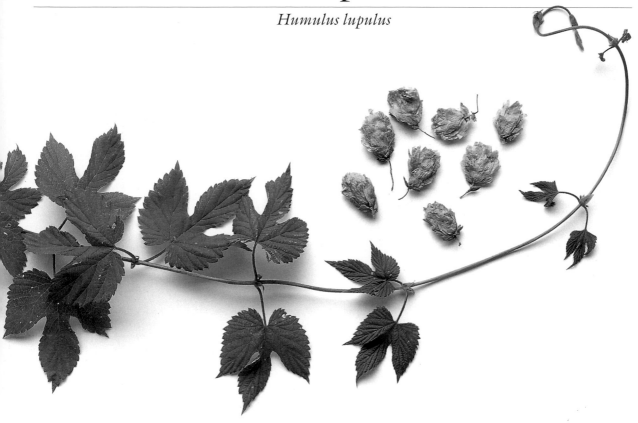

PART USED: Dried female strobiles

CONTAINS: Volatile oil, bitter-resin complex, known as lupulin, tannins, estrogenic substances, asparagin, trimethylamine, choline

KEY USES: Sedative, antispasmodic, bitter tonic, digestive, antiseptic, astringent, diuretic, anodyne, febrifuge

Note The pollen from hops may cause contact dermatitis.

Hop pillows are well known for inducing sleep, indicating the sedative action of hops – useful for relieving tension and anxiety, soothing pain, restlessness and agitation. The antispasmodic action reduces tension in muscles throughout the body, relieving spasm and colic in the gut, and makes hops a good remedy for irritable bowel syndrome, diverticulitis, nervous indigestion, peptic ulcers, Crohn's disease, ulcerative colitis and stress-related digestive problems.

The bitters in hops aid digestive function, enhancing the action of the liver and the secretion of bile and digestive juices. The tannins aid healing of irritated and inflammatory conditions and stem diarrhea, while the antiseptic action of hops relieves infections.

The estrogenic action of hops make them an excellent remedy for any problem around menopause. Hops have also been used for suppressed and painful periods – they have a depressive effect on men's libido so that beer drinking may not be the best thing for enhancing their sexual energy.

The asparagin in hops is a soothing diuretic, reducing fluid retention and hastening elimination of toxins from the system. This combined with the action on the liver have given hops a reputation for clearing skin problems. Their relaxant and antihistamine action is also useful here.

Hops have been used in creams to keep the skin soft and supple and delay wrinkling. Their antiseptic action is useful for cuts, wounds and ulcers.

Coping with change

The journey of life from youth to old age, fertility to infertility, one kind of beauty to another, and from innocence to wisdom, is inevitable; the way women experience the journey depends very much on their attitudes to life in general. There are social and media pressures – encouraged by the orthodox medical profession with their hormone replacement therapy – to pretend that we can stay young forever. If we can appreciate and enjoy the changing seasons of the year, the growth and development of children to adults, then perhaps we can learn to accept and enjoy the change in our lives as we grow older. The lines we see developing in our faces can be seen as outward signs of accumulated wisdom. We need to recognize the value of age, and accept, even welcome, its manifestations. While menopausal women may not feel that their bodies are outwardly so attractive, their inner selves can radiate the great value of accumulated experience and knowledge. Their beauty changes, it does not necessarily diminish – a wise woman of ninety can indeed be beautiful.

As physical energy decreases naturally with age, so a woman's fertility decreases, because childbearing and rearing is an arduous task, even for the young, and would be over-taxing for most women over a certain age. Youthful vigour can be replaced with serenity and reflection. After years of caring for others, perhaps even to the extent of neglecting herself, it may well be time for a woman to care for her own needs, both physical and spiritual, and to allow time for herself. Many women are delighted not to have to endure the monthly physical burden of the premenstrual phase, bleeding and its associated problems. Women after the menopause are free from the burden of cycles and their physical and emotional effects which women often feel helpless to change. Menopause also frees women from the pressures of possible pregnancy, and from having to use contraception.

It may well be a struggle to free ourselves from values of our culture and to accept, and even delight in, our age and appreciate the wisdom and power it can bring. Support and encouragement are vital in this time of possible "mid-life crisis" – from our partners, relations and friends – particularly from other women who understand how it feels. It is always important to express your troubles. This may be by talking, perhaps to a counsellor, or in taking physical exercise. It is also vital to let go of any negative emotions that may serve to undermine your journey – yoga, meditation, relaxation or T'ai chi are often very helpful. Bach Flower Remedies can be excellent (see the chart on p.246). Combine them with supportive herbs to balance the emotions and increase vitality.

The change of life

Strictly speaking, "menopause" is a woman's last period. After two years have elapsed since the last period you can be sure that the "change of life" has occurred and ovulation has ceased. The approach to menopause can start in the middle to late thirties, as the amount of estrogen produced by the ovaries begins to diminish. The last period may occur any time from the mid-thirties to the late fifties. During this time, dwindling hormonal stimulation by the pituitary gland of the ovaries interrupts the steady production of estrogen by the ovaries, and a stop-start pattern begins, often giving rise to irregular periods.

There begins during these years a general re-organization of the whole of the endocrine system; other glands, notably the adrenal glands, compensate for the less active ovaries by producing the hormones themselves, albeit in smaller amounts. The adrenals produce hormones which are stored in fat cells where they are converted into estrogen. Body weight is therefore a crucial factor at this time. The body may take a while to adjust to the lower hormone levels, but generally after five years any unpleasant side effects should cease.

Menopause can be a very difficult time for women. It is often seen as the cause of the aging process in women. However, many of the symptoms blamed on the menopause, such as middle-age spread, lines on the face and greying hair, are simply part of the natural aging process which also happens to men. Some women, under pressure from society, the media and the working world, feel they must stay young, slim, sexually attractive and bounding with energy. By contrast, aging men seem to benefit from their increasing years. They are seen as "distinguished" when silver hair appears at the temples, and "interesting" as lines carve character on the face.

Women may also experience sadness or grief as their reproductive years come to an end. Some may even feel that their useful life is over – particularly if this is reinforced by men who find them less attractive, bosses who ignore or undervalue their contributions, and children who seem to need them less and prefer to spend more time with their peers.

It is in this often stressful context that we need to look at the symptoms of the menopause – symptoms such as hot flashes, mood changes, depression, headaches, palpitations, vaginal soreness, and cystitis. There may also be irregular periods or heavy bleeding, sometimes even flooding, occurring all too frequently, often every two weeks and persisting for the same length of time. While hormonal changes can account for some problems at this time, these varying symptoms cannot all be blamed solely on the menopause.

In order to understand why stress influences our hormones, we need to understand that the female hormonal system (see p.86) is influenced by the hypothalamus. This part of the brain affects the secretion of sex hormones, and also the production of a whole range of other hormones directing the endocrine glands throughout the body. These endocrine glands control our body temperature, circulation, digestion, bone structure, emotions, mood changes, water balance, sleep and weight. It is these which are upset during menopause.

The hypothalamus is highly sensitive to stress and so if we are stressed at menopause the natural takeover process of estrogen production will be upset. We cannot lay the blame for menopausal symptoms solely at the feet of changing estrogen levels. They may be much more related to stress occurring at this time.

Once we recognize this, it may be easier for us to cope with the physical changes of menopause without feeling that they are all the fault of our aging bodies. We need to be able to discuss them openly, and without embarrassment, when it is necessary to do so.

Self-help during the menopause

A healthy diet, sufficient rest and exercise, relaxation and enjoyment will help you to cope with change and to keep your hormones balanced (see also p.88).

Take herbs to support the nervous system and help to buffer the effects of stress:

skullcap	vervain
wild oats	rosemary
wood betony	

These tonic herbs improve vitality and enhance resistance to stress:

ginseng	dang gui
cinnamon	shatavari
ginger	sage
huang qi	

Take herbs to support the adrenal glands, particularly if you suffer from stress, which depletes them, or if you are on the thin side, and therefore have fewer fat-stored reserves of estrogen. Herbs such as licorice and borage will help support the adrenal glands.

Liver remedies such as dandelion root and yellow dock root are helpful, as they will help regulate the metabolism of estrogen.

Avoid smoking as it can affect the estrogen output of the ovaries. Alcohol can also have a bad effect, so keep its consumption down.

Women who have suffered menstrual or gynecological problems caused by hormone imbalances may be more prone to menopausal symptoms if their hormone imbalance continues until menopause. It is important, therefore, to deal with any menstrual problems (see Chapter 4) when they occur, to make for an easier menopause.

Around the menopause, hormone-balancing herbs and those with an estrogen-like action will prove most helpful. Chaste tree and false unicorn root are the first choice of herbs for helping balance hormones.

These herbs have an estrogen action and will help smooth the transition from ovarian to adrenal production of estrogen:

sage	motherwort
hops	wild yam
shatavari	licorice
ginseng	calendula

If you suffer from heavy bleeding or irregular periods leading up to the menopause see Disturbances of the normal cycle on p.88.

Herbal remedies in menopause

Hot flashes and night sweats

Many women around the menopause experience hot flashes or night sweats or both. They can be occasional or very frequent, and can vary in intensity from being mildly annoying or embarrassing to being very stressful, or even suffocating. Night sweats can be so extreme as to soak your nightclothes. Flashes are totally unpredictable; they feel like a wave of heat surging through the body, often upwards to the face. They tend mostly to affect the upper part of the body. Flashes may start with tingling and be accompanied by redness and sweating. After the flush, which can last anything from a few seconds to a couple of minutes, women often feel chilled. When night sweats happen frequently in the night, a woman's sleep may be seriously affected.

If you suffer from frequent flashes try to wear your clothes in layers, so you can easily remove a jacket or sweater when you feel hot and put another on if you feel chilly. You could carry a fan to elegantly cool yourself during flashes – or keep a desk-top fan at work. Although it is important for your estrogen levels that you are not underweight, remember that body fat acts as an insulator and too much of it will slow down the body's cooling mechanisms.

Wear natural fibres where possible, because synthetic ones do not allow the skin to breathe and make sweating worse. In bed, wear an absorbent material like cotton next to your skin and make sure your bedding is cotton.

When you feel a flush coming on, try not to fight it by becoming tense, but relax into it; that way it may ease more quickly. Many women find that tension, caused by panicking about a deadline or rushing about, can actually bring on flashes. Try to avoid stress, sudden changes of temperature, and hot, crowded atmospheres.

Also avoid too many hot drinks, and spicy or fatty foods as they can increase the tendency to overheat. Cut out smoking, alcohol and caffeine as they all help to upset your hormone balance. Many women feel better and have fewer hot flashes if they reduce or cut out meat and dairy produce consumption. It may be that the hormones in these foods upset the hormone balance in women.

Make sure that you drink plenty of liquid and that your diet is high in vitamin E and selenium (for sources see Diet chart p.70). These nutrients work well together to control abnormal temperature regulation that causes flashes. Begin with 400 iu of vitamin E daily. Over the next few weeks you can increase the dose by 200 iu in a week to a maximum of 1200 iu daily. Once the flashes cease, gradually reduce the dose. (Avoid vitamin E if you suffer from high blood pressure, diabetes or heart disease; seek your practitioner's approval first.) Eat plenty of foods containing vitamin C and bioflavonoids or take a supplement (1-3 grams daily), as together they can strengthen capillary walls and so prevent the dilation that causes flushing. Supplements of B complex, calcium and evening primrose oil will also help to combat the effects of stress on your hormone balance.

By taking the above advice, combined with using herbs regularly, you should be able to stop your hot flashes and night sweats.

Use estrogenic hormone-balancing herbs such as:

false unicorn root	*blue or black cohosh*
chaste tree	*hops*
wild yam	*licorice*

Drink frequently through the day a tea of sage and motherwort, both of which are excellent for relieving hot flashes. Ginseng is often helpful.

If you feel stressed use herbs to support the nervous system such as:

lemon balm	*rosemary*
ginseng	*skullcap*
vervain	

Hawthorn added to your prescription should help to balance the circulation.

Essential oils used in massage oils or added to a relaxing bath will help to ease tension.

Choose from:

lavender	*rosemary*
rose	*ylang ylang*
geranium	

Fennel

Foeniculum vulgare

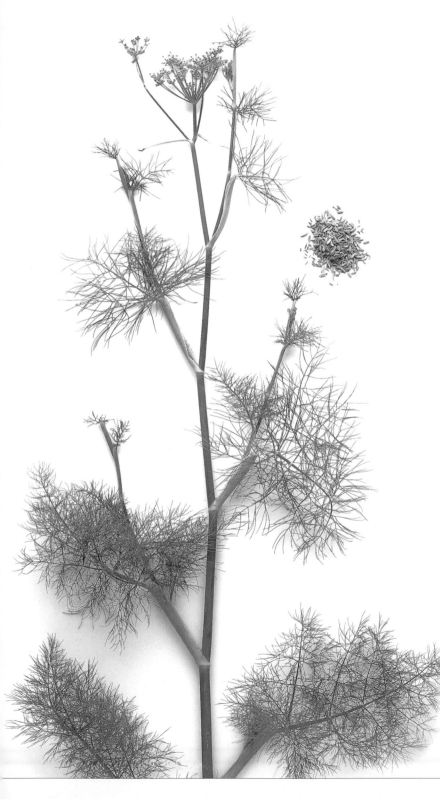

PART USED: Seeds

CONTAINS: Volatile oils, fixed oil (including petroselenic acid, oleic acid, linoleic acid), flavonoids (including rutin), vitamins, minerals (including calcium and potassium)

KEY USES: Diuretic, antiseptic, digestive, carminative, galactagogue

Fennel is a handsome feathery aromatic plant and an ancient digestive remedy. Its volatile oils increase the appetite, enhance the secretion of digestive enzymes and promote digestion and absorption. Its carminative properties relax any spasm in the digestive tract and relieve wind, colic and hiccoughs - it is one of the ingredients in gripe water. It can also be taken for indigestion, heartburn, constipation and abdominal pain, and was traditionally used in cooking to enhance digestion.

Fennel is a useful remedy for women. It has been used since the time of the ancient Greeks to promote secretion of breastmilk in nursing mothers, and when taken by the mother the volatile oils will pass to the baby to soothe digestive troubles. It has also been used to regulate the menstrual cycle and relieve period pains.

The diuretic properties of fennel help to relieve fluid retention and combined with the action of the antiseptic volatile oils, it can be used to treat urinary infections. By aiding elimination of toxins from the system via the urine, fennel makes a useful remedy for arthritis and gout. It can be used for urinary stones and gravel.

Fennel is an ancient remedy for strengthening the sight, and was used as an eyewash for soreness, tiredness, inflammation and infections of the eyes. The volatile oils in fennel have an antiseptic action, and make fennel a useful remedy for infections, particularly in the respiratory system. Dilute oil of fennel can be used in massage oils and liniments for painful joints, and on the abdomen for colic and griping. The bruised seeds, or oil applied locally, are used to relieve toothache and earache.

Depression and mood changes

Depression, moodiness, irritability, excitability, anxiety and panic attacks can afflict many women around the menopause. They most probably result from both hormonal changes and our responses to life stresses at this time. It is interesting to note that in the youth-centred cultures of the West many women suffer from these kinds of emotional problems once their fertility and youthfulness decline, while in those Eastern cultures where older women are more highly valued and respected, these problems hardly exist at all.

To provide physical support during difficult times it is important to eat a healthy diet. Avoid sugar, caffeine, alcohol and unnecessary drugs which can all deplete the nervous system and weaken resistance to stress.

Take plenty of exercise – aerobic exercise taken regularly can stimulate the secretions of endorphins (opiate-like substances) from the brain which give a sense of wellbeing and lift the spirits. Exercise increases vitality, stimulates the circulation, and calms the mind. It also releases emotions such as anger, irritability and anxiety.

You may need to take supplements of vitamin B complex, vitamins C and E, as well as evening primrose oil, calcium and magnesium which will all help support the nervous system.

There are herbs you can take regularly to lift the spirits and balance the emotions. St. John's wort is specific for depression around the menopause.

These herbs will also help lift the spirits:

lemon balm	*rosemary*
wild oats	*vervain*
borage	*cinnamon*

Skullcap, motherwort, lavender and chamomile are calming, while passionflower and valerian will help relieve extreme nervousness and panic. Bach Flower Remedies (see chart on p.246–7) are very helpful.

Essential oils of rose, geranium, bergamot, lavender and melissa can be added to massage oils or the bath to help you relax and release tensions, and to relieve sadness and depression.

Talking to others about how you feel, particularly to women who have experienced menopause, can be a great support. There may be a local self-help group where you can express your feelings. It is important to be heard and understood, to receive the support you deserve, and to recognize that you are not neurotic because you feel the way you do.

Counselling, relaxation exercises, yoga, meditation and visualization can all help you to cope at this time. Try to let go of your negativity and fear, to recognize the value of your experience and wisdom, and regain your rightful self-respect, esteem and power.

Vaginal dryness and irritation

Falling estrogen levels can cause some changes in the vagina. Estrogen maintains mucus secretion in the vagina and keeps its walls thick and moist. Lack of estrogen can make the walls thin and dry, with a tendency to crack and bleed, particularly with the friction of intercourse. Estrogen also maintains the existence of Doderlein's bacilli in the vagina and influences the pH of vaginal secretions, which keep infections at bay. Diminishing estrogen compromises these natural defences and can make women more prone to vaginal irritation and infection, known as vaginitis.

There are steps you can take to maintain the natural defences of the vagina and preserve its natural lubrication. You should avoid washing the area with soap, and be sure not to use synthetic bath preparations or detergents, vaginal deodorants or other cosmetics. Also, be careful to wash your underwear in pure soap, such as castile soap or olive-oil based soap, and avoid detergents and biological powders. Try adding a little cider vinegar to your bath – this will help maintain the natural pH of the vagina. Sea salt added to the bath will help combat infection.

Regular sexual intercourse will help to keep the vagina elastic and maintain a healthy blood supply to the area. As the vaginal walls become dry, they also tend to become thin and to atrophy, and if the area is neglected this process will speed up, creating a vicious circle – the drier and tighter the area, the more uncomfortable sex will be, so desire decreases, there is less sex, and the area becomes drier and tighter.

If vaginal dryness is a problem during sex, you need more time before penetration for arousal to stimulate your natural secretions. Sensual massage and foreplay should help, but the most important

Linden blossom

Tilia europaea

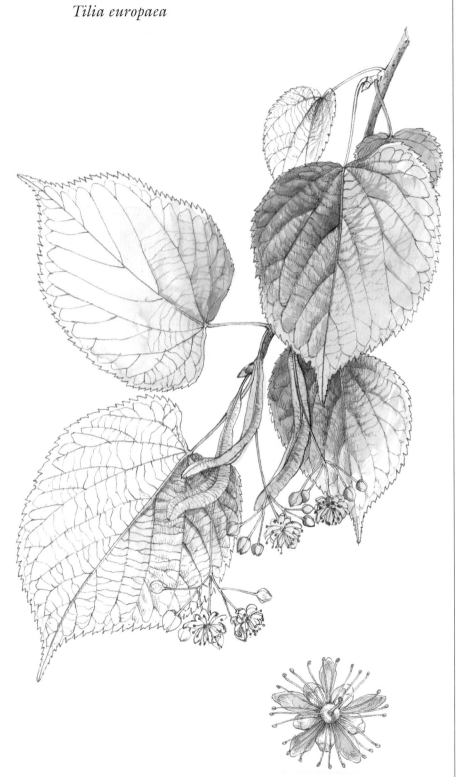

ALSO KNOWN AS: Lime flowers

PART USED: Flowers

CONTAINS: Essential oil (including farnesol), flavonoid glycosides (including hesperidin and quercitrin), saponins, tannins, mucilage

KEY USES: Nervine, relaxant, antispasmodic, diaphoretic, diuretic, astringent

Linden blossom makes a wonderfully relaxing remedy that is delicious when taken in infusion. It relieves tension and anxiety, aids sleep, calms restless and excitable children and reduces muscle tension. It makes a good remedy for conditions associated with tension including headaches, period pains, colic and cramp.

These relaxant effects combined with the beneficial action of the bioflavonoids on the arteries make linden blossom a useful remedy for reducing high blood pressure and arteriosclerosis. It also relaxes the arteries of the heart, making it useful in the treatment of palpitations and coronary heart disease.

Taken in hot infusion, linden blossom has a diaphoretic action, increasing blood supply to the skin and producing sweating. It is an excellent remedy for reducing fevers, particularly in children, and for clearing catarrhal congestion. Taken with elderflowers it will speed colds, coughs, and flu on their way. A warm to cool infusion has a diuretic action, helping to clear fluid and toxins from the body through the urinary system.

factor is desire. If you feel misunderstood or distanced from your partner you may well lose interest in sex and these problems in your relationship need to be addressed. It is a good idea to keep a lubricating jelly from the pharmacist by the bed, because even if the desire is there, some extra lubrication may be needed.

Vitamin E oil used regularly will help to lubricate the vagina, heal cracks and soreness and help keep the tissues elastic. You can open a vitamin E capsule and massage the oil with your finger into the inside wall of your vagina. Calendula cream or oil will also help heal damage to the vagina walls. Comfrey ointment or oil is also wonderfully healing, and soothes soreness and irritation. It also helps to bring moisture to the area.

Hormone-balancing herbs should be taken regularly to maintain estrogen levels and prevent vaginal changes.

Use combinations of any of the following:

false unicorn root	*sage*
blue cohosh	*calendula*
hops	*motherwort*

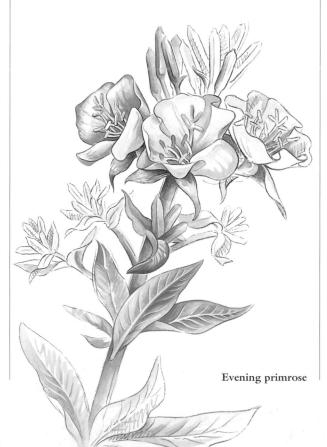

Evening primrose

Vitamins B, C, and E, as well as evening primrose oil can be taken as supplements.

Essential oils can usefully be added to massage oils, particularly for sensual massage prior to sex. Rose oil is particularly beneficial in aiding relaxation and increasing sensuality. Jasmine, geranium, lavender and clary sage can also be used.

Be sure to treat any vaginal infections which occur at this time. For herbal and dietary advice on their treatment see p.224.

Loss of libido

For some women menopause is related to a decrease in sexual desire and so in sexual activity. Vaginal changes can make sex more uncomfortable, and a lack of sexual interest contributes to the vaginal changes. In addition to this vicious circle of causes, there are often relationship problems at this time. You may feel that your partner is misunderstanding you or failing to support you at this difficult time in your life, and is part of the problem rather than part of the solution. In order for this to change, you need to talk through your difficulties, perhaps with the help of a third party such as a family counsellor.

Loss of libido may also be a reflection of how a woman feels about herself generally. If she feels unhappy about how her body looks or feels, self-conscious about changes in her body, or worried about whether she is still sexually attractive, this will affect her libido.

Taking plenty of exercise and getting in touch and in tune with your body through dance, T'ai chi, yoga or massage, may well help to change your negative perception of your body. Your partner's support in this process is very valuable. It is difficult to be interested in sex unless your partner is interested too.

One very positive aspect of sex at this time is the new freedom from the possibility of pregnancy. At last, conception is not an issue, whether you were concerned to conceive or to avoid pregnancy. There may arise a new spontaneity in your physical relationship, if you no longer need use contraception, that may help sustain the closeness and happiness between you.

There are several herbs which have a reputation as aphrodisiacs and rejuvenating tonics. They are best taken by both partners. While some of their traditionally proclaimed benefits use some poetic licence, such claims are usually based on fact.

Herbs to improve libido

Peppermint has such a strong reputation that it was forbidden to ancient Greek soldiers in wartime in case it distracted them and reduced their courage! For centuries Arab men have drunk peppermint tea to stimulate their virility.

Myrrh is considered in Ayurvedic medicine to be one of the best rejuvenating herbs to slow down the aging process. It is still used today as it was thousands of years ago to restore the female reproductive system, increase energy and to dispel repressed emotions.

Peppers, particularly cayenne pepper, increase the "fire" in the body, stimulating energy and enhancing vitality. They have long been used to increase sexual energy and fertility and to prolong life.

Rose is a traditional symbol of love, and a tonic to the female reproductive system, used to treat infertility and to enhance sexual desire. In men, roses have been used to treat lack of sexual interest and impotence. In aromatherapy oil of rose is used to treat a wide range of problems associated with the reproductive tract – including emotional problems related to sexuality causing problems such as frigidity and impotence.

Cloves are wonderfully stimulating and warming. They lift the spirits, relax tension, increase energy and have a reputation from ancient times for "stirring up lust" when eaten.

Rosemary is an excellent tonic, in the past seen as a symbol of love and fidelity. It has a rejuvenating action, and its antioxidant properties help to slow the aging process.

Ginger is another stimulating and warming spice, increasing energy and vitality and stimulating the circulation. It is used for a variety of menstrual problems, and is recommended for impotence or lack of sexual energy caused by deficiency of vital warmth in the body. It is taken as an aphrodisiac in many countries of the world.

Garlic acts as an invigorating tonic, used in the past in many places as an "elixir of youth". It imparts energy and vitality and its antioxidant properties help to slow the aging process. It has been widely acclaimed as an aphrodisiac.

Cinnamon has been used since the time of the Crusaders in love potions and as an aphrodisiac for both men and women. It is a wonderfully strengthening tonic, increasing the circulation, enhancing energy and vitality and has been used for centuries for frigidity and impotence.

Parsley was said to enhance beauty and youthfulness, and it was used in love potions for "unwilling" women for its aphrodisiac powers. It stimulates circulation and increases energy, and makes a very nutritious tonic.

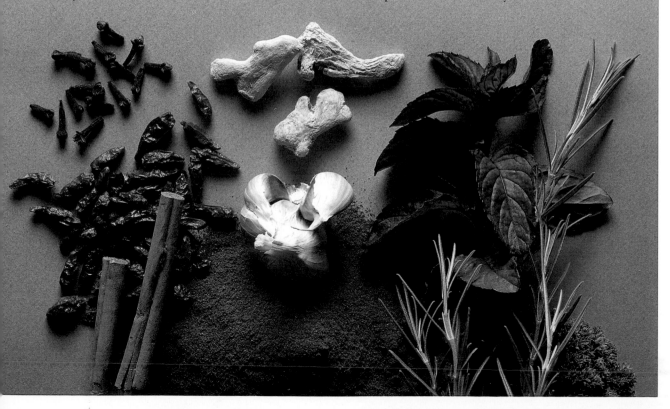

Certain foods have been famed for their aphrodisiac powers – notably watercress, onions, leeks, oats, mustard, barley and honey.

Where stress is a major factor in lack of sexual interest, add herbs to support the nervous system such as wild oats, skullcap, vervain and lemon balm to your chosen prescription.

Essential oils of rose, geranium, clary sage, geranium and jasmine can be added to baths and massage oils and can be used for sensual massage as part of your lovemaking.

Bach Flower Remedies can help relieve emotional problems related to your lack of libido (see p.246–7).

Osteoporosis

The most serious and long term problem related to lower levels of estrogen as we become older is weakening of the bones. Bone loss begins in the thirties and worsens immediately after the menopause. Signs to look out for are back pain, loss of height due to compression of the spine, muscle spasm, teeth loss and wrist fractures.

Loss of bone tissue is called osteoporosis. A woman in later life who has pronounced curvature of the upper back and a tendency to hip fracture has suffered from osteoporosis for some time.

Factors indicating risk of osteoporosis

Certain women are particularly at risk of osteoporosis. These are:

• thin women who are light boned, because women store estrogen in their fat deposits
• women who have dieted a great deal or suffered from anorexia, and thereby depleted from their diet vital vitamins and minerals necessary for hormone balance and calcium deposition
• those who only have a small amount of calcium in their diets. Vitamin D is necessary for calcium absorption so vitamin D deficiency can also be to blame
• women who have taken little exercise, particularly weight-bearing exercise such as dancing, walking, jogging and tennis. The stress on the bones encourages the laying down of calcium in them
• those who started menstruation late and had their menopause early, as they have had less estrogen in their system

• women who smoke – smoking depletes estrogen in the body and often leads to an earlier menopause
• those with female relatives with osteoporosis, as there is a genetic tendency to it
• Caucasian women; they are more at risk than black women who rarely suffer from osteoporosis
• those with a high caffeine, alcohol, and salt intake, as these can all deplete calcium and other minerals in the system
• women with malabsorption problems such as celiac disease which can cause less calcium to be absorbed from the diet
• women who take certain drugs – such as cortisone, thyroxin, antacids, tamoxifen, diuretics and phenytoin
• those with increased secretion of the parathyroid hormone (which draws calcium from the bones), diabetes, kidney or liver disease
• women who have had a total hysterectomy (where the ovaries are removed along with the uterus)

If you fall into one or more of these categories, it is worth having a bone scan to check on your bone density. Even if you appear not to be at risk, it is advisable to take preventative measures.

Prevention of osteoporosis

• Exercise regularly – at least half an hour of brisk walking every day – or choose another kind of exercise that you enjoy.
• Avoid excess alcohol, smoking, and drinks and foods containing caffeine.
• Make sure you have plenty of calcium in your diet (see diet chart p.70) and take a calcium supplement (1500 mg daily) with magnesium (750 mg).
• Take boron, found in fresh fruit and vegetables, which protects the bones from calcium loss by reducing its excretion. It increases levels of estrogen and progesterone, both required for maintaining calcium in the bones.
• Include plenty of magnesium-rich foods in your diet (see diet chart p.70). Magnesium may be as important as calcium for maintaining bone density, and is necessary for proper calcium absorption, as is vitamin D.
• Expose your skin regularly to sunlight so your body can make vitamin D.

Catmint

Nepeta cataria

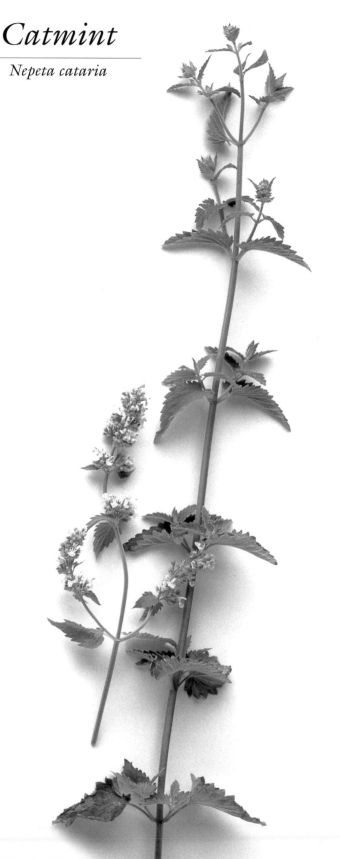

ALSO KNOWN AS: Catnip, catnep

CONTAINS: Volatile oils including nepetalactone, camphor, cryophyllenes, humulene, thymol, geraniol, tannins, bitter principle

KEY USES: Refrigerant, diaphoretic, relaxant, antispasmodic, emmenagogue, astringent

Catmint is an invaluable remedy for respiratory infections – taken as a hot tea it increases perspiration and effectively brings down fevers, and acts as a decongestant. It should be taken frequently at the first signs of colds or flu, and is also helpful in bronchitis and asthma, as well as eruptive infections such as chicken-pox and measles. It is a wonderful remedy for babies and children; being calming and relaxing it will relieve restlessness and induce sleep. Its relaxant effect is also felt in the digestive tract where it relieves tension and colic, wind and pain – excellent for babies who have wind or colic or trouble sleeping. A strong infusion will relax headaches related to tension.

Catmint can be used for other digestive problems – stomach upset, indigestion, and stress related conditions; the tannins make it a good remedy for diarrhea, particularly in children. As an enema it is prescribed for inflammatory bowel conditions, bowel infections, constipation and diarrhea.

Catmint's relaxant effects are also felt in the uterus. It can be used to relieve period pains as well as tension or stress prior to a period. It can also be used to regulate periods, and for delayed or suppressed menstruation.

A hot infusion makes a good antiseptic inhalant for sore throats, colds, flu and coughs, a decongestant for catarrh and sinusitis, and a relaxant for asthma and croup. Its disinfectant properties can be used for infected skin problems. The tannins speed tissue repair and staunch bleeding of abrasions and cuts; they aid healing of burns and scalds, piles and insect bites, and inflammatory skin problems.

• Take zinc and vitamins B and E which help maintain estrogen levels.

• Do not diet severely – it is better to be slightly plump than underweight. However, avoid eating fatty foods and too much meat as that can predispose to other health problems such as cardiovascular disease.

• Avoid bran, excess whole grains, rhubarb and spinach as these can reduce the absorption of vital minerals.

• Avoid eating excess dairy foods as a diet high in dairy foods and meat (high phosphorus foods) has been linked to osteoporosis, as has a diet high in convenience foods, which often lack vitamins E, B, and C, magnesium and zinc, and high in phosphorus which encourages bone loss.

• Take vitamin K. Research suggests that it may be vital for prevention of osteoporosis. It helps synthesize a substance called osteocalcin which attracts calcium to bone.

• Avoid constipation, which can upset the normal bacterial population of the gut. A diet high in meat, dairy produce and junk foods will encourage constipation and an over-abundance of unfriendly bacteria in the gut that has been linked to osteoporosis.

• Take herbs containing calcium (see p.123), notably parsley, dandelion leaves, nettles, kelp, and horsetail which can be added to your diet or taken regularly as a herbal remedy.

• Take estrogenic herbs which discourage calcium loss from the bones – choose from calendula, ginseng, false unicorn root, sage, hops, blue cohosh, wild yam and licorice.

• Add herbs to your prescription to stimulate digestion and absorption of minerals, and to enhance the function of the liver and gallbladder: adequate bile salts are necessary for proper calcium absorption. Choose from dandelion root, yellow dock root, calendula, rosemary, wormwood or yarrow.

Avoiding ERT and hysterectomy

Estrogen replacement therapy consists of the hormones estrogen and progesterone being used to replace the decreasing secretion of these hormones at and after the menopause. The use of ERT is widely advocated to deal with most menopausal symptoms such as hot flashes, vaginal changes, osteoporosis, low libido and mood swings. It may effectively stop these symptoms, but it does little to enable a woman to understand the working of her own body in relation to her lifestyle and emotions, and to inspire her to deal with many of the stresses occurring at this time. It may be a solution to some problems but it has some fairly serious disadvantages.

Estrogen-only ERT causes thickening of the womb lining and can predispose to cell changes that can lead to endometrial cancer (see p.239). Most ERT does now contain progesterone – but if you are having ERT check with your practitioner. Long term use of ERT has also been linked to the development of breast cancer. Its benefit in preventing osteoporosis is only evident in women on ERT for more than seven years, and research has shown that even those who have taken it for more than ten years were not protected from fractures. As soon as women stopped ERT, bone mineral density dropped dramatically, almost to the same level as in women who had never taken ERT. It appears that ERT may significantly prevent osteoporosis but only if it is taken for the rest of life.

ERT can have a variety of side effects, experienced by about 20 per cent of women who take it. They include nausea, irritability, breast enlargement and tenderness, bloating, depression, and cramps in the abdomen and legs. The therapy causes regular bleeding, similar to a period. Since this is the time to be free of such inconveniences, many women will find this annoying.

It is claimed that ERT can protect against heart disease, but this is very controversial. Taken in the contraceptive pill, estrogen is known to increase the risk of cardiovascular disease, so it is hard to believe that it behaves differently after menopause. Some studies actually suggest ERT may increase the risk. Estrogen can increase the risk of developing gallbladder disease and aggravate any existing gallstones.

ERT can aggravate some medical problems and therefore should be avoided by women with certain conditions. These include: fibroids, endometriosis, a personal or family history of breast cancer, migraine, high blood pressure, epilepsy, liver problems, and diabetes.

Alternatives to ERT

There are natural sources of estrogenic substances which are safe alternatives to ERT.

Sage

Salvia officinalis

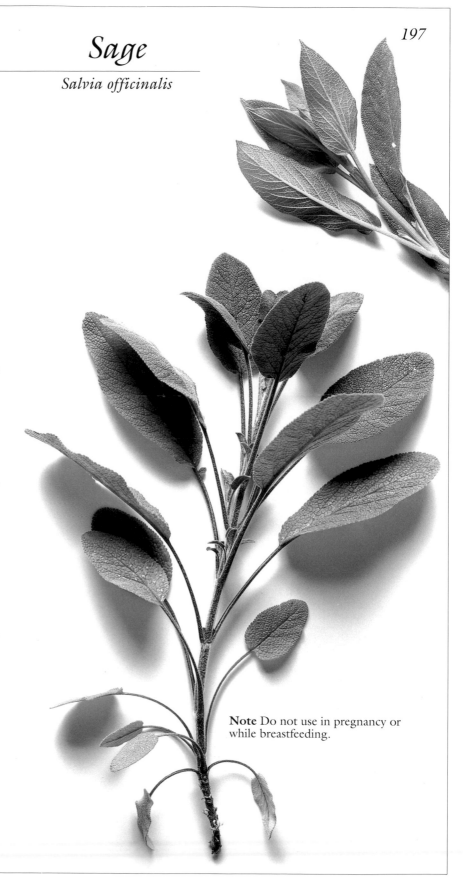

PART USED: Leaves

CONTAINS: Volatile oil, estrogenic substances, salvin and carnosic acid, flavonoids, tannins, phenolic acids

KEY USES: Antiseptic, astringent, digestive, estrogenic, antioxidant, nerve tonic, antispasmodic, bitter tonic, anti-hydrotic

Sage is one of the most valued herbs of antiquity. It is highly antiseptic, an excellent remedy for colds, fevers and sore throats and should be taken at the first signs of any respiratory infections. It relieves tonsilitis, bronchitis, asthma, catarrh, and sinusitis. Its astringent and expectorant properties help expel phlegm from the chest and reduce catarrh. The tea can be used in inhalation to disinfect the airways. Sage will enhance the immune system and help to prevent infections and auto-immune problems.

Sage makes a good digestive remedy. The volatile oils have a relaxant effect on the smooth muscle of the digestive tract, while in conjunction with the bitters, they stimulate the appetite and improve digestion. Sage encourages the flow of digestive enzymes and bile, settles the stomach, relieves colic, wind, indigestion, nausea, diarrhea and colitis, liver complaints, and worms. Its antiseptic properties are helpful in infections such as gastroenteritis. Sage is a tonic to the nervous system and has been used to enhance strength and vitality. It has a tonic effect upon the female reproductive tract, and is recommended for delayed or scanty menstruation, or lack of periods, menstrual cramps and infertility. It has an estrogenic effect, excellent for menopausal problems, especially hot flashes and night sweats. It stimulates the uterus, so is useful during childbirth and to expel the placenta. It stops the flow of breastmilk and it is excellent for weaning.

Sage has powerful antioxidant properties, helping to delay the aging process and reduce the harmful effects of free radicals.

Note Do not use in pregnancy or while breastfeeding.

Certain foods contain estrogen-like substances known as phytosterols – including:

rhubarb	oats
celery	alfalfa
soybeans	fenugreek
anise	
soya products such as tofu and miso	

Several herbs contain similar estrogenic substances. These include:

sage	hops
calendula	fennel
wild yam	licorice
false unicorn root	ginseng
motherwort	shatavari
black cohosh	blue cohosh

There is much you can do to ease the transition from hormone production by the ovaries to that by the adrenal glands, and to help your physical and emotional journey at this time of change. See Coping with change on p.186.

Hysterectomy

A hysterectomy can either involve removal of the uterus, the uterus and cervix, or of the uterus and ovaries. When the ovaries are removed it causes a premature menopause because they are no longer present to produce estrogen and progesterone. Hysterectomy is the most common major surgical operation for women and is most commonly performed because of abnormal bleeding and fibroids. A hysterectomy is a major operation; physical recovery takes many weeks or even months.

These are the usual complaints which lead to hysterectomy:

invasive cancer of the cervix
cancer of the uterus
large fibroids
endometriosis
heavy or persistent bleeding or flooding
ovary or fallopian tube disease, e.g. cysts, cancer
prolapse
pelvic infection
pelvic inflammatory disease
rarely, complications after childbirth
a ruptured uterus or massive hemorrhage

Hysterectomy can have profound effects on your identity and feelings of femininity. The number of operations is increasing, particularly among younger women. There is a view held, perhaps mostly among male gynecologists, that when childbearing age is past the uterus is redundant, prone to problems such as bleeding and disease, and some women may be better off without one. If a hysterectomy is suggested to you as treatment, it is important to understand why, and to find out about possible options. Heavy bleeding, endometriosis, pain and small fibroids may be treated without surgery. Also, there is a new laser technique available which removes the inner lining of the womb instead of the entire uterus.

Avoiding hysterectomy

Preventative medicine is vital in avoiding the development of those health problems which, if left to advance, may eventually make a hysterectomy necessary. The key to a healthy reproductive system is largely the maintenance of a correct hormone balance. There is a wide variety of factors which contribute to this, all of which are discussed on p.86. They include eating a good diet, minimizing stress and having a healthy lifestyle. Using herbs, eating certain foods and often taking supplements, is part of such a lifestyle; it is also important to balance work and leisure, activity and sleep, challenge and relaxation, exercise and rest. If you have hormone imbalances contributing to gynecological problems such as heavy or abnormal bleeding, fibroids, endometriosis and period pain, these are best treated. For treatment of menstrual problems and heavy bleeding see Chapter 4 p.88. For treatment of other gynecological problems including ovarian cysts, cervical changes, prolapse, fibroids, P1D and endometriosis see Chapter 12, p.219.

St. John's wort

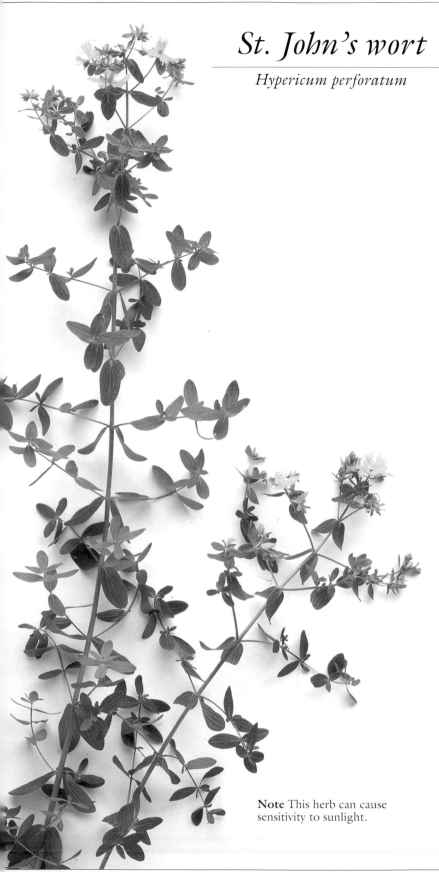

Hypericum perforatum

PART USED: Aerial parts

CONTAINS: Glycosides (including the red pigment hypericin), flavonoids, tannins, resin, volatile oil

KEY USES: Antidepressant, antimicrobial, antineoplastic, sedative, astringent, expectorant, diuretic

St. John's wort has been highly valued since antiquity for its healing powers (believed to be derived from St. John the Baptist). It is a wonderful remedy for the nervous system, relaxing tension and anxiety, and lifting the spirits – it is considered specific for emotional problems during the menopause. Its tranquilizing effect has been attributed to hypericin, which reduces blood pressure, capillary fragility and benefits the uterus. St. John's wort can be used for painful, heavy and irregular periods as well as PMS. It has a diuretic action, reducing fluid retention and hastening elimination of toxins in the urine. It has been used to good effect for bed-wetting in children. It is also useful for gout and arthritis.

St. John's wort also has an expectorant action, clearing phlegm from the chest and speeding recovery from coughs and chest infections. It has an antibacterial and antiviral action, active against TB and influenza A, and is being researched for its beneficial effect in the treatment of AIDS and HIV as well as cancer.

Its astringent and antimicrobial action is effective in the digestive tract where it can treat gastroenteritis, diarrhea and dysentery. It is also said to heal peptic ulcers and gastritis.

Used both internally and externally, St. John's wort is a wonderful remedy for nerve pain and any kind of trauma to the nervous system. It can be used for neuralgia such as trigeminal neuralgia and sciatica, fibrositis, back pain, headaches, shingles and rheumatic pain. The herbal oil soothes and heals burns, cuts, wounds, sores, ulcers and calms inflammation.

Note This herb can cause sensitivity to sunlight.

10 *Later Years*

Most of us want to live a long life, enjoying our later years as comfortably as possible, free from illness and pain. Many women in our society fear growing old, and certainly our attitude to our age will influence how well we feel both physically and emotionally. In a culture which values youth and earning ability above wisdom and experience, women in their later years often feel rejected and worthless. As our bodies age we may feel that we are losing the only asset of any value that we have. Denial of the value of age may be related to fear about infirmity and death, combined with the idea that old age is synonymous with ill health – which it does not have to be.

It is important to bear in mind that our society's attitudes to older women are cultural, and not grounded in fact. Anthropology shows that in more "primitive" societies than ours, women past the menopause often experience a positive change of status. They continue to be responsible for younger members of the community, and to have authority over them, but they also become eligible for certain roles previously denied them, such as healers, midwives, givers of initiation and holy women. In some Asian societies women can discard the veil after the menopause, in others trade and travel restrictions for women disappear, so older women take on new business enterprises or administrative work within the community which give them a new degree of power. In some societies older women continue and very often develop their sexual roles – in the Kung tribe in South Africa it is said that older women often take younger lovers and have a great deal more sexual freedom than younger women. These and other studies show that the older woman can achieve the greater authority, power and respect that her increasing years deserve. We are capable of recognizing the same power within ourselves, despite our cultural pressures.

The Russian Shirali Mislimor was asked what the secret of his long life was, and he replied:

"I was never in a hurry in my life and I am in no hurry to die now. There are two sources of long life. One is a gift from nature, and the pure air and clear water of the mountains, the fruit of the earth, peace, rest and the soft warm climate of the Highlands. The second source is within us. He lives long who enjoys life and who bears no jealousy of others, whose heart harbours no malice or anger, who sings a lot and cries a little, who rises and retires with the sun, who likes to work and who knows how to rest." At the time, he was said to be 166 years old.

Ginkgo

Ginkgo biloba

ALSO KNOWN AS: Maidenhair tree

PARTS USED: Leaves, seeds

CONTAINS: Leaves: Flavonglycosides (ginkgolide heterosides), quercetin, proanthocyanidins, lactones, terpenes, sito-sterol
Seeds: Bioflavones, minerals, fatty acids

KEY USES: Leaves: stimulant, nervine, astringent, diaphoretic
Seeds: Astringent, antifungal, antibacterial

Ginkgo is the oldest living species of tree, having survived for 200 million years, and is known as a living fossil. One tree can live as long as 1,000 years – and interestingly this fascinating tree imparts these qualities of longevity to humans. The leaves retard the aging process in the circulatory system and thus affect the arteries, capillaries, veins and heart. It improves blood flow through the arteries to the brain, alleviating vertigo, tinnitus, short-term memory loss, headaches, depression, poor concentration and other age-related disorders. It has been shown to improve neural transmission in the brain, making it a good remedy for degenerative senility.

Ginkgo also improves circulation throughout the body, useful particularly for elderly people who feel the cold in their extremities. It helps stop blood clotting and acts as an antioxidant, and a free radical scavenger, and makes an excellent medicine for arteriosclerosis, high blood pressure, angina and to prevent strokes and heart attacks. It has been seen to improve visual acuity, hearing, balance, mood, varicose veins, ulcers and hemorrhoids. It can also be used externally for hemorrhoids, varicose veins and ulcers.

The seeds (Bai gou) are used in Chinese medicine for asthma and chesty coughs associated with thick phlegm. They act as a tonic to the kidneys and bladder and have been used for incontinence and excessive urination.

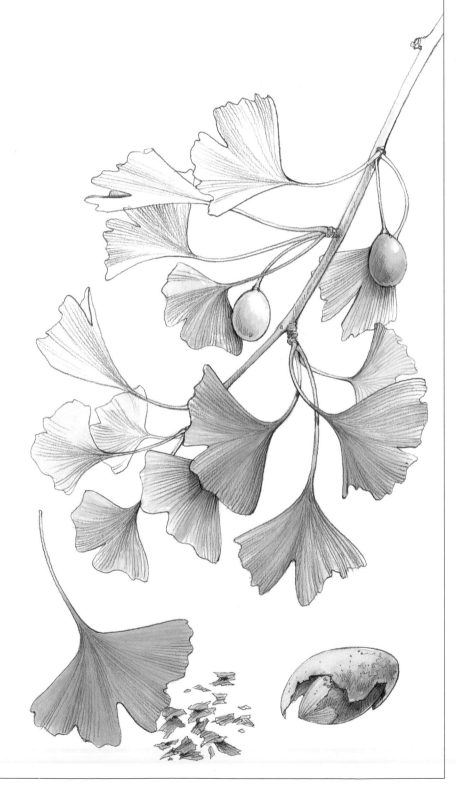

Changes in life and the body

Women form the majority of older people because we live on average for six to ten years longer than men; women over 65 are the fastest growing group in Western populations. Because women outlive men, we often have to face alone the problems that age can bring, such as losing relatives and close friends, caring for loved ones, poverty, chronic illness or infirmity, and being dependent on others for basic care. However, the very fact that there are so many women in this age group means there is a large support group of other women available, who have similar experiences, and who can care for one another.

Freed from the time- and energy-consuming activities of working, housekeeping and childbearing, older women often experience a new surge of creative energy. It can be directed into new creative activities, new interests or studies. There is also now the opportunity to serve the inner world and to develop one's spiritual life.

Older women may find time for reflection and become aware of their own needs as never before, exploring their femininity and acknowledging their feminine wisdom. As the outer eyes grow dimmer, so the inner eye brightens and clarifies. In this way many elderly women contribute enormously to the busy materialistic world in balancing its emphasis on all things physical by their recognition of more subtle worlds, and in letting go of attachment to worldly possessions, the physical body and its image.

Keeping well

To gain the most from our later years, we need to care for our bodies as best we can. Many health problems associated with old age, such as heart disease, high blood pressure, diabetes, arthritis and cancer, are not caused by advancing years; they occur in children and young adults too. It is quite possible to be old and healthy and to die healthy, but this means being healthy to start with. The same requirements for optimum health that apply to children and young adults also apply to post-menopausal women – a healthy diet, plenty of fresh air and exercise, adequate rest and relaxation and freedom from stress.

Diet in later life

The relationship between diet, health and the aging process is well established. It is quite clear that throughout life a healthy diet is of utmost importance. The origins of ill-health which lead to loss of function in later years are generally established in youth and early adulthood. It is a little late to adopt a wholesome diet and lifestyle for the first time in your sixties or seventies, but is certainly worth doing even then.

Studies of the aging process have shown that the amount of food we eat may have a significant effect on how long we live and how healthy we feel. The longest-lived people generally eat very healthily but in small amounts. Researchers have suggested that if most people ate less, and very gradually reduced their weight to 10-25 per cent below their normal weight, they would be at their point of maximum metabolic efficiency, health and longevity. They advise women to eat a diet giving about 7,524 joules (1,800 calories) a day.

Studies among the elderly have shown that many people in their later years tend to neglect their diets, for a variety of reasons, and that deficiencies of vital nutrients serve to contribute to ill-health and loss of function which in turn may prevent them from eating well.

The role of oxygen in the aging process has also been explored recently. Fats and lipids play a variety of important roles in the body. PUFAs (Polyunsaturated fatty acids) build cell walls and are vital to the structure of the brain, nervous system and blood vessels. They protect against degenerative diseases, heart and arterial problems, skin disease, senile dementia and cancer.

Oxygen can have a damaging effect on fats in the body by causing the release of free radicals: molecules that damage cells and tissues leaving destructive waste products behind. Free radical attack can cause a number of pathological conditions including cancer, arthritis, cardiovascular disease and signs of aging such as wrinkled skin. It may be that one key to the aging process is free radical damage to the fatty linings around the cell mitochondria, which produce energy. Happily there are a number of substances, called antioxidants, which can halt this very destructive aging process. The main antioxidants are vitamins A, C and E, the mineral selenium and the amino acid cysteine (for sources see p.70–74).

Antioxidants bind to the free radicals and stop them from damaging the mitochondria. It is worth taking supplements of these substances, for although your diet may be reasonable, deficiencies can be caused by malabsorption due to a variety of conditions. These include gastric and duodenal ulcers, deficient hydrochloric acid in the stomach, liver or gallbladder disease, and celiac disease.

Other substances which help protect against free radical damage are zinc, copper and manganese. These work together with vitamin E to resist free radical invasion of cells. Selenium not only protects against free radicals, it also enhances the function of the immune system, the red blood cells and the liver. It helps the body cope with the toxic chemical pollutants present in our food, the atmosphere, and any drugs we take, and helps to prevent cancer and heart disease. The amino acid cysteine, together with magnesium, also helps cleanse body wastes and detoxify toxic residues of chemicals and drugs.

Vitamin C protects the body wonderfully from damage caused not only by free radicals but also by bacteria, viruses, toxins and the waste products of metabolism. Vitamin C helps to keep collagen strong and elastic. This is the substance which holds cells together and is responsible for the stability and tensile strength of tissues throughout the body. Wrinkles, flabbiness and discoloration of the skin, as well as atherosclerosis and cardiovascular disease, are related to collagen deterioration. Vitamin C also has a stimulating effect upon the adrenal glands, which produce a number of vital steroid hormones, including estrogen after menopause. Gradual decrease in the output of these hormones is said to be partly responsible for many of the symptoms of aging. Daily doses of vitamin C can rejuvenate all endocrine glands, including the adrenals. In addition, it keeps the bowels moving, preventing constipation, and helps to keep cholesterol levels down. It protects against allergies, and aids the healing of tissues.

Beta-carotene is converted in the body to retinol, the biologically active form of vitamin A, which not only scavenges free radicals and protects the body's cells from free radical damage, it also stimulates the immune system. It thus helps the body fight off viruses and bacteria, neutralize toxins and eliminate cancer cells. Vitamin A also helps to maintain the health of mucous membranes of the mouth, digestive tract, vagina, and eyes.

B vitamins help slow down the effects of aging on the body. Together they help the liver in its detoxifying and metabolic work; they enhance the function of the nervous system and enable you to think clearly, function energetically, digest properly and keep on an even keel emotionally. Niacin helps keep cholesterol levels down and improves circulation, choline improves the memory, pantothenic acid enables you to sleep easily and withstand stress and is thought to prevent depression and extend life. Riboflavin helps cystine, vitamins C and E in their work to destroy free radicals and promotes tissue repair and energy metabolism.

Yoghurt is a very valuable item in the diet and has been prized as such for thousands of years. Live yoghurt contains bacteria including the lacto bacillus bulgaricus which has a wide range of health-giving properties.

It helps maintain the normal bacterial population in the gut and eliminates an overgrowth of putrefactive bacteria, often caused by eating too much meat and refined foods, a run down condition, or the use of antibiotics. Lactic acid in yoghurt aids synthesis of B vitamins, increases absorption of nutrients – particularly calcium – and regulates bowel function. It also inhibits infection in the bowel which can cause diarrhea, food poisoning and salmonella. Yoghurt also helps increase antibody formation and aids the immune system's fight against illness and infection. It protects against heart disease by increasing high density lipoprotein cholesterol in the body, and has a reputation for affecting brain activity, keeping the mind alert. Research has shown that live yoghurt also helps to suppress activity of enzymes in the colon that convert certain chemicals into carcinogens, so it may well be beneficial in the prevention of cancer.

Preventing constipation

A healthily functioning digestive system and bowel are vital in keeping the body free from illness. They ensure proper absorption of nutrients from the diet; the effective elimination of toxins and waste products; and they maintain a plentiful supply of beneficial bacteria in the gut, which in turn aid digestion and elimination. The digestive organs also produce important nutrients on their own, notably B vitamins.

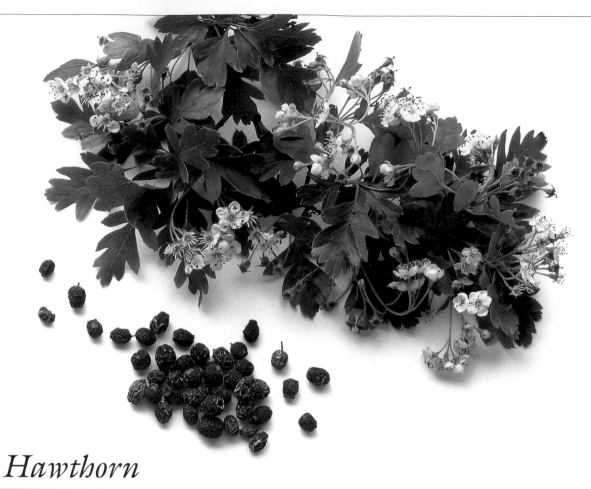

Hawthorn

Cratagus oxyacantha
Cratagus monogyna

ALSO KNOWN AS: May blossom, whitethorn

PARTS USED: Berries, flowers, leaves

CONTAINS: Saponins, glycosides, flavonoids, acids, including ascorbic acid, tannin, procyanidines, trimethylamine

KEY USES: Cardiac tonic, hypotensive, vasodilator, astringent, relaxant, antispasmodic, diuretic

Hawthorn is veritably the best remedy for the heart and circulation. The flowers, leaves and berries all have a vasodilatory effect, opening the arteries and thus improving blood supply to all tissues of the body. This helps to balance blood pressure and makes an excellent remedy for high blood pressure particularly that associated with hardening of the arteries.

Hawthorn can be used to improve poor circulation associated with "aging" arteries, poor circulation to the legs and poor memory and confusion related to poor blood supply to the brain. It opens the coronary arteries in the heart, thereby improving blood flow and softening deposits, and makes an excellent remedy for angina. It has further benefit to the heart in its action on the vagus nerve which influences the heart, so that an over-fast heart rate is slowed and heart irregularities settle down. It is

the ideal remedy for all heart conditions.

The berries have an astringent effect and can be used for diarrhea and dysentery. In addition the leaves, flowers and berries have a relaxant effect in the digestive tract and act to increase the appetite, relieve distension and stagnation of food in the intestines. They have an equally relaxant effect on the nervous system, relieving stress and anxiety, calming agitation, restlessness and nervous palpitations and inducing sleep in those suffering from insomnia. They also have a diuretic effect, relieving fluid retention and dissolving stones and gravel, and can be used during the menopause for debility or night sweats.

A decoction of the berries can be used as an astringent gargle for throats and a douche for vaginal discharges.

The most important factor in regular bowel habits is diet. A wholefood diet, rich in whole grains, fruits, vegetables, nuts and seeds will provide plenty of fibre to help keep the bowels moving. Lack of fibre is a major cause of digestive problems, including constipation, colitis, diverticulitis and bowel cancer, as well as other problems such as varicose veins and hemorrhoids.

The bowel is a passageway for carcinogens such as toxins and pesticide residues from food, as well as bile acids. Dietary fibre increases the bulk of the stool, diluting these carcinogens and speeding them on their way, giving them less contact with susceptible cells in the bowel lining. Fibre also helps to regulate blood sugar.

Exercise in later life

Oxygen is vital for the normal healthy functioning of every cell in the body. Our organs, muscles, brain and nerves function at optimum capacity only when supplied with adequate oxygen – our sedentary lives may well force cells to fulfil their vital tasks with a constant deficiency of oxygen, contributing significantly to lack of function and ill health. Vigorous daily exercise which accelerates heartbeat, respiration and perspiration is therefore vital for bringing the maximum amount of oxygen into tissues and organs. Exercise such as dancing, swimming, bicycling and brisk walking are perfectly adequate. A few early morning exercises will get the blood flowing and help you to feel awake, alert and energetic.

Regular exercise also keeps the heart and circulation healthy, lowers the risk of heart attacks, strokes and high blood pressure, maintains bone density and helps you relax. Aerobic exercise stimulates the secretion of endorphins (opiate-like substances) from the brain, which enhance the immune system and give you a sense of wellbeing, lifting the spirits wonderfully. Sunlight has a similar effect, so exercise outside when possible.

Exercise also keeps your weight down, and keeps the chest and lungs healthy, helping to prevent colds and coughs and other respiratory infections. It keeps the bowels functioning well and the digestive tract healthy. As exercise stimulates the flow of blood, with its nutrients, to the skin, it maintains the skin's collagen content, helping it retain elasticity and stay less wrinkled. It also helps keep you warm in the winter.

The mind also needs exercise. By working the brain you stimulate circulation of blood and nutrients to it, and this helps to keep the nervous system healthy and helps to prevent memory loss and confusion. Stimulate the mind by reading, thinking, memorizing things, playing games such as chess which stimulate the analytical mind, discussing and problem-solving. These activities will all keep the brain active.

Emotional support in later life

As we grow older, keeping in touch with our friends and family is important. It provides interest and love in our lives and helps us be aware of our own feelings and sense of self.

Friendship and love are valuable not only to our happiness and sense of fulfilment, but also because they enhance physical health. Where elderly people lack human companionship, a faithful dog or cat is a good substitute. The benefits of keeping a pet have been proven by research. It shows that not only does walking a dog ensure the benefits of regular exercise, but also the affection between owner and pet helps regulate blood pressure, decreases the risk of heart attacks and strokes, and aids relaxation.

Sharing our time and energy with others is deeply rewarding, but it can also be painful. We may see friends and relatives become unwell and die, and the closer the bonds the more we will feel their loss. The death of a husband or wife after many years of companionship, and the prospect of living alone, must be particularly hard to endure. To cope with such pain in life requires the emotional support of friends and relatives with whom we can express our grief, and also the physical support of a good diet and plenty of rest, so that we are not totally exhausted by the effects of emotional stress.

Grieving is a normal, important process after bereavement or other great loss. Each person will grieve in their own way and needs to have both time and space to go through the process. After the initial shock and numbness, it is better to allow your emotions out; try not to suppress your feelings with tranquilizers and anti-depressant drugs. The grieving process can take several years, and during it we may learn to come to terms with death, helping to prepare us for our own journey to whatever comes after this life.

Food and herbs to enhance wellbeing

In addition to maintaining a good, healthy diet you can continue to use herbs for many of the minor complaints of later life.

There are several herbs which have been used since ancient times to increase strength and energy, and for their rejuvenative powers.

Such rejuvenative herbs include:

ginseng	myrrh
cayenne	rosemary
sage	ginger
thyme	dang gui
garlic	cinnamon
shatavari	

Foods with similar properties include:

cloves	cardamon
oats	honey
parsley	watercress
onions	leeks
barley	carrots
lemon	cabbage
potatoes	

Several of the aromatic herbs contain antioxidant substances which prevent damage from free radicals and help to retard the aging process.

Herbs which contain antioxidants include:

rosemary	sage
thyme	garlic
ginger	

Foods which contain antioxidants include:

cabbage	carrots
lemons	potatoes in their skins

Several herbs have a beneficial effect upon the heart and circulation, helping to maintain a healthy blood supply to the body and brain, reducing the build up of atherosclerosis and helping to prevent arteriosclerosis, high blood pressure, heart attacks and strokes.

Herbs which benefit the circulation include:

garlic	ginger
cayenne	ginkgo
hawthorn	linden blossom
dandelion root	

Onions, potatoes, carrots, barley, oats, leeks and olive oil have similar properties.

There are also herbs which strengthen the nervous system, help to balance the emotions and enable relaxation. Such herbs can be taken to help relieve stress and tension, to support you through difficult times and to help ensure restful sleep.

These herbs will strengthen the nervous system:

rosemary	sage
oats	vervain
ginseng	

These will enhance relaxation:

chamomile	skullcap
linden blossom	catmint
lemon balm	rose
passionflower	

To help prevent and treat sluggish bowels, and ensure proper elimination of toxins, you can use herbs that enhance the function of the bowels. Choose from burdock, licorice, dandelion root and linseed.

If you are prone to infections, use herbs to stimulate the immune system.

Immunity stimulating herbs include:

thyme	echinacea
ginger	garlic
myrrh	rosemary
sage	calendula

These foods have the same effect: lemons, cabbage, cloves, parsley, carrots, honey, mustard, leeks, onions, and watercress.

If you feel the cold and suffer from poor circulation, hot teas of ginger, cinnamon, cloves, and black peppercorns will be very helpful. Adding plenty of garlic, onions, leeks, radishes, spices and pepper to your food will also stimulate blood flow and keep you warm. Avoid cold food and drinks.

Wood betony

Stachys betonica

PART USED: Flowering herb

CONTAINS: Tannins (up to 15%), saponins, alkaloids (betonicine, stachydrine, trigonelline)

KEY USES: Digestive, circulatory stimulant, nerve tonic, vulnerary, astringent, liver remedy

The name betonica comes from the Celtic *ben* meaning head, and *tonic* meaning good – referring to its use for conditions associated with the head, particularly for inveterate headaches. It relieves those related to poor circulation to the head by improving the circulation; those related to a sluggish liver by enhancing the liver's action, and those related to tension because it is a relaxant. It was taken internally and powdered for snuff for headaches, and when mixed with powdered eyebright, used to clear congestion in the head from colds and catarrh.

Wood betony acts as a tonic to the nervous system, relieving tension, anxiety and depression, and soothing pain, particularly that of neuralgia as in sciatica. It has also been used for arthritis, gout and rheumatism. It has a beneficial effect on the digestive tract and liver, and can be used for indigestion, nervous dyspepsia, spasm and colic, wind, heartburn, biliousness, liver and gallbladder problems. The tannins help to astringe the gut, making it useful for diarrhea. Its astringent effect is also useful when treating colds and catarrh. When taken as a hot tea, wood betony stimulates the circulation and helps to throw off colds and other infections – particularly those affecting the head. Trigonelline has been reported to lower blood sugar, making wood betony useful to diabetics.

The tannins in wood betony make it a useful astringent used externally to stem bleeding, speed repair and repel infection of cuts and wounds, sores, ulcers, varicose veins and hemorrhoids. It can also be used for bruises, sprains and strains, and was used in a lotion to beautify the skin.

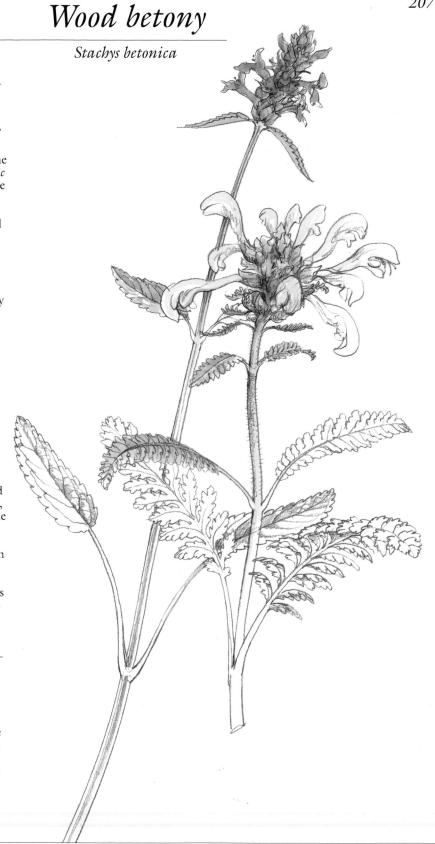

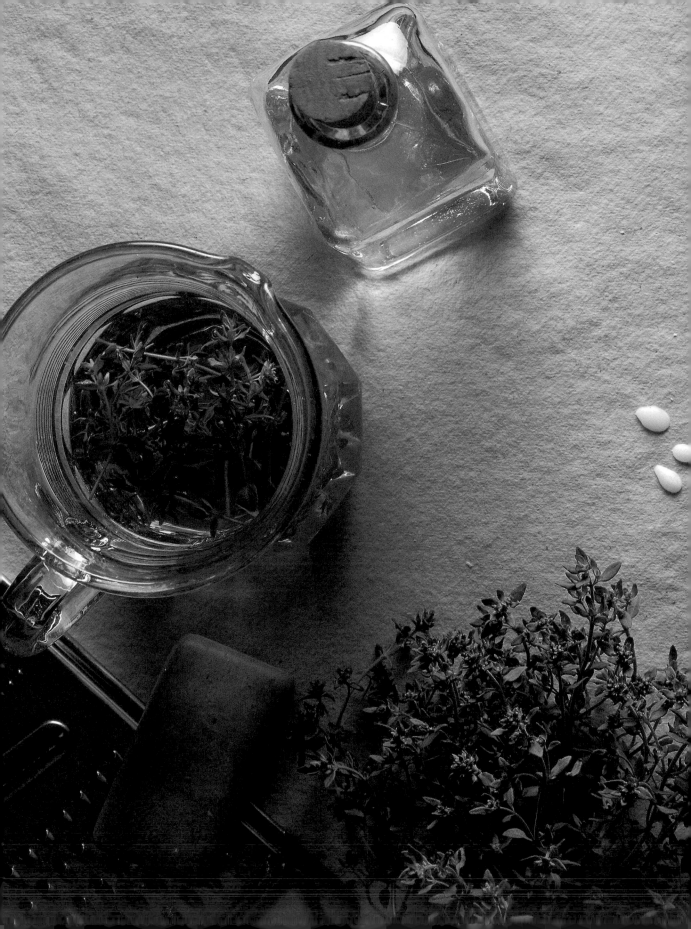

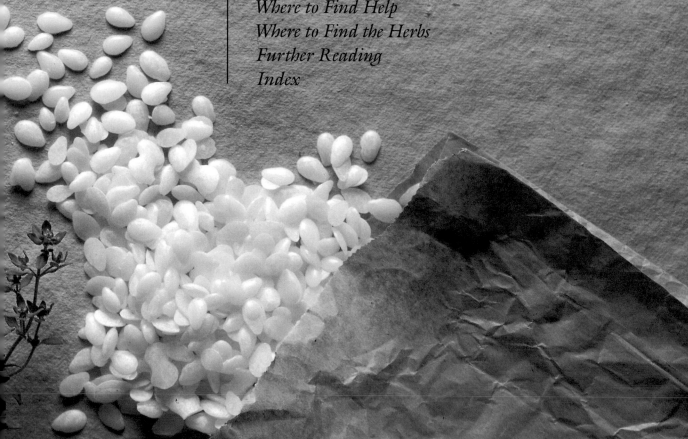

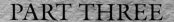PART THREE

Practical Problem Solving

First Aid
Healing Yourself
Beauty Treatments
Housekeeping Herbs

11 First Aid

Herbs can be used to treat everyday ailments and minor accidents. Every household should have a cabinet well stocked with herbs ready for use, and if possible a supply of fresh herbs from the garden in the spring and summer. First here are suggestions for the contents of your first aid cabinet.

The First Aid Cabinet

Essential oils
lavender
rosemary
thyme
tea tree

Dried herbs
linden blossom
elderflowers
peppermint
yarrow
chamomile

Other remedies
slippery elm powder
echinacea tincture
calendula tincture
St. John's wort tincture and oil
myrrh tincture
distilled witch hazel
Rescue Remedy: drops and cream
homeopathic arnica
comfrey ointment
calendula ointment
hypericum-calendula tincture and ointment

Have also in the house
aloe vera plant
fresh root ginger
local, organic honey

Abrasions and minor cuts

It may be best to avoid making a drama of children's minor accidents resulting in cuts and scrapes; the fuss makes any injury seem worse than it is.

• A couple of drops of Rescue Remedy, taken under the tongue, or one tablet of homeopathic arnica taken immediately works wonders for minor shock.
• Clean the area with herbal antiseptic to prevent infection and aid healing.

Use 4-5 drops of tincture of any of these in a little warm water, or decoctions or infusions of the herbs:

golden seal   calendula
St. John's wort   myrrh
witch hazel

If the area feels very painful, bathe it regularly with diluted St. John's wort tincture or an infusion of peppermint or lavender.

Use a few drops of the following essential oils in boiled water; they are antiseptic, pain-relieving and healing:

lavender   peppermint
eucalyptus   tea tree
geranium

These ointments are suitable for minor cuts and abrasions:

St. John's wort
calendula
comfrey
Rescue Remedy cream

• If the cut is quite deep, apply pressure to the area to stop the bleeding. If the sides are gaping open, bring them together firmly with finger and thumb. Bind the wound with surgical tape, then cover with dressing and bandage. Seek medical advice quickly, as a stitch or other means of closing the skin may be needed, and the sooner it is done, the better the cosmetic result. If the cut or abrasion is relatively minor, it is best left uncovered.

Honey applied directly to a deep wound and bandaged firmly generally prevents infection. It absorbs moisture, and few bacteria can live without moisture.

If fresh parsley is crushed and the juice applied to cuts, it will speed healing and encourage the rapid formation of pus.

The juice from crushed St. John's wort leaves can also be applied directly.

Use the following either as teas, to soak lint for application to wounds, to beat into cold cream, or to use as poultices:

comfrey   slippery elm
cabbage   rosemary
plantain leaves   elderflowers

Bites and stings

Dog bites
• Treat for shock if necessary, using Rescue Remedy, or arnica tablets.
• Cleanse the area in running water.
• Apply salt water or antiseptic herbs or oils.

These are suitable antiseptic herbs:

thyme   lavender
calendula   plantain
St. John's wort

• A poultice of fennel seed tea will draw out the poison.
• You can also bind cabbage or violet leaves over the bite. Cover with cotton bandages. Between changes, bathe it with a strong brew of rosemary.

Note Dog bites, cat bites, and especially human bites, often require antibiotic treatment. If the wound is deep, seek medical advice on tetanus.

Insect bites
To relieve swelling and pain, and to prevent infection and promote healing, use any of the following:

pulp of raw onion or garlic
cucumber juice
lavender oil
distilled witch hazel
crushed basil leaves
sage infusion
*rosemary oil: 1 teaspoon in half a
    pint of light beer*
tea tree oil
eucalyptus oil
melissa oil

Remove a bee sting by pressing it out sideways with a thumbnail rather than pulling, to avoid pressing in more poison. Apply bicarbonate of soda or honey to neutralize the acid in the poison.

Note If there is a known allergy to bees, adrenaline should be given. If there is very rapid swelling that starts to affect the lips, tongue, throat and therefore breathing, this is an emergency and the patient should be taken to hospital.

Remedies for bee and wasp stings:

lemon juice
vinegar
crushed plantain leaves
crushed garlic or sliced onion
witch hazel
lavender oil
urine
cinnamon oil

The bites of ants are relieved by applying:

garlic   *raw onion*
cucumber juice

Apply to mosquito bites:

lavender oil   *lemon juice*
witch hazel   *fennel seed tea*
cider vinegar   *crushed basil*
sliced onion

To relieve a jellyfish sting apply:

alcohol   *ammonia*
vinegar   *papaya*
urine

To prevent any bite becoming infected take echinacea internally three to six times daily.

See p.272 for advice on repelling insects. Mosquitoes can be kept away by applying oils of lavender or citronella, or by burning aromatic herbs. If your summer evenings are ruined by these insects, try this as a remedy.

Suitable aromatic herbs are:

rosemary   *sage*
lavender   *peppermint*

Healing oil for bites, wounds and chilblains

*1¹/₂ tablespoons powdered rosemary,
    rue, woundwort, or basil*
1 cupful salad oil
1 teaspoon vinegar

Place ingredients in a jar, stand it in a container of sand, and place in sunlight. Shake it daily. After five days drain off the oil and pour into another jar, add more herbs and repeat the whole process twice. The last time, leave herbs to macerate for 14 days. If sunlight is not available, use a warm oven over several days.

Boils and carbuncles
A boil is a local inflammation of a hair root or a cut caused by bacterial infection. A carbuncle is a cluster of boils on one site. Boils are the body's natural way of ridding itself of noxious poisons. If you suffer frequently from boils, you need a general reassessment of your diet, lifestyle, or both, with a view to enhancing your body's resistance. It may also be that there is a particular focus for sepsis in the body such as a dental

abscess or chronically diseased tonsils. Diabetes is a cause of recurrent boils.

Make sure your diet is rich in fresh fruit and vegetables as vitamin C is essential in fighting infection. Take plenty of garlic.

Herbs to treat the immune system:

echinacea
huang qi

Herbs to fight infection:

myrrh	*dandelion root*
thyme	*burdock*

Here are two treatments which, applied externally, will draw out and discharge the toxins from boils and carbuncles.

Mix equal parts of honey and cod liver oil, and apply on lint, renewing the dressing every five hours. Honey draws to the site body fluids containing antibodies which help overcome infection.

Alternatively, make a hot poultice of slippery elm to which a few drops of either lavender or eucalyptus oil have been added.

Bruises and sprains

Sprains occur when the ligaments around joints, such as wrists and ankles, over-stretch and sometimes even tear.

• Support the sprained joint with a bandage.
• Use ice packs; a packet of frozen peas is ideal.
• Apply cold compresses for half an hour to contain bruising.

Use any of the following:

distilled witch hazel
comfrey: apply bruised leaves directly
arnica: 2-3 drops of tincture in half a pint of water
hyssop: bruise the leaves until the juice runs, and place on the painful part
calendula, yarrow, St. John's wort:

use 1-2 tsp of tincture in a little water as a cold compress, or apply fresh leaves
cabbage: bind the leaf over the painful part

Useful poultices for bruises and sprains are also made of chopped parsley, or fresh cranesbill leaves, held in place by a bandage.

To reduce discoloration and pain, cover the bruise with the inner side of banana skin, or pulped mallow leaves, held in place with a cold, wet bandage.

If you bruise easily you may be deficient in vitamin C and bioflavonoids.

Consult your practitioner if pain has not considerably improved after 24 hours; the underlying bone may be broken.

Burns and scalds

These can safely be treated at home if only a small area is affected and only the top layer of skin is burnt. Do not puncture blisters from burns. If burns become more painful, or infected, consult your practitioner.

• Immerse the area immediately in cold water for at least ten minutes or until the pain subsides.
• Apply every 15 minutes a remedy to minimize swelling and prevent infection.

Use one of the following:

undiluted lavender oil
undiluted vitamin E oil
comfrey ointment
St. John's wort oil
fresh aloe vera juice
distilled witch hazel compress
comfrey infusion compress
calendula flowers chopped and wrapped in gauze strip
the grated pulp of half a raw potato

See p.214 for other remedies.

Arnica

Arnica montana

ALSO KNOWN AS: Leopard's bane, wolf's bane, mountain tobacco, mountain daisy

PARTS USED: Dried flowers or extract. Homeopathic ointments and other preparations available

CONTAINS: Volatile oil (including terpenes, thymol, thymol methyl ether), palmitic, linoleic, linolenic and myristic acids, resin, arnicin (a bitter principle), helanalin, tannin, steroid (arnisterin, arnidiol), flavones, betain, inulin, phytosterol

KEY USES: Analgesic, expectorant, anti-inflammatory, nervine, local stimulant, diaphoretic, emollient, diuretic, antibacterial, vulnerary

Arnica is a wonderful medicine. It increases resistance to infection, including listeria and salmonella, and speeds healing after surgery, dental extractions and injuries of all kinds. It can be taken, generally in homeopathic doses, for mental and physical shock, bruises, sprains, pain and swelling and fractures. It also has a reputation for resolving fevers, stimulating the circulation and reabsorbing internal bleeding.

Arnica can be used externally as a dilute tincture or in a cream to speed healing of wounds, bruises, sprains and swellings. It is wonderful for calming children who may have fallen over, bumped their heads, or knocked themselves. Applied over any unbroken surface it will ease pain, relieve rheumatic joints, and painful, swollen feet. Diluted one part in ten with calendula it can be used for skin rashes and other inflammatory skin problems.

Note Arnica should not be taken internally except in homeopathic doses, or using one drop of tincture stirred into a glass of water. Large doses taken internally can cause severe irritation to the mucous membranes of the stomach and bowel. If the tincture is applied neat to broken skin it may cause an allergic reaction.

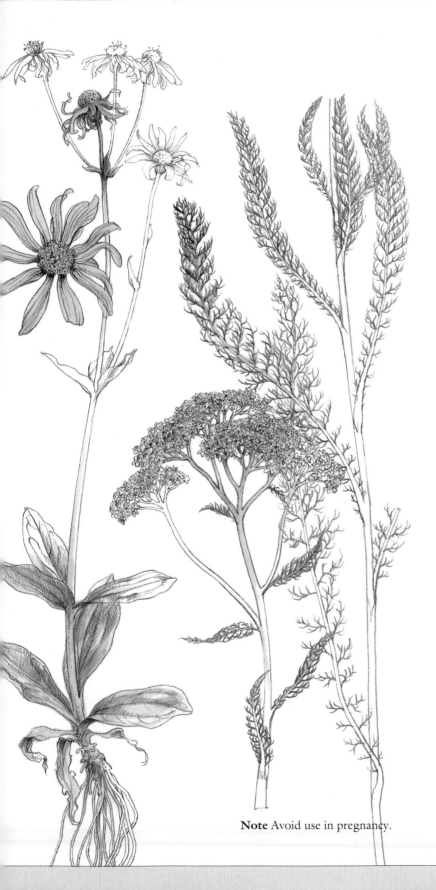

Yarrow

Achillea millefolium

ALSO KNOWN AS: Nosebleed, millefoil

PART USED: Aerial parts

CONTAINS: Volatile oil, coumarins, lactones, amino acids, sterols, bitters, flavonoids, tannins, saponins, salicylic acid, sugars, cyanidin

KEY USES: Astringent, vulnerary, anti-inflammatory, antiseptic, digestive, bitter tonic, antispasmodic, diaphoretic, hypotensive, diuretic

Yarrow is a highly versatile remedy, with anti-inflammatory and antiseptic volatile oils, and astringent tannins. The resins are also astringent and antiseptic, while silica promotes tissue repair. These properties promote healing of cuts and wounds, burns and ulcers, and inflammatory skin conditions. In the digestive system, yarrow stimulates the appetite, enhances digestion and absorption; its astringent properties curb diarrhea and dysentery, and stem bleeding from the lining of the gut. The antiseptic and anti-inflammatory properties treat infections and inflamed conditions such as gastritis and enteritis, the bitters stimulate liver function, while its antispasmodics relax tensionin cramp, wind, colic or nervous dyspepsia.

Taken hot, yarrow is excellent for helping to throw off fevers and infections such as colds, flu, coughs, and sore throats. It clears heat and toxins from the system by causing sweating. As a tonic to the circulatory system, yarrow helps improve varicose veins, hemorrhoids, phlebitis and thrombosis, and reduces blood pressure. Yarrow's diuretic action aids the elimination of fluid and toxins from the system via the urine. It also relieves cystitis, irritable bladder, stones, and gravel. It helps relieve painful joints and clear the skin. Yarrow contains sterols which have a hormone-like action and help to regulate the menstrual cycle. It reduces heavy bleeding and uteric congestion, and relieve heavy periods. It is also a tonic to the nervous system.

Note Avoid use in pregnancy.

egg white beaten stiffly
egg white and olive oil whisked
   together, applied in layers allowed
   to dry between applications
grated comfrey root, held in place
   with gauze
grated carrots or leeks
melon flesh
glycerine
black tea
honey: apply gauze soaked in honey
   and cover with bandage
elderflower tea or cream
chickweed infusion

Any of these remedies will help relieve pain and aid healing. Re-apply when the pain returns.

• Raise the affected part slightly to slow the blood flow and ease the pain.
• Once the pain has diminished, cover loosely with a clean, dry dressing. Avoid using fluffy material which may stick to the burn; if it does, soak with a warm golden seal or echinacea decoction.

Chilblains

The onset of chilblains is related to circulation problems, often made worse by becoming cold, a poor diet, a sedentary occupation and wearing tight shoes. It may help to take plenty of exercise and wear warm clothes.

You can warm the feet with a mixture of powdered cayenne pepper and talcum or arrowroot powder. Use it to dust the feet before dressing.

To improve the circulation, take hot foot baths with a decoction of 1 oz ginger and two sticks of cinnamon in two pints of water. Soak the feet occasionally in salty hot water.

Take plenty of garlic and ginger in your diet to improve the circulation.

Salve for chilblains:

Crush some primrose leaves and beat them into melted lanolin and honey with a few drops of thyme oil. Apply the salve warm and cover the feet with large cotton socks.

Another treatment is to apply crushed snowdrop bulbs, or sliced onion. Cover one side of the onion with salt and put the fresh side on the chilblains. Cover with a clean bandage.

Other treatments for chilblains:

rosemary oil
lavender oil
peppermint oil
undiluted Friar's Balsam (on
   unbroken chilblains)
garlic oil or juice
tincture of myrrh
nettle juice

Chilblains may indicate a lack of calcium and silica.

Sources of these in the diet include:

yoghurt	cheese
soybeans	almonds
millet	sesame seeds
lemons	oats
spinach	parsley
figs	green vegetables

Cold sores

These are caused by the virus herpes simplex. A first attack may bring swollen glands, a feeling of being unwell, and painful mouth ulcers. Subsequent attacks occur mostly when people are run down, and start with a tingle and itch. Then tiny blisters form, mainly around the nostrils and lips. They break open after a time, weep, crust over and disappear. Scratching spreads the virus and can lead to bacterial infection.

The virus lives permanently in the nerve endings of many adults and children. Babies can be infected by the virus, and it can complicate other inflammation or infections such as eczema.

The cold sore virus can be activated by a rise in skin temperature, perhaps caused by a fever, or by sunshine.

The following may also activate the virus:

poor diet
dietary triggers such as chocolate,
   peanuts
mental or physical stress
rubbing or chafing of the skin
menstruation
depleted immunity from being run
   down

To treat cold sores it is important to raise the level of the immune system, thus helping the body to combat viral attack. You can also adjust your diet, reducing intake of the amino acid arginine which predisposes to the virus, and increasing that of lysine, which helps control it. (See also Herpes, p.227.)

Arginine is high in:

gelatine	chocolate
carob	coconut
oats	peanuts
soybeans	wheat flour
wheatgerm	

Lysine is high in:

chicken
beans and beansprouts
brewer's yeast
most vegetables and fruit except
   pears

To help the immune system, take plenty of garlic and foods rich in:

vitamin C	bioflavonoids
B vitamins	calcium
magnesium	

While you have cold sores, do not indulge in kissing and use separate facecloths and towels from those of other members of the family.

Be sure to take plenty of exercise, to stimulate the lymphatic system.

These herbs will support the lymphatic system and the immune system:

echinacea   nettle
golden seal   wormwood
cleavers   calendula
plantain   myrrh
bayberry   poke root
burdock   dandelion root
huang qi   licorice

These can be used externally :

melissa oil
lavender oil
calendula tincture
myrrh tincture
golden seal tincture

Fainting

The classic remedy for faintness – to sit with the head between the knees – returns blood to the head; lying down does this too. After a faint, let the subject lie still, but raise the legs to encourage blood flow to the brain. Once the subject regains consciousness, give small sips of water or ginger tea made with root ginger. Make sure there is as much fresh air as possible.

Take teas of rock rose flowers, or wild rose flowers if they are available; take honey and ginger, and drink teas of elderflowers or rosemary.

Hay fever

If you suffer from hay fever, start immune enhancement to decrease your susceptibility to hay fever two months before the season starts by taking ginseng, huang qi, or echinacea and eating some comb honey daily, though not if you are allergic to bee stings.

When symptoms first appear, fast for one or two days on fruit.

Inhale vapour from a basin of hot water to which a few drops of melissa or chamomile oil have been added. This will soothe the mucous membranes and quieten the allergic reaction.

These herbs will relieve symptoms:

echinacea   elderflowers
peppermint   nettles
chamomile   yarrow

There are dietary measures you can try, such as eliminating wheat or dairy produce, or both, from your diet. Take extra vitamin C, zinc, vitamin A and calcium.

Try a steam inhalant using a pint of hot water with one teaspoon of this mixture:

30 ml Friar's Balsam
2.5 ml eucalyptus oil
6 drops peppermint oil
5 drops lavender oil
5 drops pine oil

Headaches

Use the essential oils of lavender, peppermint, or rosemary as inhalants or in compresses.

The essential oils of lavender, rosemary or peppermint can be massaged into the head at the site of the pain.

These herbs can be taken as teas or tinctures to relieve headache:

chamomile   hops
wood betony   skullcap
peppermint   lavender
rosemary   pulsatilla
linden blossom   vervain
feverfew

Heat rash

It is important to recognize sunstroke when dealing with both sunburn and heat rash. When the body becomes severely overheated the cooling mechanism of the skin fails, and it becomes hot and dry. The body temperature can

rise dangerously, giving rise to feelings of dizziness, nausea, weakness, and fever, often with a severe headache.

Treat for shock, as above, and seek medical help. Cool the body with cool water until the temperature drops, but avoid over-chilling. Give water to drink with half a teaspoon of salt to every glass.

Nettle is a good remedy for heat rash; apply it as a poultice made of nettles soaked in warm water, or as a compress using the nettle infusion. Cold compresses using lavender oil are also effective.

Nosebleeds

Nosebleeds which occur after a blow to the head may be a sign of a fracture; seek medical help immediately.

The usual cause of nosebleeds is the rupture of blood vessels on the inner surface of the nose, brought on by hard nose blowing, sneezing, a knock, a foreign body, or an infection.

Hold the sides of the nose firmly together just under the bony part, well above the nostrils, for five to six minutes to allow a clot to form. When the bleeding stops, don't blow or sniff as this could dislodge the clot and start the bleeding again. Apply a cold compress to the back and sides of the neck. Lean the head forward. Calendula tincture or oil of cypress on cotton wool will quickly stop a nosebleed. Hold it under the nose and gently sniff.

If nosebleeds happen often, consult your practitioner. If no cause can be found, you can take extra bioflavonoids and vitamin C, or rutin tablets to strengthen capillary walls.

Use the following as astringents to stop the bleeding. Apply by sniffing gently from a piece of cotton wool:

witch hazel   St. John's wort
yarrow

Scalds, see *burns*

Shock

There are two kinds of shock: an emotional shock which accompanies bad news and deep stress, and medical shock which follows trauma such as a car accident.

For the first kind of shock, take one or two drops of arnica tincture stirred in a glass of water, or homeopathic arnica tablets. Rescue Remedy is also appropriate here. For this kind of shock, and stress, take teas or tinctures of lemon balm, chamomile, or skullcap.

Medical shock of the kind which can follow a serious injury requires urgent medical attention, though both arnica and Rescue Remedy are useful if there is no possibility of internal injury.

Splinters

Never ignore splinters, as the wound may become septic. Seek medical assistance if the splinter is large, especially if it is glass. Use an antiseptic to wash the area. Try to pull the splinter out with tweezers. Sterilize a fine needle in a flame and use it to ease out the splinter. Heat also helps draw out splinters.

You can apply a hot poultice made with:

slippery elm   bread
comfrey ointment   bran

Alternatively, apply hypericum-calendula ointment covered with a plaster to draw out the splinter.

If the wound becomes infected, treat with crushed garlic, not in contact with the skin but wrapped in a cloth then used as a bandage. Leave it for two days and then replace it daily.

Alternatively in cases of infection you can apply calendula tincture, or the essential oils of lavender, lemon, or tea tree.

Sprains, see *bruises*

Stings, see *bites*

Sunburn

When treating sunburn look out for symptoms of sunstroke (see under Heat rash, p.215), which can be serious.

Relieve the pain of sunburn by taking a cool bath to which a few drops of lavender oil have been added. Apply Rescue Remedy cream when the skin is dry.

These will also relieve the pain:

fresh cucumber juice
goat's milk with a little honey
buttermilk and honey
dock leaves laid over the area

Infusions of the following may be taken as cold teas and used for bathing the area:

nettle   peppermint
chickweed   chamomile
calendula

The essential oils of bergamot or lavender can be added to a cool bath or applied to the skin in a base oil.

The following can also be applied to relieve soreness and burning:

calendula tincture mixed with olive oil
St. John's wort oil or ointment
dilute nettle tincture or ointment
aloe vera juice
fresh live yoghurt
solution of sodium bicarbonate

It may help the skin to resist sunburn if you take vitamin B complex some time before exposure. See p.259 (Herbs for Beauty) for other sunburn treatments.

The best preventive measure against sunburn is to avoid being in the midday sun, or if you must go out, using a sunblock and covering up the body.

Toothache

If the pain is caused by a cavity, apply a little clove oil to the site until you can see your dentist. Echinacea is also anesthetic; take it as a mouthwash and swallow it. Yarrow, peppermint, or dried hops taken as infusions will soothe the pain.

Travel sickness

Travel sickness is nausea and vomiting which occur when there is disorientation; this happens when the brain receives conflicting messages – the eyes indicate that the world is still while the ears tell the brain it is moving. The normal relief is to look at the horizon, outside the vehicle, to confirm via the eyes that the world is indeed moving underneath you. Don't read. Have plenty of fresh air.

Ginger is excellent for nausea, so chew fresh root ginger or crystallized ginger, drink ginger beer or ginger tea, or take ginger tincture as drops in water. Teas of meadowsweet or peppermint can also be sipped every few minutes.

Wounds and deep cuts

Medical help is needed for deep wounds. Deep wounds carry the risk of tetanus. If you are unsure when you last had tetanus immunization, find out. A booster is needed ten years after the first immunization.

The advice at the foot of p.210 applies here. Place the injured part under running water for about five minutes. Then apply wet cloths or large dock leaves sprinkled with witch hazel.

The fresh leaves of these can be laid over surface cuts; bind them with cloth and change three times daily, exposing to the air between changes.

cabbage   kale
lettuce   comfrey

Plantain

Plantago major

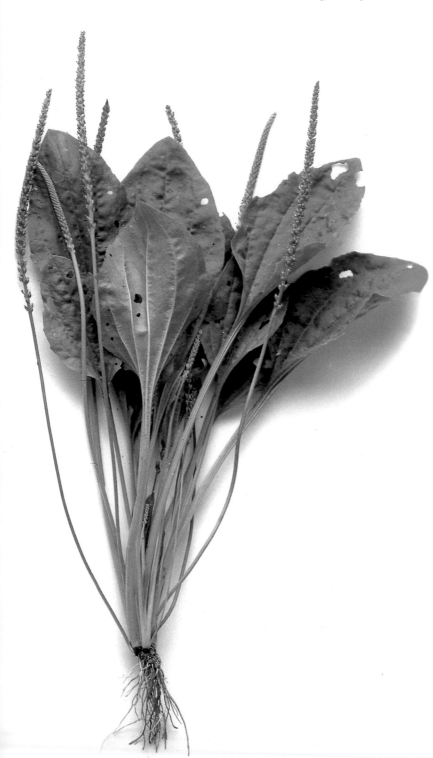

ALSO KNOWN AS: Broad-leaved plantain, ribwort, snakeweed

ALSO: *Plantago psyllium*, Psyllium plantain or fleaseed; *P. lanceolata*

PARTS USED: Leaves, *P. psyllium*: Seeds

CONTAINS: Leaves: mucilage, glycosides, tannins, silica. Seeds: 30% mucilage, monoterpene alkaloids, glycosides, fixed oil, fatty acids, tannins, sugars

KEY USES: Leaves: Demulcent, refrigerant, detoxifying, astringent, vulnerary, decongestant, expectorant, antiseptic, diuretic. Seeds: bulk laxative

Plantain is famous as a wound healer and an antidote to poisons. It clears heat, congestion and toxins from the body, useful in treating fevers, infections and skin problems. Its mucilage has a soothing effect particularly in the respiratory, digestive and urinary systems. It protects their mucous linings from irritation and relaxes spasm in asthma and colic; it soothes the cough reflex, relieving harsh, tickly, and nervous coughs. The tannins are astringent, useful to reduce swelling and inflammation, staunching bleeding and encouraging healing, explaining its traditional use for TB, bleeding in the stomach and bowels, vomiting of blood, diarrhea and colitis, and for excessive menstrual bleeding.

Plantain depresses the secretion of mucous, particularly in the respiratory system – useful when treating colds, catarrh, sinusitis, bronchial congestion and allergic conditions such as hay fever and asthma. Its expectorant action clears phlegm from the chest. It can be used for catarrhal congestion in the middle ear, glue ear and ear infections. The antiseptic action of plantain augments its success as a remedy for respiratory complaints such as colds, sore throats, tonsilitis and chest infections. It also helps clear stomach and bowel infections, as well as urinary infections, cystitis, prostatis and urethritis, soothing and reducing the pain and irritation of colic. Plantain is a useful remedy for prostatic enlargement.

12 *Healing Yourself*

The natural biological functions and rhythms that characterize women, and which are responsible for menstruation, fertility, conception and childbirth, are naturally prone to imbalances and disruption. A variety of factors in a woman's life, such as stress, overwork, lack of exercise and relaxation, poor diet and sexual problems, can disrupt the smooth running of the system. They can upset the hormone balance, reduce immunity, influence circulation to and from the reproductive system, increase tension and congestion and thereby contribute to the range of gynecological problems that plague so many women.

It is often in the treatment of such problems that women feel particularly vulnerable: they concern the most private parts of the body. Most women prefer to be treated by other women, who are more likely to empathize with the experience and possible causes of the problem.

Many women nowadays are becoming increasingly knowledgeable about their bodies, and through self help involving a healthy diet and lifestyle, are working as far as they can to prevent illness. When imbalances and ailments do occur, they try to view them from a holistic perspective; that is, they look on symptoms not simply as an isolated, local problem, but as a manifestation of disharmony on a more general level.

Throughout history women have used plants to regulate hormone balance, and enhance the function of the reproductive system. Herbs have also been used to aid healing when problems arise. There are many herbs which act on the reproductive system, relieving congestion, increasing circulation to and from the area, resolving heat and inflammation, relaxing tension and pain, and many which have a balancing effect on female hormones. There are uterine tonics that tone and strengthen the tissues in the reproductive tract and maintain their health and efficient functioning. Some herbs relax tension. Some contain steroidal saponins which closely resemble human hormones and are greatly beneficial where gynecological problems are related, as they often are, to hormone imbalance. Using a good diet, a healthy lifestyle and the therapeutic use of herbs, the majority of gynecological symptoms that so many women suffer can be relieved. Equally important, through understanding how they arose, women may come to a greater knowledge of themselves and their bodies.

Gynecological ailments and treatments

Benign breast problems

Many women suffer from breast problems such as tenderness, aching, lumpiness, and other difficulties, and it is reassuring to note that about 90 per cent of all such breast problems are benign. However, it is best to investigate any breast problems quickly, as malignant conditions can mimic benign ones.

Benign Mammary Dysplasia (BMD)

This is also known as fibrocystic breast disease, chronic cystic mastitis, fibroadenosis or cyclical mastalgia. It is characterized by tenderness and lumpiness of the breasts; one or more painful masses may be felt in one or both of the breasts. The tenderness, size of the breasts and size of the lumps fluctuate according to the menstrual cycle, being worst in the week before the period. Women between the ages of 20 and 40 are mostly affected, and generally as one gets older the lumps become more definite. Some women have at times such tender breasts that they cannot bear them to be touched and need to wear a bra at night for support and protection.

Contributing factors to BMD

Mammary dysplasia is related to estrogen levels, particularly with over-stimulation of the breast tissue by estrogen and prolactin – it does not occur in post-menopausal women. It is aggravated by methylxanthines in coffee, cola, chocolate and tea, and eliminating these from the diet has a direct effect on reducing the size and pains of cysts in the breasts during the week before menstruation. Note that decaffeinated coffee still contains methylxanthines.

Research indicates that women who suffer from tender breasts and cysts have lower levels of selenium in their bloodstreams than other women, as do women with breast cancer.

Low thyroid function and the low iodine levels associated with it may contribute to breast problems. Thyroid hormone helps the liver's metabolism of estrogen and low thyroid levels are therefore associated with excess blood estrogen.

Excess fat in the diet is also implicated. Studies have shown that reducing dietary fat can substantially reduce breast problems, blood estrogen and prolactin levels, as well as blood cholesterol and weight.

Women with constipation, particularly those with fewer bowel movements than one every other day, are more prone to benign mammary dysplasia than others. This is because of the accumulation of harmful bacteria in the gut and poor excretion of estrogen. This is more of a problem with those who eat meat.

Stress plays a major part in upsetting hormone balance and so could contribute significantly to breast problems.

Self help for BMD

○ Avoid tea, coffee, cola and chocolate.
○ Cut out junk food, including refined foods and sugar, avoid excess alcohol, eat plenty of fresh fruit and vegetables.
○ Eat a low fat diet, reduce dairy products.
○ Stop smoking.
○ Eat only organic meat, to avoid residues of growth-stimulating hormones, only free-range chicken, fish or combinations of vegetable proteins, grains, nuts, seeds, beans and pulses.
○ Ensure your bowels are emptied daily, by seeking treatment if necessary (see p.121).
○ Eat live yoghurt every day, or take supplements of lactobacillus to help maintain the correct bacterial population of the bowel.
○ Essential fatty acids are vital to normal hormone balance, so as well as adding to the diet pure unrefined virgin oils (olive oil, sunflower and sesame oil) take a 500 mg daily supplement of evening primrose oil or gamma linoleic acid in some other form such as borage or blackcurrant seed oil capsules.

Supplements of vitamin B6 are often helpful as B6 helps the metabolism of essential fatty acids.

Vitamin E has significantly reduced breast pain and benign cysts in many women. Take between 300 and 1200 iu daily; preferably at night.

Herbal remedies for BMD

To help maintain normal thyroid function take kelp daily.
To balance estrogen levels take chaste tree or false unicorn root, or both, daily.

Add herbs to aid liver function and the elimination of toxins and excess estrogen from the body, such as burdock, dandelion leaf, yellow dock root, or calendula.

If the breasts are particularly painful add black cohosh.

To aid lymphatic drainage and clear congestion of the breast, use calendula leaves or poke root.

If you feel that stress is a contributory factor, add skullcap or vervain to your prescription.

Massage your breasts gently every day to increase the circulation to and from them and to stimulate lymphatic drainage. Use dilute oils of lavender, cypress and rose singly or in mixtures, and add a few drops of essential oil to your baths.

Breast abscess

An abscess develops from a bacterial infection in the breast tissue, which normally enters through a cracked nipple. A crack can occur in a nipple through breastfeeding or irritation and inflammation caused by rubbing of clothes on the nipple – such as "jogger's nipple". The development of an abscess may indicate a depleted immune system.

Symptoms of breast abscess

swelling, pain, throbbing and redness of the breast
hardness and raised temperature in the breast
fever and malaise
tender, swollen lymph nodes under the arm
a pus-filled abscess which gradually works to the surface

Self help for breast abscess

○ While breastfeeding, treat promptly any tenderness, swelling of the breast (see p.172) or cracks which occur in the nipple (see p.171) to avoid the development of mastitis (see p.172) or a breast abscess.
○ Seek treatment if you are constipated (see p.121). Constipation can contribute to a toxic system.
○ If you are diagnosed as having an abscess, take a multimineral and multivitamin supplement and vitamin C (5 g daily), to help the body's fight against infection.
○ Avoid sugar, junk foods, tea,

coffee, alcohol and fatty foods.
○ Make sure you eat a light diet containing plenty of fresh fruit and vegetables. A brown rice and vegetable fast for three to four days may be helpful.
○ Draw out the infection with a hot Epsom Salts compress. Dissolve the salts in water and apply as a compress at night.

Note If you suspect you have a breast abscess, you should visit your practitioner. If neglected, an abscess could lead to the development of toxemia.

Herbal treatment for breast abscess

At the first signs of an abscess take echinacea and garlic every two hours to enhance the immune system. Combine this with herbs to clear toxins and congestion from the breast and stimulate lymphatic drainage – cleavers, poke root, calendula, dandelion root and burdock. Black cohosh is useful where there is a lot of pain.

Once the abscess has developed and is throbbing (indicating the presence of pus), it is best to encourage the pus to come to the surface by applying hot compresses or poultices of herbs to the area for an hour three times daily. Plantain, flax (linseed), and slippery elm have-drawing properties. A hot bread or a cooked onion poultice may also prove useful. Add a few drops of essential oils to the above poultices or to hot water for compresses. Rosewood, geranium, lavender, tea tree, eucalyptus or chamomile will help reduce infection as well as inflammation.

Alternatively, dilute 15 drops of oil in 20 ml of base oil and massage the breast gently twice daily.

If you have a fever, go to bed and take linden blossom or chamomile tea through the day.

Endometriosis

Endometriosis occurs when endometrial tissue, which normally lines the inside of the uterus, grows in other sites in the pelvis, such as on the ovaries or the fallopian tubes. It can also grow on the bladder and intestines.

The patches of endometrial tissue respond to menstrual hormones just as does the lining of the uterus, growing and then bleeding. However, the blood is not able to escape from the body in the normal way of menstruation, and instead forms congestion in the pelvis. Pain and inflammation can lead to a build up of scar tissue and adhesions between the pelvic organs – such as ovary to uterus, uterus to bowel. Because of this endometriosis is likely to cause infertility. "Chocolate cysts" filled with blood can form where there is regular bleeding at sites of endometriosis.

Symptoms of endometriosis

very painful periods
pain with sexual intercourse
infertility
cyclical bowel disturbance
heavy menstrual bleeding

Diagnosis of endometriosis

Endometriosis is normally diagnosed by laparoscopy, during which a small incision is made near the navel and a small lighted instrument like a periscope inserted to inspect the abdominal organs.

Causes of endometriosis

There are several theories about the factors that can lead to endometriosis.

It may be related to an imbalance of hormones, with over production of estrogen being at fault. It stops after the menopause and is most common in women who delay childbearing, begin sexual intercourse late, and who have few or no children. During pregnancy it goes into remission, which can last for some time afterwards.

There may be genetic factors involved as it tends to run in families.

It may be caused by menstrual blood and tissue from the uterus flowing backwards up the fallopian tubes into the pelvic cavity during spasms.

Endometrial tissue may be carried through the lymphatic system and deposited elsewhere – in rare cases endometriosis has been found in the lungs.

Endometrial growths sometimes appear in scar tissue from previous pelvic surgery, so surgery may spread existing endometriosis.

Endometriosis may form on misplaced remnants of prenatal tissue (that formed before birth).

Stress appears to be a major factor contributing to hormonal imbalance and endometriosis. Particularly significant is when stress is related to sexuality, lack of confidence, anorexia, difficulty with intimate relationships, break up of a relationship, sexual problems, or a history of sexual abuse.

There may be a link between chronic candidiasis and endometriosis, as many endometriosis sufferers have had a history of vaginal thrush, or over-use of antibiotics and often symptoms of allergy associated with candida.

Herbal treatment of endometriosis

Internal Hormonal balancing herbs are called for, to reduce oversecretion of estrogen. These include chaste tree, false unicorn root and lady's mantle. Other hormonal regulators and tonics to the reproductive system can be used, for example raspberry leaf and partridge berry.

If there is a lot of pain, use pelvic relaxants or analgesics (pain relievers) such as pulsatilla, chamomile, motherwort, cramp bark, wild yam or blue cohosh.

Where there is much pelvic congestion or heavy bleeding, or both, astringents such as witch hazel, golden seal, oak bark or beth root should be helpful.

Where there is stress use supportive herbs such as vervain, skullcap, oats and the Bach Flower Remedies (see p.246–7) that are specifically indicated.

You may have an overburdened liver which cannot deal efficiently with sex hormones and their breakdown, so herbs to enhance liver function should be included in your prescription. Choose from rosemary, dandelion root or calendula.

Saw palmetto can block the action of FSH (see p.86) that increases endometrial tissue.

If there are signs of candida or thrush treat accordingly (see p.226).

External Essential oils of geranium, rose, cypress and clary sage will help to relieve stress and to resolve issues surrounding femininity and sexuality; they will also help balance hormones. Dilute the essential oils in a base oil such as almond oil for massage to the abdomen or back, and add them undiluted to baths, sitz-baths, hand and foot baths, and vaporizers. The essential oils of chamomile and lavender can also be used in this way for their gently relaxing effects.

Meditation, relaxation techniques, and counselling or psychotherapy may all be helpful in resolving issues surrounding endometriosis. Seek professional help if you feel there are unresolved emotional problems from your past.

Dietary measures for endometriosis

○ Avoid caffeine completely.
○ Avoid alcohol and all junk foods.
○ Take supplements of vitamins E, B complex and C, zinc, and evening primrose oil. Selenium ACE can also help. Calcium and magnesium (500 mg) in the second half of the cycle can help reduce cramping and PMS symptoms.

Bladder and kidney disorders

The urinary system performs the vital task of producing and excreting urine, so cleansing the body of waste products. The system helps to maintain a constant internal environment by governing the water and chemical composition as well as the acid-alkali balance of the body.

It is important to drink plenty of liquid each day to assist the kidneys in their cleansing work, to flush through toxins and the waste products of metabolism, and to prevent them from causing irritation of the urinary tract.

Urinary tract infection

Urinary tract infections occur commonly in women, and are frequently caused by bacteria (E coli) from the bowel affecting the bladder. They creep round from the anus, helped by wiping from back to front rather than vice versa after urination or a bowel movement. They affect women much more than men, mostly because of anatomical differences: the urinary passage to the bladder, the urethra, is much shorter in women.

Vaginal infections such as thrush and chlamydia can also be related to urinary tract infections. Infection can affect the urethra, then pass into the bladder, causing cystitis. From the bladder it can pass along the urethra to affect the kidneys, causing pyelonephritis. A urinary infection may be low grade and cause few symptoms, but more commonly it produces a variety of uncomfortable symptoms.

Symptoms of urinary infections

an urge to pass water frequently
possibly, pink or cloudy urine indi-
     cating the presence of blood
urgency in passing water
pain, burning, or stinging on pass-
     ing water

The presence of a urinary infection can be confirmed by urine analysis. However, cystitis symptoms can occur where there is no evidence of bacteria in the urine. They occur intermittently in some women and chronically in others.

Causes of cystitis symptoms

Drinking too little causes very concentrated urine which can contain substances which irritate the urethra or the walls of the bladder. It also means that toxins and micro-organisms are not flushed through the system as frequently or effectively as they should be, leaving them to irritate the bladder, or develop into infection.

Incomplete emptying of the bladder can leave a residue of urine containing irritants and bacteria which can multiply and cause inflammation or infection.

Chemical irritants such as soaps, bubble bath, talcum powder, perfumes or vaginal deodorants may set up inflammation of the urethra. Chlorine from swimming pools and biological washing powder may also be to blame.

Contraceptive devices can cause problems. Spermicidal cream can cause irritation; a

diaphragm can put pressure on the bladder causing incomplete emptying, the pill can cause hormonal changes which can make the bladder or urethra more sensitive than usual.

Sexual intercourse can cause bruising to the urethra which is situated just above the vaginal opening. This can lead to inflammation or introduce infection (which is why it is called "honeymoon cystitis" when it is related to sexual activity). The urethra is affected by other movements or vibrations such as motorbike, horse or even bicycle riding, for the same reason.

You may be particularly sensitive or allergic to various foods which irritate the nerve endings of the bladder. Foods or drinks such as chlorinated water, orange juice, alcohol, sugar, coffee, tea, vinegar, spices, gluten and milk products can all be to blame.

Hormonal changes during pregnancy, causing relaxation to the smooth muscle throughout the urinary system, slow the flow of urine through the dilated tubules and bladder. The more stagnant urine encourages the growth of bacteria and infections easily arise.

During the menopause hormone changes can also lead to more relaxed muscle tone with the same results.

Extremes of either cold or heat can result in irritation of the bladder.

Thrush can also cause cystitis.

Cystitis can accompany other health problems such as diabetes, multiple sclerosis, fibroids, stress, kidney stones, prolapse and endometriosis.

Self help for cystitis and urinary infections

If you have a tendency to infection or irritation of the urethra and bladder, the following measures should be helpful.

○ Always wipe from front to back after urination or a bowel movement. Try to avoid the spread of fecal bacteria from the anus during sex. It helps to wash the area beforehand. Passing water after sex will help to flush out any bacteria which may have been introduced into the urinary system, so drink some water beforehand.
○ Use KY jelly or some other kind of lubricant to avoid bruising during sex. Remember that petroleum-based products should not be used with condoms or a diaphragm (cap).
○ Drink plenty of liquid to keep the system flushed out particularly before and after sex, and at least three to four pints daily.
○ Keep the anal area as clean as possible by bathing it with natural unscented soap, and after each bowel movement if you have a tendency to recurrent cystitis.
○ Empty your bladder as soon as possible when you feel the need.
○ Avoid the use of vaginal deodorants, perfumes, soaps or any other chemicals.
○ Do not wear tight fitting clothes or underwear and avoid synthetic materials as they provide a moist, warm environment, loved by bacteria and other micro-organisms.
○ If you use the pill, the diaphragm, spermicidal gel or condoms, try a different method of contraception for a while to see if the tendency to cystitis diminishes. You may need to discuss this with the family planning clinic.
○ It is best to wear sanitary pads rather than tampons while menstruating as the strings of tampons could spread bacteria from the anal area. Make sure you change your protection very regularly.
○ Make sure your diet and lifestyle are healthy, and that you allow yourself time for plenty of rest and relaxation.

Stress, overwork and tiredness can all depress the immune system and increase the tendency to infection.

○ Avoid sugar, tea and coffee, excessive orange juice and alcohol. It is best to stop smoking as this also compromises your immunity.

○ Drink plenty of unsweetened cranberry juice as this flashes out the urinary system and helps to prevent infection, apparently by stopping bacteria from adhering to the bladder walls.

○ Make sure that you treat vaginal infections promptly and any other systemic infection that could lower your immunity.

During a cystitis attack

At the first signs of irritation start drinking about half a pint of liquid every 20 minutes for the following three to four hours. After your first drink, take half a glass of apple juice to which you can add one teaspoonful of bicarbonate of soda (unless you have heart problems or high blood pressure) which helps to make the urine more alkaline and so reduces stinging and irritation.

Repeat every hour on the first day, less on the second and stop after the third. After that, drink either herbal teas or barley water (see p.138), or alternate the two, choosing from: plantain, horsetail, chamomile, corn silk, meadowsweet, or raspberry leaves, or a combination of any of these. They should be drunk lukewarm or cold.

Fill two hot water bottles and place one on your back and the other, wrapped in a towel so that it does not burn, between your legs while you rest.

Whenever you pass water, wash yourself gently using water to which a drop of lavender or thyme oil, or infusions of any of the above herbs have been added. Dab dry, don't rub.

Hot compresses of chamomile infusion can be applied over the abdomen, or you can sit in a large bowl or shallow bath of chamomile tea, which is wonderfully soothing.

Avoid tea, coffee, alcohol, orange juice and spicy or acidic foods such as tomatoes, strawberries, sour fruit, rhubarb or spinach.

Drink cranberry juice, leek and onion soup and eat plenty of garlic, raw if possible.

Dilute oils of frankincense, bergamot or fennel may be helpful used externally. A few drops of essential oil can be added to the bath water or used in a compress over the bladder and lower back.

Kidney infection

It is important to treat a urinary tract infection as soon as it arises, otherwise, in some instances, cystitis can creep from the bladder up the ureters to the pelvis of the kidney and become pyelonephritis, a much more serious and unpleasant problem. This infection of the kidney can also develop independently of cystitis and is characterized by pain in the lower back, fever and shivering, lethargy, headaches and possibly some discomfort on passing water. Untreated kidney infections, especially if they become chronic, may cause kidney damage, leading to water retention, high blood pressure and eventual kidney failure. During pregnancy a kidney infection can cause premature delivery.

The treatment of kidney infections is similar to that for cystitis; drink lukewarm to cold herbal infusions frequently throughout the day. Herbs may also be needed to bring down a fever and thereby help to keep you more comfortable. Hot infusions of linden blossom, chamomile or yarrow can be drunk freely.

Herbs to boost immunity such as garlic and echinacea should also be taken every two hours in acute conditions and three times daily for chronic problems.

Note Always check that your kidney infection has cleared by taking urinary specimens to your doctor. Your kidneys are fundamental to your health and infection can be silent and symptomless. It is best to seek help from a qualified herbalist when treating kidney disease.

Prolapse

When the ligaments and muscles that normally hold the uterus and vagina in place become weak with age or after childbirth, the uterus or vagina or both slip downwards. In uterine prolapse, the uterus bulges into the vagina and can cause pressure on the bladder or rectum. In vaginal prolapse, which is more common, the walls of the vagina become weak and surrounding structures such as the bladder and rectum push into them.

Causes of prolapse

Childbirth In normal circumstances, childbirth should not weaken the ligaments which support the uterus; they should simply move aside as the cervix dilates to allow the baby to be delivered. If the birth is very fast and the baby is pushed out before the cervix dilates fully, or if there is a forceps delivery, the ligaments may be damaged and weakened. There may also be excess strain on the ligaments in a multiple birth.

Tears in the ligament are repaired with scar tissue which is not as strong as normal ligament. It may hold up until menopause when, because at this stage muscles start to lose their tone, the prolapse becomes evident.

As far as the vagina is concerned, even normal childbirth causes such stretching of the vagina that it can be left weakened in places. If the front wall of the vagina is weakened the bladder may push into it (cystocele) and if the back wall is affected, the rectum can bulge into it (rectocele).

Gravity With age, our muscles and ligaments gradually weaken, especially if the tone of these structures has not been maintained by sufficient exercise.

The normal forces of gravity cause constant pressure downwards on all the abdominal organs, which can eventually cause prolapse.

Chronic constipation and straining at stool will increase this downward pressure and further weaken muscles and ligaments. A chronic cough can do the same. Overweight or obesity also increase the tendency to prolapse, because the extra weight puts pressure on all the muscles in the abdomen.

Symptoms of prolapse

heavy dragging in the lower
   abdomen
pain with sexual intercourse
backache
stress incontinence
difficulty emptying bladder
frequent urination
discomfort passing stools
difficulty passing stools
frequent urinary infections
vaginal discharge

Another symptom of prolapse may be a feeling of something coming down in the vagina. It may be possible to feel a slight bulge inside the vagina if you feel with your finger. If prolapse is complete, a part of the uterus or the vagina can protrude outside the vagina and feel sore. It may be inflamed or ulcerated and is prone to infection.

Self help for prolapse

○ If your prolapse has not developed too far, pelvic floor exercises (see p.161) may help substantially. They need to be practised every day without fail and their strengthening effect on the muscles will be gradual, so try not to be discouraged if success is not immediate.
○ It is best to act at the first sign of prolapse, to avoid it progressing so far that surgery is the only alternative. This is particularly important if you have not finished having a family as surgery could damage the uterus; also, a future childbirth could undo the operation.
○ To help tone your muscles sit in a bowl of cold water every day for 30 seconds.
○ If you have chronic constipation, this should be treated (see p.121), or if you have had a cough for a while, visit your practitioner to ascertain its cause and then treat it.
○ Avoid tight clothes as they may increase the risk of prolapse. If you are overweight try to put this right by changing your diet or taking more exercise.
○ Avoid standing for long periods. Daily exercise is important to increase the general circulation which will ensure adequate blood supply to the pelvic muscles and ligaments.
If the prolapse has progressed too far for these measures to help, you may be fitted with a pessary by your practitioner. Often this is a temporary measure while you wait for surgery.

Herbal remedies for prolapse

Uterine tonics, such as lady's mantle, beth root, false unicorn root, sage or raspberry leaves taken internally can help to tone up your uterine muscles. Astringents such as bayberry, horsetail or shepherd's purse should be combined with specific uterine herbs.

After the menopause, lack of estrogen leads to atrophy of the pelvic ligaments causing prolapse. So estrogenic herbs such as sage, hops, calendula, wild yam or ginseng can be helpful.

If there is soreness in the vagina or of the cervix, chickweed used locally as a douche or ointment is soothing and healing. A daily douche of a mixture of horsetail, bayberry and sage made up as tea will help local tone of the vagina, and help prevent soreness or infection.

Pessaries made of glycerine and gelatin containing astringent herbs, such as golden seal and witch hazel, are also useful.

Massage the lower abdomen and lower back with dilute oils of rosemary and lemon, or put a few drops in the bath every day.

Vaginal and vulval infections

The vagina, like other orifices in the body, has in normal circumstances an efficient defense system which helps to prevent infection despite the numerous potentially harmful micro-organisms that could invade the area.

The vagina is self cleansing, secreting mucus from its walls and producing a clear, slightly sticky discharge, which can be creamy in appearance. The vaginal secretions are acid with a pH of around four, which repels most infections. The acidity is maintained by benevolent bacteria called Doderlein's bacilli which live in the vagina and are sustained by estrogen. They convert glycogen, present in vaginal secretions, to lactic acid, and act effectively against hostile bacteria. These are some of the beneficial organisms that are destroyed by antibiotic treatment.

Infections in the vagina generally produce a vaginal discharge which differs from the normal. However, it should be borne in mind that a normal vaginal discharge can increase at certain times – during teenage years, during pregnancy, around ovulation and during sexual arousal. If at other times your discharge appears different in its amount, colour or texture or smells unpleasant you may well have an infection.

If you suspect you have a vaginal infection let your practitioner take a swab for laboratory analysis. If your infection is one that is sexually transmitted, self-help measures and herbal treatment should go hand in hand with orthodox treatment to ensure that the infection is brought under control. Untreated, some vaginal infections can have very serious consequences. They can move up into other areas of the reproductive system and lead to pelvic inflammatory disease (PID), causing chronic abdominal pain and internal scarring that can jeopardize fertility.

Factors contributing to vaginal infection through lowered resistance

poor diet
unhealthy lifestyle – insufficient exercise, fresh air, rest or relaxation
sleep problems, lack of sleep
infection elsewhere in the body
drugs such as steroids, the pill, antibiotics
anemia
stress, exhaustion
over-frequent washing in soap
use of deodorants or perfumes around the vagina
tight jeans, underwear or synthetic fabrics surrounding the area

Self-help for vaginal and vulval infections

Your partner should also seek treatment, since men can harbour infecting organisms in the urethra or under the foreskin and can re-infect you once you have recovered.

○ Always be as scrupulous as possible about personal hygiene. Make sure you wipe from front to back and never vice versa – to avoid bacterial contamination of the vagina from the anus. Be aware of cleanliness before, during and after sexual intercourse. Pass water after sex to help wash away micro-organisms from the entrance of the vagina.

○ Avoid using vaginal cosmetics which may contain irritating chemicals or upset the delicate balance of bacteria or the vaginal pH – no vaginal deodorants, scented lavatory paper, perfumed douches, tampons, for example, and avoid washing the area with soap.

○ Wear cotton underwear and avoid tight underwear, synthetic materials, and tight jeans which inhibit circulation to the area and create moist, damp conditions ideal for infections to thrive in. Expose the area to the air when you can and sleep without underwear on.

○ Eat plenty of whole grains, nuts and seeds, unrefined cold-pressed oils, fresh fruit and vegetables. Eat organic where possible. Avoid junk foods, fried foods, sugar and caffeine.

○ Make sure you have plenty of rest and sleep, and take lots of exercise in the fresh air. Pelvic floor exercises (see p.161) will help increase circulation to the area. If you feel run down or under stress, this may well contribute to the development or continuation of the infection. Yoga or meditation practice may be helpful. Follow advice for stress management (see p.50).

○ Add a cupful of vinegar to the bath water from time to time to help maintain the acid pH of the vagina. You can also take a teaspoon of honey and cider vinegar in hot water regularly.

Herbal and dietary treatment for vaginal and vulval infections

Internal Bacteria and viruses are constantly present in our bodies, awaiting their opportunity to multiply when conditions are right and when our immune mechanisms are not robust enough to see them off. It is important to enhance general resistance and to treat underlying conditions contributing to lower resistance, such as stress, a toxic system, or other infection elsewhere in the body.

Take echinacea, astragalus or myrrh, or both, to enhance immunity and to combat infection, three times daily in chronic infections and every two hours in acute problems. Take garlic (fresh or in capsules) daily. Add herbs that are cleansing and detoxifying to the reproductive area – thyme, cleavers, golden seal, poke root or calendula.

You may need to add herbs to the mixture you have chosen to address the cause of your vaginal infection. If you are stressed and run down add vervain or skullcap to restore the nervous system, and dang gui or astragalus as general tonics. If your bowels are congested, your tongue coated and you feel generally congested and depleted, use cleansing herbs to detoxify the system, such as yellow dock, burdock or dandelion. Astringent remedies are helpful where there is a heavy discharge, such as lady's mantle, beth root or oak bark.

A useful prescription would be:

echinacea 2 parts
beth root 2 parts
cleavers 2 parts
golden seal 1 part
thyme 2 parts

External Golden seal, myrrh, bayberry, thyme, rosemary, marjoram, calendula and cinnamon can be used in dilute tinctures or teas, or as lotions, to apply to the vaginal area, or as douches two to three times daily. You can also mix them into a base of aqueous cream if that would be easier for you to apply. Try a sitz-bath of infusions of any of these herbs.

If there is a profuse discharge, add astringent herbs to your mixture for a lotion, douche, cream or bath. Beth root, lady's mantle, witch hazel and oak bark are all suitable.

Yoghurt can also help to re-establish the natural bacterial flora of the vaginal area, and applied liberally it is particularly soothing when there is itchiness and soreness. Use a soothing cream if the vulval area feels sore or is very itchy – chamomile, comfrey and chickweed are particularly useful.

Prescription for vaginal douche or lotion:

tincture of calendula 20 ml
tincture of golden seal 20 ml
tincture of myrrh 10 ml
essential oil of chamomile
   2 drops
essential oil of marjoram
   5 drops
essential oil of tea tree
   5 drops

Dilute 1 teaspoon in 1 litre of water for use as douche twice daily. Alternatively, dilute a quarter to half a teaspoonful in enough water to soak a tampon in and insert it for 1 hour 2 - 3 times daily.

Until your infection is completely clear and you feel quite well, take foods or supplements to support the system such as:

multimineral and multivitamin
   tablet
vitamin E (in wheatgerm,
sunflower seeds, eggs) to increase
   your resistance to infection
vitamin C (in fresh fruit and vegetables)
a zinc supplement or foods high in zinc (such as pumpkin seeds) to help repel infection and speed healing of damaged tissue
iron-containing foods (see p.120–121)
cranberry juice (unsweetened) to acidify the system
plenty of water or herbal teas to help eliminate toxins through the urine and stools. You should also cut out tea which inhibits iron absorption (iron deficiency predisposes towards chronic vaginal infection).

Vaginal thrush
Candida albicans

If the normal defense mechanisms which operate in the vagina are disturbed, yeast-type fungi which normally live in the vagina and anus have an opportunity to multiply unchecked, and this gives rise to a thrush infection.

Possible causes of thrush

change in hormone balance
the contraceptive pill
steroids
antibiotics
spermicides
diabetes and pregnancy (both conditions increase the glycogen in the vaginal secretions creating an ideal medium for the fungus to flourish)
use of vaginal cosmetics, deodorants, douches, soaps
sexual transmission
an underlying weakness of the immune system caused by general depletion, poor diet, unhealthy lifestyle
another infection in the vagina, such as chlamydia (making the area susceptible to recurrent thrush infection)

Symptoms of thrush

a white, cheesy discharge that smells yeasty
itchiness or soreness in or around the vagina
discomfort with sexual intercourse
burning on passing water
possibly a rash

Vaginal thrush may be a symptom of more widespread infection through the body, known as chronic candidiasis. This is caused by an overgrowth of the candida fungus in the bowel, in turn caused by an upset in the normal bacterial population which should check the growth of micro-organisms. Candida causes irritation and inflammation of the gut wall, making it more permeable, and allowing possible allergens from the diet, as well as toxins from the bowel, to pass into the bloodstream. This affects both the immune and endocrine systems and can cause allergy to intestinal yeasts.

The tendency to chronic candidiasis is increased by:

stress
low thyroid function
oral contraceptives
pregnancy
pollution, hormones and preservatives in food
antibiotics

Possible symptoms of chronic candidiasis

vaginal thrush
anal irritation
abdominal bloating and wind
bowel disturbances such as diarrhea or constipation, colitis, Crohn's disease, irritable bowel syndrome
muscle or joint pain
nasal congestion or rhinitis
mood swings, depression, irritability
lethargy, fatigue, poor memory and

concentration
cystitis symptoms
skin problems such as acne
headaches or migraine
sweet craving
PMS
endometriosis
low libido
food allergies
MS symptoms
ME
cold, damp feelings on the skin

Symptoms are often worse on cold damp days, or in a room where there might be mould.

Herbal treatment for chronic candidiasis and thrush

Take echinacea three times daily in chronic cases of vaginal thrush, and every two hours in acute attacks, to boost the immune system. Add to your prescription herbs which have antifungal properties, such as calendula, thyme, golden seal, cinnamon and rosemary.

You may need to add herbs to your mixture taken internally to address the cause of the thrush infection. If you feel it is related to stress, try to address its causes, and add herbs such as skullcap, vervain or oats to support the nervous system. If you feel that your system is generally depleted add dang gui or ginger.

Use a douche of teas or dilute tinctures of thyme, calendula, golden seal, chamomile or myrrh once a day. Alternatively use a tincture of golden seal, calendula and thyme with oils of tea tree or thyme or both, as a lotion.

Make the mixture in the following proportions:

calendula tincture 20 ml
thyme tincture 20 ml
golden seal tincture 10 ml
tea tree or thyme oil 5 drops

Use half a teaspoonful diluted in enough water to soak a tampon. Insert the tampon for an hour. Do this night and morning until the symptoms clear.

Chamomile cream or chickweed ointment is very useful to soothe itching and irritation.

If you feel that your system is generally toxic or your bowels are congested take cleansing remedies such as yellow dock, cleavers, poke root or burdock.

Self help for vaginal thrush

○ Avoid sex until all signs of infection clear. Check that your partner also treats himself in case the infection is passing between you.
○ Use no cosmetics around the vagina or vulva and do not wash with soap.
○ Avoid tight fitting clothes that encourage a warm, damp atmosphere.
○ Eat a healthy diet, with plenty of whole grains, nuts and seeds, unrefined oils and fresh fruit and vegetables. Eat organic as much as possible. Eliminate junk food from your diet, along with sugar, alcohol, tea, coffee, fatty foods and additives.
○ Wherever possible, seek alternative treatment for any infections which may develop so that you can avoid antibiotics. Add sea salt to your bathwater – enough to make the water taste salty. Bathe the vagina with a solution of one teaspoonful of sodium bicarbonate to one pint of warm water. You may need to put this in a douche bag.

Note Never douche if you are pregnant.

○ Sit in a bowl of dilute vinegar or lemon juice to correct any pH imbalance, and maintain an acid environment. Use one part of vinegar or lemon juice to three parts water. Apply live, unsweet

ened natural yoghurt with a clean finger or an applicator.
○ Seek alternatives to spermicides, the pill, and the diaphragm.
○ Avoid using tampons.

Yeast-free diet

If you have symptoms of chronic candidiasis, it is best to avoid any foods containing yeast and to eliminate sugar (which feeds yeast) from your diet.

So avoid the following:

sugar, molasses, honey or any sweetener and foods containing them
cheese
alcohol and fermented beverages, including medicines made with alcohol
vinegar, mustard, pickles, mayonnaise, ketchup and other sauces, salad cream
soy sauce
mushrooms
dried fruits
foods flavoured with citric acid
bread
vitamin supplements with yeast, such as brewer's yeast, B vitamins
yeast extract
foods and drinks containing malt

To help combat yeast infection in the body eat plenty of garlic, cold pressed olive oil and live yoghurt. Take supplements of yeast-free B complex, multiminerals and vitamins, anti-fungal caprylic acid, garlic perles, acidophilus and evening primrose oil.

Genital herpes

Herpes Simplex II is a virus that gives rise to the genital herpes infection. It is generally transmitted by sexual intercourse or intimate contact when the virus is active and the infection evident. After an initial infection the virus lives dormantly in nerve endings and can be reactivated when you are run down, for example by illness such as a cold or flu, by tiredness or physical or emotional stress. It may be reactivated by certain dietary items. It may also be related to a change in skin temperature and extremes of heat or cold, and can occur pre-menstrually. Weeks or years can go by between one outbreak and another.

Symptoms of genital herpes

Herpes causes small fluid-filled blisters which are red and can be very painful. They erupt on or around the vagina, the anus or buttocks, and can also appear on the thighs, after a day or two of tingling or pain along the surrounding nerves. The blisters usually last for a few days, during which time the virus is highly contagious, and causes much discomfort, particularly when sitting. Then scabs form as the blisters dry up and eventually disappear. The first eruption is generally the most unpleasant, and can be accompanied by swollen glands in the groin, muscle aches, malaise and fever. The blisters and pain can last for up to three weeks.

There is an association between genital herpes and cancer of the cervix though one does not necessarily cause the other. However, if you do have genital herpes it is important to have smear tests annually. Genital herpes is a particular problem during pregnancy, in case the virus is active at the time of the birth. If the baby comes into contact with the virus as it travels down the birth canal it can cause blindness and severe illness. If you have genital herpes during pregnancy it is best to have cultures taken twice a week after the 36th week. If they are negative it should be safe to have a vaginal delivery, if not it may be advisable to have a Caesarian. Make sure you tell

your obstetrician or midwife if you have genital herpes.

The herpes virus, called Herpes Simplex I, also causes cold sores around the mouth or nose. It is now thought that this infection can be transmitted to the genital area where it becomes genital herpes. So if you get cold sores, leave them well alone and always wash if you touch your face. Genital herpes is on the increase; it is thought that around 25 per cent of sexually active adults have had the virus and have had outbreaks. Many more than this have been found to carry the antibody without any evidence of the infection, showing that they must have been exposed to the infection, if only via cold sores.

Prevention of genital herpes

Never have sexual intercourse if your partner has an active infection and avoid oral sex if you or your partner have cold sores. Since it is now thought to be possible to become infected without evidence of an acute infection, it is best to practise safe sex as a general rule.

Try to avoid becoming stressed, tired and run down from overwork or an unhealthy lifestyle of excesses. Yoga, meditation and counselling may be helpful in stress management. Also the use of herbs and correct diet will help to support the nervous system (see p.53).

Take plenty of fresh air and exercise to enhance the immune system and keep yourself healthy.

Diet for genital herpes

There are two amino acids which have been shown to influence the outbreak of infection once you have initially contracted the virus. Lysine has the ability to inhibit attacks while arginine predisposes to them, so it is advisable to eat a

diet high in lysine and low in arginine.

Lysine containing foods:

potatoes	yoghurt
cottage cheese	milk
fresh vegetables	prawns
beansprouts	legumes
soy beans	brewer's yeast
eggs	poultry
meat	fish

Arginine containing foods:

chocolate	peanuts
cocoa	carob
brown rice	oatmeal
raisins	sunflower seeds
sesame seeds	popcorn
eggplants	tomatoes
green peppers	mushrooms
cashews	pecans
almonds	sugar
coffee	tea
coconut	chick peas
hazelnuts	walnuts
brazil nuts	

Self help for genital herpes

○ Try to work out which foods (or anything else) trigger attacks. Eat a generally healthy diet, low in sugar, caffeine, and fats and avoid junk foods.
○ Tannic acid in black tea is a natural anesthetic; place a tea bag soaked in hot water over the area to soothe the pain. Bathing the area with diluted bicarbonate of soda is also very soothing.
○ Expose the area to the air as much as you can to keep the sores dry and encourage them to heal. Vitamin E oil or wheatgerm oil can be gently dabbed on the sores to speed healing.
○ Avoid excess heat, saunas and sunbeds.
○ During acute attacks add a few spoonfuls of sea salt to the bath water to help relieve the soreness.
○ Take supplements of lysine (500 mg daily to keep the infection away and 500-1000 mg two

Huang qi

Astragalus membranaceus

ALSO KNOWN AS: Astragalus, milk vetch, huang ch'i

PART USED: Root

CONTAINS: Linoleic acid, linolenic acid, betaine, choline, glycosides, isoamni-tine, kumatakenin

KEY USES: Stimulant, tonic, diuretic, immunostimulant, antimicrobial, cardiotonic

Huang qi is one of the most famous Chinese tonic herbs, considered by some to be a superior tonic for younger people than ginseng. It is particularly beneficial as an energizer for young, physically active adults. Astragalus is a wonderful tonic to the immune system – in Chinese medicine it is said to energize the outside of the body and tonify the protective energy known as the Wei Chi'i which flows just beneath the skin, which protects the body from external "pathogenic factors", such as cold, damp, wind, and heat.

Huang qi also acts to balance fluids in the body and prevent fluid retention. Particularly when combined with dang gui (see p.32) it acts to stimulate the circulation. It dilates blood vessels, lowers blood pressure, and acts as a heart tonic, increasing the endurance of fatigued hearts.

Huang qi helps to restore a defective immune system, and speeds recovery in those who have undergone chemotherapy or radiation therapy. It has been shown to enhance the function and increase production of white blood cells, and to promote adrenal cortex and bone marrow function which are depressed in cancer patients. It increases resistance to viral infection and is being looked into as a possible treatment for HIV and AIDS. Huang qi acts to reduce "T-suppressor cells" which inhibit immunity and tend to be found in large numbers in AIDS patients and the elderly. For this reason it may help delay the aging process and have rejuvenative properties. It has been shown to have antibiotic properties and to reduce toxicity in the liver.

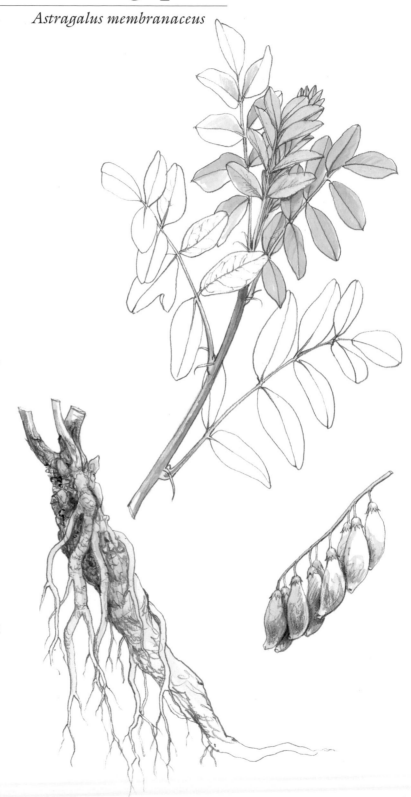

to three times daily when it is active). Take a multimineral and vitamin supplement to help boost immunity.

○ Eat foods high in zinc, vitamins A, B, C and E to raise resistance to infection.

Herbal treatment of genital herpes

Internal To enhance the function of the immune system take herbs such as astragalus, echinacea and garlic. Add cleansing herbs to aid elimination of toxins from the system, such as burdock, dandelion root, nettles and yellow dock, and herbs to stimulate the lymphatic system such as cleavers, calendula and poke root.

To direct the action of the prescription, add specific herbs for the reproductive system such as partridge berry, raspberry leaves, lady's mantle or false unicorn root.

The following recipe can be used during infection and for a week or two afterwards:

equal parts of:
peppermint   echinacea
cleavers   burdock
lady's mantle
with ½ part of unicorn root

External You can use a variety of herbs applied to the trouble spot to speed the healing of the blisters, soothe the pain and discourage secondary infection. Use an infusion or dilute tincture of any of these: echinacea, golden seal, myrrh, calendula and St. John's wort to bathe the area, or add to bath water.

Dilute essential oils can be dabbed gently onto the blisters; oils of melissa, clove, lavender, tea tree, thyme, and St. John's wort applied neat will help soothe pain. Make a lotion to dab on by mixing 10 drops of essential oil

with one teaspoon (5 ml) of lavender tincture. Add a tablespoon (15 ml) of water and use three to four times daily.

Distilled witch hazel will speed the clearing up of the blisters and help to dry them; dab it on several times daily. Once the blisters have dried you can apply comfrey tea, oil or ointment to complete the healing. Vitamin E oil would also be useful here.

Genital warts

Genital warts are becoming increasingly common. They are caused by the Human Papilloma Virus (HPV) and there are eight types, some of which remain internal and invisible.

Two of the most common types may be connected to changes in the cervix. It has been shown that women who smoke are more likely to develop precancerous changes of the cervix if they have genital warts, probably because smoking depletes the immune system. The pill is also thought to contribute to cervical changes in women who have the wart virus.

Genital warts are sexually transmitted; where there are symptoms these can develop between three weeks and nine months after exposure to infection. They appear initially as small, hard spots around the opening of the vagina, in and around the anus, or on the cervix where they are rarely visible. Genital warts are painless, and can grow to resemble a tiny cauliflower. Some warts are flat and very hard to see or feel, except with an expert eye. Sometimes the warts itch, and if they affect the urethra can cause pain on urination.

Self help for genital warts

○ If you have genital warts it is important to have annual cervical

smears because of the possible risk of cervical changes.

○ Make sure that your partner seeks treatment also so that you do not become re-infected.

○ Avoid taking the pill.

○ It is important not to smoke.

○ Practise safe sex by using a condom.

○ If you have a vaginal discharge or infection seek treatment, as this can encourage the development of warts.

Herbal and dietary treatment for genital warts

Internal Herbs to enhance the body's vitality and its fight against the wart virus are called for, as well as herbs to detoxify the system. Echinacea, astragalus and garlic enhance the immune system and should be taken three times daily. Burdock, dandelion root, nettles, plantain and cleavers will aid cleansing of the body. Thuja is a specific herb for warts and should be added to your recipe.

A useful recipe to be taken three times daily as tea or tincture can be made from equal parts of:

cleavers   nettles
kelp   peppermint
burdock   dandelion root
echinacea

External Several herbs can be used directly on the warts. If they are of the visible kind, use a mirror to help you apply the remedy, or bathe the area twice daily.

Use these herbs:

tincture of thuja
oil of tea tree
fresh elderberry juice
yellow juice from fresh greater
    celandine
white juice from dandelion stalks or
    unripe figs
lemon juice

raw garlic
inner sides of broad bean pods

Continue until the warts disappear.

To raise the body's immunity and to help fight off the virus make sure you have plenty of fresh fruit and vegetables to provide iron and vitamins C and A; seafood, beans or nuts to provide magnesium; yeast extract or brewer's yeast for B vitamins; eggs, nuts and seeds to provide zinc and unrefined oils to provide essential fatty acids. Take supplements of garlic perles, vitamin C, a multimineral and vitamin supplement and cod liver oil.

Propolis tincture can be taken, ten drops in water two to three times daily. Propolis is an antiseptic material which bees collect from tree sap to plaster over the hive to keep it clean and protected from infection. Certain substances from propolis, such as flavonoids, help the body to make antibodies and enhance the work of white blood cells in warding off infection.

Note Because of the potential seriousness of genital warts, herbs and diet should be used as an adjunct to orthodox treatment.

Chlamydia

Chlamydia is an increasingly common infection which is transmitted sexually and involves a bacteria-like parasite called *Chlamydia trachomatis* which lives inside the cervical cells.

Unfortunately, the infection often produces no symptoms so that it may go undetected for years, and affecting the uterus and fallopian tubes, sometimes leading to pelvic inflammatory disease and infertility. It is possible that the inflammation caused by chlamydia allows the HIV virus (which can lead to AIDS), into the bloodstream more easily.

There are usually no symptoms of chlamydia.

Symptoms of chlamydia (if any)

vaginal discharge, either scanty or
   copious, greeny or yellow
soreness
rarely, pain on urination
rarely, frequency of urination
rarely, bleeding after sexual intercourse or smear test

Once it has ascended higher into the reproductive tract it may cause endometritis or salpingitis (see Pelvic inflammatory disease). There may be abdominal pain, pain with sexual intercourse or bleeding between periods. Chlamydia is rarely diagnosed unless another condition is being investigated.

A man infected with chlamydia may not be aware of any symptoms although he may develop a bout of mild urethritis. or NSU (non-specific urethritis). Because of this, chlamydia may be passed unwittingly from one partner to another by unprotected sex. In women it can affect the lining of the vagina, the urinary tract, mouth, eyes, rectum and cervix. Those with cervical erosion are more susceptible.

The contraceptive pill can lower resistance to the infection as the hormone it contains creates the right environment in the vagina and around the cervix for the infection to proliferate.

Chlamydia infection can cause the vagina to be more susceptible to other infections, such as thrush, or other bacterial infections which may also contribute to pelvic inflammatory disease (p.232). This is more likely in women who use IUDs. It is worth being tested for chlamydia, especially if you are hoping to conceive. The infection can be passed to the baby during delivery.

You can read more about vagi-

nal and vulval infections on p.224.

Trichomonas vaginalis

Trichomonas is a protozoa which, like thrush, is ever-present in the vagina, intestines, anus, urethra, bladder and cervix. In normal circumstances it is held in check by the local defense mechanisms and causes no problems. As in other vaginal infections, when resistance to infection is lowered the micro-organisms seize their opportunity to proliferate.

Trichomonas is generally transmitted sexually but because it can live outside the body for several hours at room temperature in the right moist conditions, it is possible to catch it from other sources, such as wet bathing costumes, underwear, damp towels or flannels used by an infected person, and even lavatory seats.

Trichomonas also thrive in a particularly acid environment so that symptoms can be worse before a period when the pH of the vagina tends to be lower.

There are few symptoms specific to trichomonas, so it is often mistaken for other infections, many of which are present at the same time.

Symptoms of trichomonas (if any)

greenish yellow, frothy, foul-
   smelling discharge
discharge may be thick and white
   and mistaken for thrush
itching and inflammation of the
   vulva
blood stained discharge

If you suspect you have trichomonas, visit your practitioner. Diagnosis can be made by taking a swab. If infection is present it is important that your partner is also treated, despite the fact that he probably will not exhibit any symptoms, to prevent re-infection. If it is left untreated, trichomonas can lead to Pelvic inflammatory disease, which in turn can lead to infertility.

Gonorrhea and Syphilis

These infections are grouped with herpes, chlamydia and trichomonas because they are all sexually transmitted diseases (STDs).

Gonorrhea involves the bacteria gonococcus, and unfortunately rarely produces symptoms in women. Sometimes between two days and three weeks after exposure there may be a yellow-green discharge, vaginal irritation or cystitis symptoms which can easily be mistaken for something else. In men, it causes a burning sensation when passing water in the early stages, and pus may be passed from the penis.

Gonorrhea often accompanies chlamydia or trichomonas, so if you are diagnosed as having one infection, you should be tested for the other. If one is treated and not the other, the infection may be masked and can cause further problems in the reproductive system, especially in the case of gonorrhea.

If gonorrhea is left untreated it can spread to vital structures such as the uterus and fallopian tubes and lead to Pelvic inflammatory disease (PID). This can cause blocked tubes, infertility and increase the risk of an ectopic pregnancy (see below).

Gonorrhea can also affect the heart, the meninges, the eyes and can cause arthritis. A baby can contract the infection at birth as it passes down the birth canal, also affecting the baby's eyes, sometimes causing lasting damage.

Syphilis is more rare than gonorrhea and even more difficult to detect. It is a systemic infection involving treponema (pallidum) which has an incubation period of two to four weeks. It starts with a small, painless sore known as a chancre. This reddens and ulcerates, containing fluid that is highly contagious. The glands in the groin may be swollen and tender. The chancre normally appears in the genital area, but also it may affect the mouth or the fingers. It heals within six to ten weeks.

If syphilis is untreated, it develops into secondary and tertiary stages, eventually affecting the whole system and particularly the heart and nervous system (including the brain). If caught at an early stage and treated with large doses of antibiotics it can be successfully controlled.

Pelvic inflammatory disease (PID)

Pelvic inflammatory disease is a general term used to describe acute or chronic infections which affect the uterus, fallopian tubes, ovaries or the surrounding tissues. It is also known as pelvic infection or salpingitis.

The condition is often caused by sexually transmitted diseases (STDs) such as chlamydia (see p.231) or other infections entering via the vagina and travelling upwards. Often such infections go unnoticed and untreated. Complications following childbirth, surgery in the abdomen or pelvis, infection following a miscarriage or termination, or the fitting or presence of an IUD, may also be responsible.

PID is more likely to occur in younger women who have frequent sexual intercourse, or who have had several different partners, increasing the risk of infection. During ovulation, menstruation and childbirth when the cervix is more open, the risk of infection is greater.

Symptoms of Pelvic inflammatory disease

irregular or heavy menstrual bleeding
spotting between periods
profuse, often bad-smelling vaginal discharge
flu-like symptoms, chills and general malaise
pain with sexual intercourse or bleeding after sex
lower back pain and or leg pain, pain in lower abdomen
frequency of urination, pain when passing water
abdominal swelling, nausea or diarrhea, poor appetite

In an acute infection there may be a fever and severe abdominal pain. Chronic or recurrent infections tend to be less intense and characterized by relapses and remissions.

It is very important to treat the first signs of such an infection promptly, since pelvic infection can cause an abscess, peritonitis and the development of scar tissue in the reproductive tract, particularly the fallopian tubes, that could lead to an ectopic pregnancy or infertility.

Unfortunately a low grade infection may not produce symptoms intense enough to warrant treatment, or may be mistaken for something else such as period pains, and often remains undetected, causing infertility from scarring for no apparent reason.

Self help for Pelvic inflammatory disease

It is important to treat all signs of PID promptly.
○ If having sexual intercourse with a new partner or a partner who has other partners, make sure you practise safe sex to avoid infection.
○ Watch for any of the listed symptoms following childbirth,

miscarriage or a termination, any gynecological examination (such as D and C), removal or fitting of an IUD.

○ Have bed rest until all the symptoms have cleared. Avoid sexual intercourse until you are fully recovered.

○ Your partner may also need to be treated if the infection is sexually transmitted.

○ Avoid using an IUD, douches or tampons.

○ Make sure your personal hygiene and that of your partner is scrupulous.

○ Take plenty of exercise to ensure good circulation to and from the pelvis. Gentle yoga or T'ai chi may be particularly helpful.

Herbal and dietary treatment for Pelvic inflammatory disease

Take regular baths or sitz-baths in warm water to relax the abdominal muscles. Add a few drops of essential oil of lavender, rosewood, rosemary or geranium to the water to relax you and help fight infection.

Massage the lower abdomen and back with dilute essential oils daily.

Take echinacea internally every day, every two hours in acute infection and four times daily in chronic or recurrent infections. You may need to maintain this treatment for several weeks, or even months.

Thyme, myrrh, parsley, or poke root will also help fight the infection and build up the immune system. Add herbs with an affinity to the reproductive system to direct the action of the antiseptic herbs. These include blue cohosh, lady's mantle, calendula or false unicorn root.

Make sure your diet is high in fresh fruit and vegetables, and avoid sugar, junk foods and caffeine. Cut down on milk products. Avoid smoking and alcohol.

Take supplements of vitamins A, C, and E and zinc to help build up the immune system and aid tissue healing.

Recovery is likely to be slow and initially may have to go hand in hand with orthodox and antibiotic therapy to curb the infection.

Bacterial infections

These are also known as non-specific vaginitis (NSV), bacterial vaginosis or anaerobic vaginosis. The most common causes of these infections are bacteria called *Gardnerella vaginalis* or *Mycoplasma hominis.*

Gardnerella is commonly transmitted sexually, and is in fact the most common sexually transmitted disease (STD) in women. It rarely creates symptoms in men. Gardnerella symptoms are a watery, grey, fishy-smelling discharge which is often worse after sex or at the onset of menstruation. There may be other infections present, so gardnerella is hard to diagnose without a swab and is often mistaken for thrush.

Non-specific bacterial infections generally give rise to the following symptoms which may also be found with gardnerella.

Symptoms of bacterial infections

cystitis symptoms
lower back pain
swollen glands in the groin
vaginal discharge made up largely
   of pus which is thick, white or
   yellow. There may be traces of
   blood
itching and irritation of the vulva
   which may be severe

All bacterial infections need to be treated promptly to prevent spread of the infection up the reproductive tract to the uterus and fallopian tubes. Here they may be implicated in the development of pelvic inflammatory disease (see p.232), which can lead to infertility and increase the likelihood of an ectopic pregnancy.

Fibroids

Fibroids are benign, non-cancerous growths in or on the walls of the uterus. There may be a single fibroid or more commonly several, often developing on stalks.

Fibroids vary in size from that of a small pea to the size of a seven-month fetus, and are very common, particularly in women aged between 35 and 40. Since they are estrogen-dependent, they shrink after the menopause and often grow during pregnancy. When small, they often cause no symptoms and are only discovered on uterine examination. If large, they tend to give rise to heavy, prolonged periods and may prevent conception, cause miscarriage or obstruct childbirth, when a Caesarean may be necessary.

Fibroids have a tendency to occur in women who are overweight and this may be related to estrogen levels, as estrogen is stored in the fat. They have been found to be commoner in women with gallstones, and those who do not have children.

Symptoms of fibroids

heavy, prolonged periods
bleeding between periods
iron deficiency – anemia due to
   blood loss
painful periods
pressure on the bladder, causing
   frequency of urination, incontinence, urgency in urination or
   cystitis symptoms
enlarged abdomen
pain during sexual intercourse
backache
constipation

If the stalk of the fibroid becomes twisted it can cut off its blood supply, causing "red degeneration" of the fibroid which subsequently leaves behind a hard "womb stone". If this occurs there can be abdominal pain, vomiting, fever and malaise.

Self help for fibroids

○ Keep your weight down and reduce fat intake.
○ Make sure you have a good diet with plenty of whole grains, fresh fruit and vegetables.
○ Avoid caffeine, alcohol, junk foods, sugar and additives to prevent future accumulations of toxins which may be a contributory cause of fibroids.
○ Ensure a daily bowel movement – constipation will cause accumulations of toxins in the system. If you need help with constipation, see p.121.
○ Take plenty of exercise to ensure a healthy circulation to the pelvis. Yoga may be helpful.

Herbal treatment for fibroids

Use hormone balancing herbs such as chaste tree or false unicorn root.

Add tonics to the reproductive system such as lady's mantle or partridge berry.

Relaxants to the uterus – cramp bark, pulsatilla, wild yam or blue cohosh – should help reduce spasm and pain.

Circulatory remedies such as yarrow, dang gui, cinnamon, or ginger will help blood supply to the area and ensure adequate nutrition and removal of wastes from the uterine area.

To help cleanse toxins from the system, add depurative herbs such as dandelion root or calendula.

If menstrual bleeding is heavy, use beth root or geranium to help prevent anemia. If you need iron in your diet, see p.120.

Ovarian cysts

Ovarian cysts are generally fluid-filled sacs which develop on or near the ovaries. Sometimes they are dermoid, that is, made of tissue similar to that of teeth or hair. They are often small and cause no symptoms. If they are large or numerous the condition is called polycystic ovary disease. The cysts can press on organs such as the bladder, or interrupt normal hormonal function. Cysts can appear and disappear within weeks or months.

Symptoms of ovarian cysts

If cysts are large or numerous they can cause:

swelling in the lower abdomen
pain with sexual intercourse
pressure on the bladder which can cause urgency to urinate or frequency of urination, or cystitis symptoms

If polycystic ovary disease interferes with ovarian function it can cause:

irregularity or absence of periods (amenorrhea) and infertility
extra body hair, indicating a hormonal imbalance
pain when ovary is examined

A clear diagnosis is generally made by laparoscopy.

Note Ovarian cysts can cause severe acute abdominal pain, nausea and fever. If this occurs, contact your practitioner immediately. A cyst is subject to twisting, hemorrhage, or rupture, and can cause an acute abdominal emergency with a risk of peritonitis.

Self help for ovarian cysts

○ To clear from the system toxins which contribute to ovarian cysts, make sure you have a healthy diet, with plenty of fresh, if possible organic, fruit and vegetables, whole grains, nuts, and seeds.
○ Avoid tea and coffee, junk food, white flour products, sugar, fatty and refined foods.
○ Drink plenty of pure, filtered water or herbal teas to ensure you pass toxins out via the urine.
○ Take vigorous exercise, so that you sweat and help elimination of toxins through the skin.
○ Make sure you have at least one bowel movement daily. If you suffer from constipation it is important to treat it (see p.121).

Herbal and dietary treatment for ovarian cysts

Take kelp daily to ensure normal thyroid function. Low thyroid function causes an excess of estrogen which is related to ovarian cysts.

To restore estrogen levels take hormone balancing herbs such as chaste tree or false unicorn root.

Add tonics to the reproductive system to restore normal function – either partridge berry, false unicorn root or blue cohosh.

If there is pain add pulsatilla or black cohosh.

To help the liver's metabolism of estrogen add dandelion root. If there are urinary symptoms use horsetail or uva ursi. Rub dilute oils of either cranesbill, rose, lavender, clary sage or neroli, or mixtures of these, gently on the abdomen and add a few drops to the bath.

A cold sitz-bath for a couple of minutes each day will help ensure a healthy circulation to the pelvis.

Supplements of vitamins B complex and E will help re-establish hormone balance and the liver's metabolism of estrogens.

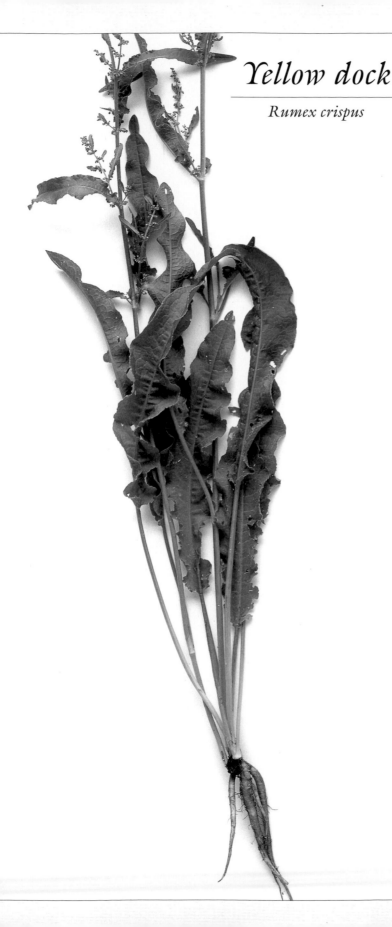

Yellow dock

Rumex crispus

PART USED: Root

CONTAINS: Anthraquinone glycosides, tannins, iron

KEY USES: Alterative, purgative, cholagogue, astringent, diuretic, tonic

Yellow dock has a powerful cleansing effect in the body. It provokes a bowel movement within a few hours of taking it, while also reducing any excess activity of the gut, and soothing any irritation of the gut lining, making dock a gentle bowel cleanser for long term treatment of sluggish bowels. It can also be used for bowel infections and to heal peptic ulcers. It soothes irritation in the respiratory tract. Its bitter glycosides stimulate the liver, enhancing bile production, making it a good remedy for a sluggish liver, a weak digestion, distension and wind. The root has diuretic properties, increasing urine production and elimination of toxins via the urinary system. It can be used for gout, cystitis, water retention, urinary stones and gravel.

Yellow dock makes an excellent remedy for skin problems such as weeping eczema, psoriasis, nettle rash, boils and abscesses. It has the effect of mobilizing congested blood and lymph and pulling toxins out of the tissues, as well as ensuring their elimination and can be used wherever there is congestion, heat and inflammation. It makes an excellent addition to prescriptions for arthritis, gout, rheumatism, and chronic lymphatic congestion. It has also been used for irregular periods, heavy bleeding and menstrual pain, as well as fibroids in the uterus.

Dock roots contain iron and provide an excellent remedy for anemia. This, with its tonic effect on the liver, has given dock a wide reputation as a revitalizing remedy, for general debility, mental lethargy, headaches, convalescence, low spirits and irritability.

The cooling and healing actions of dock make it an excellent external remedy for all kinds of inflammatory skin conditions.

Cancer, HIV and AIDS

Cancer and precancerous changes

Cancer is both a very challenging disease and a very emotive subject. The very thought of it may be frightening, and our feelings when confronted with it overwhelming, yet through it we may have the opportunity to understand ourselves and our bodies in more depth and actually use it as a tool for our transformation.

Cancer may force us to look in greater depth and detail at our diet and lifestyle, our relationships, our work, our emotional attitudes and mental outlook. Those with cancer need a great deal of help and support, be it through meditation, yoga, counselling, psychotherapy, healing, or other therapies, to enhance our understanding of ourselves and our condition. This is the time to put ourselves first and not keep putting off the time that we will truly care for ourselves. The time is now.

It is becoming increasingly clear that cancer has no single cause, but is probably the result of a combination of factors, which may be physical, physiological, genetic, emotional or environmental. Our body cells are constantly changing and responding to these kind of influences. Malignant changes can occur in certain cells and these, when we are healthy, are killed by our body's marvellous defense system. It is when our defenses are severely compromised that malignant growths occur.

More and more research is showing what havoc is wreaked on our immune systems by substances in our foods. Car fumes, tobacco smoke, water fluoridation, industrial waste, asbestos and radiation are all well-known carcinogens. Within us all, however, is the potential power to destroy cancerous cells, which explains the "spontaneous remissions" that many experience. It is this healing capacity that we need to explore, to strengthen or regenerate our immune system so as to fight off the disease.

What is cancer?

Cancer is abnormal reproduction of cells. Normal cells reproduce throughout our lives, to replace those that are worn out, to repair injured ones and to allow growth of the body in a controlled and orderly way.

Changes in cellular tissue cause certain cells to grow, divide, and reproduce in an uncontrolled way – much more rapidly than normal cells – and eventually to produce a lump, known as a tumour. A tumour can either be benign or malignant. A benign tumour remains confined to one area and the cells are not cancerous. A malignant tumour may spread its cells to other parts of the body.

As the tumour grows, the cells invade surrounding tissues and can also be carried via the blood and the lymphatic system to other areas, where new growths, know as metastases, may develop. Once cancer is diagnosed, by analysis of cells taken from the tumour, orthodox treatment normally involves surgery to remove the tumour and the area around it, radiotherapy to kill the cancer cells, or chemotherapy using drugs to kill the cancer cells. One or all of these treatments may be used at any one time.

Unfortunately both radiotherapy and chemotherapy not only destroy cancer cells, they also affect the white blood cells in the body, the mainstay of the immune system necessary for the body to fight off disease, including cancer.

Breast cancer

Cancer of the breast is the most common of all cancers in women and tends to afflict those who have a relative with breast cancer. However, there are many other factors which influence the development of cancer which you can do something about, unlike your genetic inheritance.

Factors influencing the development of breast cancer

High fat consumption is a contributory factor. Toxins such as drugs, pesticides and herbicides are stored in animal fat and women who eat fatty meat obviously also consume these toxins, which are then stored in the fat tissue. Since fat makes up a large proportion of breast tissue, a woman's breast becomes a storehouse for toxins. Dietary fat stimulates the secretion of prolactin, a pituitary hormone, which may contribute to breast cancer.

Research has shown that obese women have a higher chance of developing breast cancer than other women, because estrogen is stored in body fat and estrogen contributes to breast cancer.

Low intake of vitamins A, C, and E, selenium, folic acid, iron, zinc and magnesium have been shown to be linked with cancer.

Certain food substances, such as the nitrosamines derived from foods containing nitrites such as bacon, hot dogs, salami and sausages, as well as saccharine and sugar intake can contribute to breast cancer. Hydrogenated or partially hydrogenated oils are also under suspicion.

Heavy drinking may contribute to breast cancer. Vegetarians have been shown to suffer less from breast cancer than meat eaters. This may be related to toxins in animal fats as well as to the fact that meat eaters have higher levels of prolactin than vegetarians.

Women who started taking the pill before the age of 25 and who took it over more than four or five years have been shown to have an increased risk of breast cancer. The same is true for women who took estrogen replacement therapy (ERT) for five to ten years or more.

Women who began their periods early and who had a late menopause, and those who have never had children, are more prone to breast cancer. Women who had their first child over the age of 30 are at higher risk than those who had their first child before the age of 22.

Women who have had cancer elsewhere, or in one breast, are more at risk. The incidence of breast cancer increases with age and is most common between the ages of 50 and 65.

Stress is also an important factor in breast cancer.

Symptoms of breast cancer

a lump or change in the shape or size of the breast
thickening or dimpling of the skin
enlarged veins
a retracted nipple, if this is not normal
discharge from the nipple
non-cyclical pain, particularly when past the menopause
swelling of the upper arm, in the armpit or above the breast

Helping to prevent breast cancer

Check your breasts once a month, a few days after your period finishes so that any cysts in the breast that come and go with the period do not cause unnecessary concern. Post-menopausal women can check at any time.

Go through the same routine every month so you can spot changes. First look at your breast in the mirror to make sure there are no changes in shape, size, texture, or colour of the breast. Then lie down and feel each part of the breast with the flat of your fingers for any lumps or bumps or changes in skin texture.

Do not smoke and keep your alcohol intake low.

Make sure your diet is excellent, with a predominance of fresh fruit and vegetables, organically grown for preference, whole grains, nuts and seeds, beans and pulses, oily fish and unrefined vegetable oils.

Avoid fatty food, keep your meat intake as low as possible, avoid junk food and refined carbohydrates, particularly sugar. Keep well away from known carcinogens such as smoked meats, sausages, peanuts, additives, saccharine and hydrogenated oils.

Make sure you have plenty of vitamins A, E, C and D in your diet (see Diet chart on p.70) as these have been shown to help convert abnormal cancer cells back to normal healthy cells. They also enhance the function of the immune system in its battle to destroy abnormal cells.

Beta carotene in carrots, cauliflower, brussels sprouts, cabbage and broccoli for example has been extensively shown to inhibit the growth of cancer cells. Vitamins C and E help to protect the stomach, bowel and bladder from the carcinogenic effects of certain foods. Vitamins A, C, and E and selenium have antioxidant

properties. They inhibit deterioration of cells caused by "free radicals" which contribute to the development of cancer and in this way help prevent it. Make sure your diet also contains plenty of essential fatty acids.

A high fibre diet, with plenty of whole grains and vegetables not only prevents constipation, but also hastens the removal of carcinogens from the bowels and diminishes their chances of absorption into the system. Fibre also enhances the elimination of estrogen via the bowels, thereby helping to prevent excess estrogen in the system from contributing to breast cancer.

To avoid contaminants in water it is best to drink bottled and filtered water.

Avoid taking the contraceptive pill and the use of estrogen replacement therapy (ERT).

Take plenty of exercise and make sure you get fresh air, rest and relaxation and adequate sleep. If you are overweight it is worth seeking help to bring your weight under control.

If you are stressed, take time off to relax and let go of tensions and anxieties. If you are troubled by any particular emotional problems, or you are holding on to unresolved or unexpressed emotions which are troubling you, try to deal with them and let them go. This may be facilitated by relaxation, yoga, hypnotherapy, counselling, meditation or psychotherapy – or simply by allowing yourself to share your troubles with a friend.

If you are putting yourself under any unnecessary pressures, try to let go of them and spend at least one hour daily doing or being just what you want to. Give that hour to yourself, put yourself first for a change, even if it means just lying on the sofa listening to music or reading a good book, or luxuriating in a warm aromatic bath.

If you are aware of any health problem which may compromise your general health, it is important to seek treatment. Although localized cancers have generally been interpreted as local problems it is more probable that disease in one area of the body is much more to do with generalized systemic imbalance or ill health.

Pre-cancer and cancer of the cervix

The cervix is the neck of the uterus where it opens into the vagina. Like the skin and mouth, this is an area of the body where precancerous changes can be detected. If such changes are diagnosed, there is time to reappraise both health and lifestyle, and to treat the immune system so as to help ward off cancer.

Cervical dysplasia

Abnormal cell growth, or dysplasia, in the cervix can be identified by a cervical pap smear test. It is best to have a test once every 18-24 months if you are between the ages of 20 and 60, but once a year if you are at risk. This is particularly important if there have been previous treatment for cell changes, or genital warts. The results of cervical smears vary according to the extent of change in the cervical cells.

Temporary changes in the cervical cells can be caused by infection or inflammation of the cervix. If your test reveals precancerous changes with accompanying infection or inflammation, it is important to seek treatment for these and then have another test.

Factors in cervical changes:

The earlier in the teenage years a woman commenced sexual intercourse, the higher the risk.

The more sexual partners she has had, the higher the risk, maybe because of the higher risk of contracting sexually transmitted diseases.

Certain viruses increase the likelihood, particularly genital herpes and genital warts.

The use of oral contraceptives can depress immunity, in this way predisposing to cervical changes.

Low levels of vitamins A, C, and E, folic acid, selenium, zinc, and beta carotene, have all been associated with changes in the cervix.

Having an underactive thyroid can increase the risk.

Smoking, including passive smoking, is a factor, and so is stress.

Having your first baby in your teens increases the risk, and the more pregnancies you have, the higher the incidence of cervical changes.

Women with partners who work with chemicals such as tar, machine oil, dust, asbestos, coal and metals are at greater risk, if their hygiene is poor.

Abnormal pap smear test

If your pap smear test is abnormal there are several things you should do. First, make sure your diet is excellent. Follow all the dietary advice on p.68.

Take supplements of vitamins C, B6, A, and E, iodine, selenium, and zinc. Women taking 10 mg of folic acid daily for three months have been able to reverse moderately severe cervical changes. A good multivitamin and mineral supplement should cover all of these.

Stop smoking. Take plenty of exercise in the fresh air, ensure that you allow time for rest and relaxation and that you get enough sleep.

Drink only filtered or bottled water.

Although orthodox therapy involves local treatment, it is important to bear in mind that cancer is a systemic condition, regardless of where it is found, and is an indication that the body's defenses are severely compromised.

Cancer of the cervix

Cervical cancer can cause bleeding in between periods if you are still menstruating, or at any time if you are post-menopausal. You may have bleeding after sex or a smelly vaginal discharge.

The average age of women with cervical cancer is 45 although recently many younger women have developed it.

To help prevent cervical cancer

○ Use a condom to protect the cervix from genital warts, herpes, trichomonas and even sperm. It is significant that cancer of the cervix is about four times lower in women whose partners have had a vasectomy.
○ Ensure that your partner washes his penis carefully before sex as well as his hands, particularly if you do not use a condom and if he works with any of the risk chemicals (see above).
○ Avoid using the contraceptive pill.
○ Make sure you (and your partner) seek prompt treatment for vaginal or cervical infections (see vaginal infections p.224), and have any genital warts removed if other treatment is unsuccessful.
○ Have regular pap smear tests.
○ Ensure you have a healthy diet and lifestyle and take the supplements recommended to reverse abnormal changes in the cervix.

It is important to look at the relationship between mind and body. Stress and unresolved emotional problems may well be undermining your immune system. Several studies on the interaction between emotions and the development of cervical cancer found that women with this kind of cancer tended to experience emotional difficulties in their lives.

Uterine cancer

Cancer of the endometrium, the lining of the uterus, is most common in women between the ages of 50 and 70. It tends to grow slowly and stay within the uterus, rather than spreading as other cancers can.

Factors associated with the development of uterine cancer

overweight, obesity – tending to increase estrogen levels in the body which can influence the growth of some uterine cancers
diabetes
having no children increases the risk slightly
having had breast cancer
excess estrogen from hormone replacement therapy
starting periods early and having a late menopause, increasing the years that estrogen circulates in the system
polycystic ovaries
hypertension
nutritional deficiencies – too much fatty food and not enough fresh fruit, vegetables and whole grains, fibre, beta carotene, selenium, vitamins E, A and D
an underactive thyroid – often due to iodine deficiency contributing to excess estrogen

Symptoms of uterine cancer

bleeding between periods in menstruating women
vaginal bleeding at any time in post-menopausal women
excessive bleeding before, during or after a period
bloody vaginal discharge

There may, of course, be other explanations for such symtoms. A diagnosis is confirmed by analysis of cells from the endometrium taken by a uterine biopsy.

Ovarian cancer

The ovaries are small oval-shaped organs which produce the sex hormones progesterone and estrogen and which also release eggs.

Factors associated with development of ovarian cancer

the more pregnancies a woman has, the less risk of ovarian cancer
the highest risk is in women who have not had any children
post-menopausal women over 50 have a greater tendency to develop this cancer than younger women
high fat intake increases risk, as docs obesity
deficiencies of vitamin A and beta carotene
the contraceptive pill is thought to protect against ovarian cancer
hormonal imbalances may contribute to the risk
women who have had breast cancer, or cancer of the bowel or rectum are at greater risk
radiation

Symptoms of ovarian cancer

These symptoms only appear once the cancer is well developed.

pain in the lower abdomen
swelling of the abdomen and a bloated feeling
mild indigestion, or nausea
constipation or diarrhea
poor appetite
loss of weight
possible shortness of breath
there may be bleeding between periods, or in post-menopausal women, at any time

Diagnosis can be made after either an ultrasound or CAT scan or laparoscopy.

Treatment of cancer

Part of the reason why cancer holds so much terror for women is that it may develop in their sexual or reproductive organs and that orthodox treatment, particularly surgery, may mean losing valuable parts of them that are closely related to feelings of femininity, attractiveness and sexual identity.

There may also be a fear of loss of sexual or sensual pleasures and shame about the illness itself. The most positive way to approach cancer treatment is through prevention, and by enhancing the function of the immune system in as many ways as possible. Since it is said that 80 per cent of carcinogenic influences are environmental it may be that this is more of a political question, since a change in environmental policies involves changes in social, political and economic conditions, so many of us may want to join and support environmental groups and campaign for the necessary changes. It would be good if our children had fewer risks.

In the meantime however, there is much we can improve in our own environment.

Self help to prevent cancer

○ Stop smoking and drinking.
○ Stop using synthetic chemicals in our homes and gardens and where possible at work.
○ Eat a healthy diet, avoid known carcinogens such as nitrates and nitrites.
○ Eat organic food as much as possible. The more demand that is created, the more shops are likely to stock them at competitive prices.
○ Drink unpolluted water – most tap water has nitrates and fluoride among other toxic chemicals.
○ Cut down on fatty food and if you are overweight it is important to seek to remedy this.

○ Avoid X-rays wherever possible and ultraviolet light from strong sunlight and sun beds.
○ DO NOT take synthetic hormones in the form of the pill or ERT.
○ Treat any vaginal infections, particularly viruses, promptly.
○ If you have any other chronic illness or infection, allergies or feel generally run down, you should seek treatment.
○ Take plenty of regular, aerobic exercise.
○ Make sure you get enough rest, relaxation and sleep.
○ Examine the stresses in your life and your response to them.

Stress and cancer

The relationship between the mind, the emotions and the body has been well researched, especially in the field of cancer. Many women who develop cancer apparently have a tendency not to express their emotions in the normal way, and as a result these emotions can build up and manifest through the body. We all have sources of negative emotions, and we all need outlets for them.

Women who suppress their anger have, for instance, raised levels of immunoglobin IgA in their bloodstreams which is related to breast cancer and its spread to other parts of the body.

However, this is not to blame the personality for cancer, but only to recognize that some traits may contribute to the illness and can be remedied. Any regime to prevent or treat precancer or cancer therefore needs to pay attention to the mind and the emotions, and to the development of the spiritual self.

It is important to seek whatever help you feel to be most appropriate to help you to break free of the past, to embrace the present and live in it as fully as possible.

Diet and cancer

A healthy diet is one of the best ways to protect against cancer and enhance the immune system's fight against it.

Certain food substances called antioxidants have been shown to have anti-cancer properties and should be eaten regularly.

vitamin A and beta carotene
vitamin C
vitamin E
selenium
B vitamins
folic acid
essential fatty acids

For foods containing these substances, see Diet chart on p.70.

Herbs and cancer

There are several herbs which have been found to have anti-cancer properties which can be used either to help prevent or treat cancer.

Use any of these in conjunction with orthodox treatment:

yellow dock	*plantain*
garlic	*huang qi*
nettle	*echinacea*
myrrh	*burdock*
cleavers	*poke root*
thyme	*blessed thistle*
St John's wort	*calendula*
greater horsetail	

Herbal treatment should begin with a cleansing programme which is best carried out only if you are strong enough and with the help of an experienced practitioner.

A useful general cleansing mixture is made with equal parts of burdock, cleavers, yellow dock, calendula and echinacea. Add a little licorice and peppermint according to taste and take as tea or tincture three times daily.

There are certain herbs with a reputation for having anti-cancer properties and an affinity for particular areas of the body.

For the breast they include:

poke root	*cleavers*
calendula	*dandelion root*
yellow dock	

For the uterus and cervix they include:

calendula	*myrrh*
plantain	*burdock*
rose	

For changes in the cervix herbs can be used locally two or three times daily as a douche or in tincture form and applied via an applicator or on a tampon. If you use an applicator lie down for ten minutes afterwards, to ensure the herbs have a chance to reach the cervix. If you use a tampon insert it soaked in dilute tincture, using half to one teaspoon of tincture in some water.

Use equal parts of:

golden seal	*thuja*
myrrh	
calendula and rosewater	

For malignancies which are related to estrogen excess, such as tumours in the breast and uterus, you can include hormone balancing herbs in your recipe, such as chaste tree and false unicorn root.

When using herbs to prevent or treat cancer, it is always very important to support the nervous system. Herbs with a nervine action such as wood betony, skullcap, vervain, wild oats or rosemary can be added to your prescription.

The appropriate Bach Flower Remedies could also help you through these difficult times (see chart on p.246–7).

For those who feel run down, tired, lethargic and weak, there are some wonderful herbs which have famous tonic properties, help to impart strength, support the nervous system and invigorate the immune system.

These include:

ginseng	*garlic*
ginger	*huang qi*
myrrh	*clove*
cinnamon	*thyme*
rosemary	

Herbs to relieve the side effects of orthodox treatment for cancer

Any of the above herbs can be used preventatively and as treatment, alongside other treatment. Other herbs as well as foods can prove very useful to help combat side effects of orthodox treatments, to support the body, speed the healing process and restore vitality.

The herbalist can help relieve side effects of radiotherapy and chemotherapy such as nausea, vomiting, poor appetite, tiredness, liver upsets and skin problems. Herbs can also help protect the immune system against damage during orthodox cancer treatment.

For nausea and vomiting use these as teas or tinctures:

cinnamon	*peppermint*
ginger	*chamomile*

Apparently marijuana and cannabis can effectively reduce nausea and vomiting caused by chemotherapy. Several drugs have been made in recent years based on cannabis and used with cancer patients. The herb is said to work better when eaten rather than smoked.

To protect the digestive tract and heal it from the effects of radiotherapy and chemotherapy, take aloe vera juice or capsules, agar agar or other alginates from seaweeds, slippery elm or iceland moss.

To protect the liver take:

dang gui	*yellow dock*
rosemary	*burdock*
dandelion root	

To protect the immune system and restore vitality during chemotherapy and radiotherapy:

echinacea	*ginger*
ginseng	*garlic*

Other Chinese herbs such as ligusticum and codonopsis are famous for their immune-enhancing properties. These, along with huang qi, have been shown to protect glandular function, improve blood production and increase the chances of survival in advanced cancer cases in China. Using these herbs with cancer patients in the USA has been shown to restore the immune system in 90 per cent of cases and to speed recovery and lengthen life expectancy.

Another Chinese herb, Siberian ginseng (*Eleutherococcus senticosus*), has been shown to increase tolerance of anticancer drugs, improve vitality and increase life expectancy. It enhances immunity and improves resistance to unwanted damage in orthodox cancer treatment.

Korean ginseng (*Panax ginseng*) enables the body to cope better with stress, both mental and physical, including that from radiation and chemotherapy. It has been shown to increase survival rates in cancer patients, to restore the blood, and reduce tiredness, illness and debility.

Radiation treatment can cause burning and hair loss. If you apply wheatgerm oil or vitamin E oil to the area before and after each radiation treatment, this will help prevent burning, and reduce pain and scarring. Use it twice daily in the intervals between treatments as well.

If burning does occur, aloe vera gel will speed healing and soothe pain and inflammation. The best way to use aloe vera is straight from the plant – they grow easily as pot plants.

Supplements of vitamin E and beta carotene will help minimize side effects including hair loss.

Radiation therapy and chemotherapy cause drastic reduction of several vitamins in the body which may deplete the system and increase side effects, including vitamins A, C, E, and B complex as well as folic acid. These can be taken as supplements before and after treatment and will help to protect the body from the harmful effects of these treatments.

Also take supplements of antioxidants, which are vital in helping protect the body against damage caused by radiation. Antioxidant substances include vitamins A, C, E and selenium. Several herbs also have antioxidant properties, including thyme, rosemary, garlic and ginger.

Acquired immunodeficiency syndrome (AIDS)

AIDS is a syndrome characterized by a weakened and deficient immune system that lays the body open to a multitude of problems. As far as we know it involves infection with the HIV virus, which is present in body fluids of an infected person, including the blood, menstrual blood, semen, urine, vaginal and rectal secretions. It is mainly transmitted sexually and via contaminated blood. for example on the shared needles of drug users.

Wild oats

Avena sativa

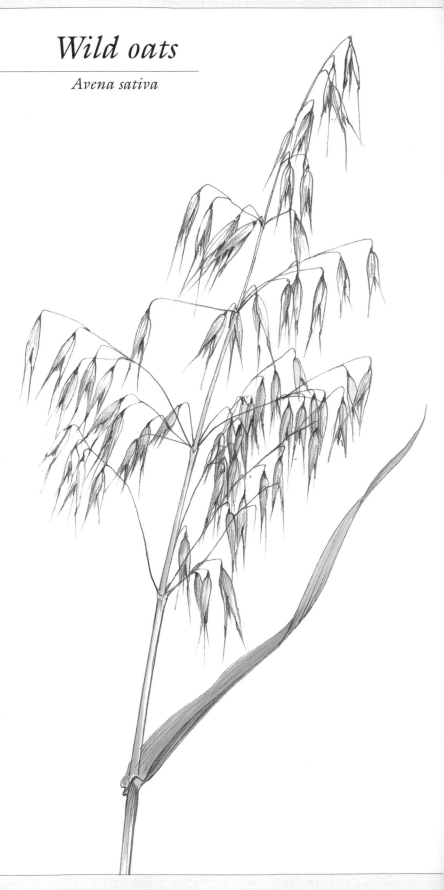

PART USED: Grain

CONTAINS: Starch, alkaloids, saponins, flavones, sterols, vitamin B, protein, fats, minerals

KEY USES: Nervine, tonic, antidepressant, hypoglycemic, nutritive, demulcent, vulnerary, lowers cholesterol

Oats are a wonderfully nutritious remedy, full of protein, calcium, magnesium, silicon, potassium, iron and vitamins. Their body-building nutrients help make strong bones and teeth and are vital to a healthy nervous system – oats have traditionally been used as a nerve tonic to treat depression, debility and nervous exhaustion. They are helpful when withdrawing from tranquilizers and antidepressants. While being stimulating and energy-giving, they are also relaxing and aid sleep. Since oats are easily digested they make an ideal food for the chronically sick, convalescents and when recovering from childbirth. They have a reputation as a uterine tonic and for helping to overcome sterility and impotence, stimulating the thyroid and influencing sex hormone production. Oats have the ability to regulate estrogen levels.

Oat fibre can significantly lower blood cholesterol, helping to combat cardiovascular disease. It can be helpful for high blood pressure, obesity, varicose veins and hemorrhoids.

Oats have been used as a soothing remedy for irritated conditions of the digestive tract, and for problems such as diverticulitis, irritable bowel syndrome, gastritis and constipation. Oat fibre produces bulkier stools and speeds their passage through the gut, reducing the exposure of the gut lining to irritants and carcinogens. This is why oat fibre is said to help prevent cancer of the bowel. Oats are also thought to protect against cancer generally.

Another exciting discovery is that oats are helpful to diabetics as they lower blood sugar. They are also useful for fluid retention.

The most likely ways for the infection to enter the body are by infected semen entering the vagina or anus. It can be absorbed through the mucous membrane of both, particularly if there are ulcers or tears in the walls of the vagina or on the cervix or the walls of the anus. It can also pass pass between people in menstrual blood. It can, rarely, enter during oral sex, especially if there are ulcers or sores in the mouth, or bleeding gums.

Infected body fluids can enter the bloodstream of another person through a graze or cut on the skin, though this is very unlikely as the infected body fluids must actually enter an open wound. They can also enter the bloodstream by injection with an infected needle. A blood transfusion for loss of blood during surgery or an accident, or blood clotting agents for a hemophiliac may carry the virus, though these are now carefully screened in most countries. It is possible to pass infection from a pregnant women to an unborn child either through the placenta or during the birth. The virus is also found in breastmilk.

The HIV virus is more easily transmitted from men to women than vice versa. Not all those who are exposed to the virus actually develop AIDS.

The HIV virus is a retrovirus which is unusual in that it has an affinity for and enters certain cells in the immune system known as T4 cells. Here it alters the genetic code of the T4 cells making them produce more of the virus instead of more T4 cells, and in this way the virus becomes well and truly embedded in the body's cells and remains there forever. The infected T4 cells are now able to make more virus which can then invade more T4 cells, and so the virus multiplies.

However, there are certain factors which must either trigger this process, which when unchecked lead to the development of AIDS. It is not definite that all those who are infected with the HIV virus actually go on to produce AIDS symptoms.

Factors which may increase the risk of this happening include:

malabsorption of food
stress
weakened immunity through poor
    diet, unhealthy lifestyle, ortho-
    dox drug therapy, such as
    antibiotics, particularly cancer
    treatment
recurring illness, or history of other
    illness
previous history of sexually trans-
    mitted disease, such as syphilis
alcohol and smoking
drug use
repeated exposure to the HIV virus
pregnancy may act as a trigger
exposure to certain infections, such
    as salmonella and herpes

On initially being infected with HIV you may not have any symptoms and within 12 weeks you should produce antibodies to the HIV virus. After that time an HIV test should show positive. In some cases it takes much longer to produce antibodies and in some instances they take about six months. It may be years before any symptoms become evident.

Self help for AIDS prevention

The most effective form of self help is to protect yourself as far as possible from developing HIV infection.

The more you know about your sexual partner(s) the better. Check whether he has been or is an intravenous drug user, if he is a hemophiliac, whether he has had or has many other sexual partners, which can obviously increase the risk of infection, whether he has had or has a gay relationship. His lifestyle even of 10-15 years ago is relevant. The fewer sexual partners you have the lower the risk of infection. Some countries carry a higher HIV risk than others, so if your partner comes from or has had a relationship with someone from Africa, the Caribbean, South America, the U.S.A. or the Middle East, the risk of infection is greater.

Be aware of possible contamination from dentists, ear piercers, tattooists, acupuncturists and electrolysis practitioners. Ensure they use disposable needles or that instruments are properly sterilized by bleach or autoclaving. Never share needles if you ever inject drugs, and do not share anybody's toothbrush or razor.

Avoid blood transfusions as far as you can. They are probably safe in the U.S.A. and U.K. but if you know you are due for an operation which may require a transfusion, you can give your own blood in advance to be safer.

Practise safe sex, which means preventing any body fluids from your partner entering your body. That includes semen, blood, urine, and feces. Remember that the linings of the vagina and anus are more absorbent than other parts of the body. Use condoms for contraception, and if you have oral sex make sure neither partner has bleeding gums, cracked lips or mouth ulcers.

If you are caring for others with HIV prevent any body fluids from entering through your skin. Cover cuts or grazes with waterproof plaster, or wear plastic gloves if you have cuts or any inflammatory skin condition such as eczema on the hands. Use bleach for cleaning up any spilled body fluids and wash soiled clothing on a very hot wash in the washing machine after immersing in disinfectant. Most normal domestic contact such as sharing towels, crockery and cutlery, hugging and touching is perfectly safe.

Support the immune system as far as you possibly can through healthy diet, plenty of aerobic exercise and fresh air, adequate sleep, rest and relaxation. Treat minor infections promptly, try to avoid stress and seek help for any long term emotional problems which are causing stress. Practise relaxation, yoga, meditation or any other energy restorative therapy to bring peace into an otherwise probably very hectic life.

Therapy if you are HIV positive

The first thing you will need is a great deal of support from family, friends and counselling services. There are many different HIV and AIDS helplines (see Appendix), and you should contact one as soon as you can.

You need to enhance the immune system by following the guidelines above and by taking certain foods, food supplements and herbs which are especially useful in the treatment of chronic viral infections (see the advice on p.225).

Essential fatty acids are vital to normal function of the immune system. They are found in fatty fish, unrefined cold pressed vegetable oils, beans and pulses, nuts and seeds. Take supplements of cod liver oil and Evening Primrose oil daily. Make sure you get plenty of antioxidant substances in your diet, including vitamins A, E, C, and selenium. B complex vitamins in brewer's yeast and yeast extract are useful.

If you have candida or a yeast infection you will need to obtain yeastfree B vitamins. A multimineral and vitamin supplement will help provide other substances the immune system needs such as iron, calcium, magnesium, zinc

and iodine. These combined with an excellent diet will also help protect against side effects from any prescribed drugs you may be taking.

A high protein diet is necessary to build up the immune system, although a cleansing, light diet is helpful while there are infections present. Eating yoghurt, garlic and unrefined olive oil, and cutting down on meat and meat products will help the normal bacterial population in the gut to flourish and so reduce the likelihood of gut infections and diarrhea.

Make sure you have a high proportion of fresh fruit and vegetables in your diet, preferably organically grown.

Garlic, onion, leeks, radish and horseradish contain substances which protect the liver from damage by chemicals and drugs and are rich in selenium, a natural antioxidant.

Cider vinegar and honey taken daily in a little hot water will help prevent infections in the mouth, throat and digestive tract. Cider vinegar in water also makes a good douche for thrush and other vaginal infections. Propolis helps fight off infection by stimulating the immune system to make antibodies. It helps white blood cells to destroy infecting organisms.

Foods such as cabbage, cauliflower, brussels sprouts, broccoli, spring greens and lemons help the liver in its breakdown of toxins and drug substances.

Avoid the use of the following:

sugar
fatty foods and meat
tobacco
refined cooking oils
alcohol
fried foods
junk foods
caffeine
refined carbohydrates
antibiotics, unless vital

Herbs for the immune system:

echinacea   *golden seal*
garlic

Dang gui helps to protect the immune system and activate different kinds of white blood cells and antibody-forming cells in the spleen.

Licorice regulates the function of white blood cells and promotes antibody production.

Panax ginseng increases the number of white blood cells, which fight infection, and makes them more effective. It increases the energy and efficiency of the liver and spleen in their immunological efforts and is excellent for those who are feeling very debilitated and weak from illness. It is not recommended during acute infection or inflammation, as it can drive the infection deeper.

Aromatic spices including ginger, cinnamon, cloves, and cardamon all include volatile oils which are strongly antimicrobial and help to ward off infection. They are all excellent strengthening herbs, which help to relieve debility and weakness, improve vitality and support a worn down nervous system. Use them in cooking and as massage oils.

Antioxidant substances present in thyme, garlic, ginger and rosemary will help protect the liver from any orthodox drugs necessary. Astragalus increases vitality, helps to stop debilitating sweating and promotes healing and repair. It has an antiviral action. St. John's wort has recently been the subject of research on its antiviral properties and particularly against retro-viruses.

Many clinical trials using St. John's wort extract are being carried out with HIV and AIDS patients and so far results look promising. Lemon balm has also been shown to be active against a number of viruses including Herpes Simplex. Other herbs in the same family, such as thyme, hyssop and rosemary, may well act as antiviral agents also.

Herbs to detoxify the system and cleanse waste products from the body should also be used. These will help minimize side effects from any orthodox drugs you may be taking by protecting the liver and enhancing their elimination from the body.

Bitters will help remove toxins from the liver and protect it from damage by drug therapy.

Suitable bitters include:

rosemary	dandelion root
golden seal	wormwood
myrrh	yellow dock root

Dang gui has also been shown to increase the breakdown of drug substances in the liver. Blood purifying herbs such as cleavers, poke root, plantain, and burdock can also be used.

Diuretic herbs will hasten the excretion of toxins and wastes via the urinary system:

burdock	cleavers
corn silk	dandelion leaf

Herbs to support the nervous system (see p.52) are essential. Add to your prescription tonic herbs such as skullcap, vervain, ginseng, wild oats, cinnamon and rosemary.

For depression, lethargy and weakness choose rosemary, lemon balm, St. John's wort, celery seed, borage, wild oats, ginger or cardamon.

For tension or insomnia try passionflower, hops, linden blossom or chamomile.

Nutritional herbs will help restore energy and vitality and provide raw materials for repair. These are parsley, kelp, garlic, oats, nettles, dandelion leaves, and borage.

Malabsorption of food and a leaky gut, allowing waste products, foods and bacterial poisons to pass into the bloodstream can occur in HIV infections. Digestive remedies such as tormentil, oak bark, dandelion root, rosemary and chamomile may be helpful.

Recently there has been speculation as to whether or not HIV is the sole cause of AIDS. Some believe it may be related to syphilis as the advanced symptoms are similar and people with AIDS often also have syphilis. Others feel that unhealthy lifestyle, medical history, repeated infections and use of drugs may well be to blame.

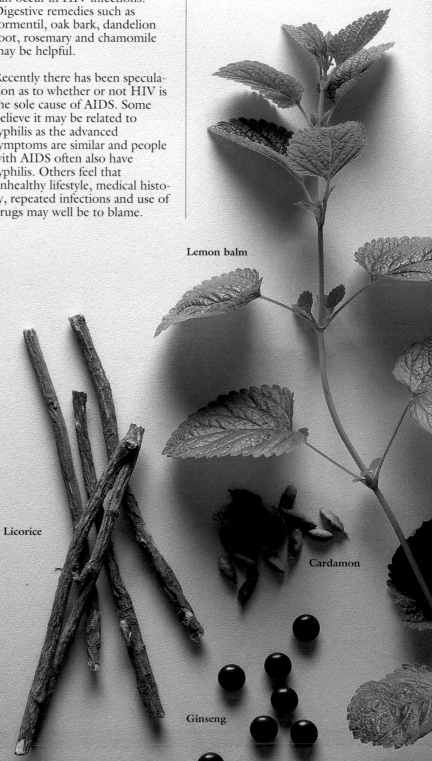

Lemon balm

Licorice

Cardamon

Ginseng

The Bach Flower Remedies

The Bach Flower Remedies are prepared from the flowers of wild plants, bushes and trees and are aimed at helping to resolve emotional and psychological disturbances, which are at the root of many physical imbalances.

For Fear

Rock Rose for fright, panic, terror, hysteria. A remedy for emergencies, even when there appears to be no hope.

Mimulus for fear of everyday known things, such as illness, death, old age, pain, darkness or being alone. Also for shyness and fear of others. These fears are kept inside and are revealed to others.

Cherry Plum for fear of being overstrained or losing control of the body, mind or emotions, such as uncontrollable anger and other impulses which may cause harm to oneself or others, including suicidal tendencies.

Aspen for vague fears of the unknown, a sense of foreboding, nightmares or terror of approaching misfortune for no apparent reason. One is often afraid to talk about these fears to other people.

Red Chestnut for overconcern or fear about the welfare of others, especially loved ones, during times such as illness, journeys, when away from them. Often one does not worry for oneself.

For Uncertainty

Cerato for doubt about one's ability to make decisions and judgements, and for constantly seeking advice from others and often being misguided.

Wild Oat for those who feel dissatisfied in their way of life, but have difficulty in determining what path to follow, though their ambition is strong.

Gentian for people who are easily discouraged, in whom small setbacks can cause depression, self-doubt, and despondency, even though generally they are doing well.

Gorse for great hopelessness, feelings of despair and futility. For giving up believing that any more can be done for them. If pushed or to please others, they may try various treatments with little real hope of improvement.

Hornbeam for those who feel they need strengthening and help physically or mentally to bear the burden life has placed upon their shoulders. For the "Monday morning" feeling, not feeling up to facing the coming day, the pressures of everyday life.

Scleranthus for indecision, inability to choose between two things, changing one's mind; energy and mood swings. For people who are quiet and tend not to talk about their difficulties to others.

For Insufficient Interest in Present Circumstances

Clematis for people who have a tendency to daydream, think about the future, and do not live fully in the present. For lack of concentration, making little effort in everyday life, and for living in hope of happier times ahead.

Chestnut Bud for those who do not learn from observation and experience and constantly repeat the same experiences and make the same mistakes, before their lesson is learnt.

Honeysuckle for those who live in the past, and do not expect happiness as they have enjoyed before. For nostalgia, homesickness, reminiscing.

Wild Rose for those who resign themselves to their present circumstances, and make little effort to find joy or happiness. For uncomplaining apathy.

Olive for complete mental and physical exhaustion brought on by ordeals. Daily life seems hard, without joy, and wearisome.

White Chestnut for persistent unwanted thoughts and ideas, which, though thrown out, return when there is not sufficient interest in the present to fully occupy the mind. For mental arguments, preoccupation, obsessive thoughts which cause mental torture, and an inability to relax or concentrate fully on work or leisure in the day.

Mustard for periods of sadness, gloom or even despair, which descend for no apparent reason, making it impossible to feel happiness or joy.

For Loneliness

Water Violet for very quiet people who appear aloof, and prefer to be alone. They are independent and self-reliant, often bright and talented, and do not tend to get involved in other people's affairs. They radiate peace and tranquillity to those around them.

Impatiens for those who think and act quickly, and so want everything done without delay. They are often happier working or being alone so that they can go at their own speed, for they are often impatient or irritated by others who do things more slowly.

Heather for people who need to discuss their affairs with other people and so seek the company of anybody who will listen. They become very unhappy if they are left alone for any length of time.

For Being Oversensitive to Ideas and Influences

Agrimony for cheerful, jovial people who hide their troubles behind their humour, not wishing to burden others with them. They will go to great lengths to avoid arguments or disharmony, and may turn to alcohol or drugs to stimulate themselves and help cope cheerfully with pain or anxiety.

Centaury for kind people who find it hard to say "no", being over-anxious to please and serve others and tending to work harder on other people's behalf than on their own particular calling or interests. They are easily exploited.

Walnut for breaking links with the past and helping adjustments to new phases (such as new relationships, jobs, houses), balancing emotions in transition periods (such as starting school, puberty, marriage, menopause) or even death of a loved one. The remedy helps protect one from outside influences which may cause one to stray from a chosen path.

Holly for people who are overcome by negative emotions such as anger, jealousy, envy, and suspicion. They suffer much inside, often when there is no real cause.

For Despondency or Despair

Elm for diligent people, who are doing good work, often helping others, and following a vocation, but who feel overburdened or over-extended at times, which causes depression or despondency.

Crab Apple for cleansing. For people who feel self-disgust or contamination, feelings of shame or low self-esteem, concentrating obsessively on one shameful aspect of themselves and ignoring others. For detoxification of the body, and cleansing of wounds, whether emotional or physical, internal or external.

Larch for people who do not consider themselves as good or as capable as those around them. Even though they may be perfectly able and accomplished, they lack confidence and expect failure, so that often they do not try hard enough to succeed.

Sweet Chestnut for those who feel that the anguish is so great it is unbearable, they have reached the limits of their endurance, and there is nothing left but dark despair.

Star of Bethlehem for great distress and unhappiness following shock, such as bad news, the death of a loved one, or an accident.

Willow for those who feel bitter or resentful about their misfortune, and, as a result, take less interest in the things in life they used to enjoy doing. They feel that life is unjust and unfair.

Oak for those who never give up, despite setbacks, misfortunes or illness. They keep trying one thing after another, determined to reach their goal, and never losing hope.

Pine for people who blame themselves and feel guilty. Even when they succeed, they are not satisfied with their efforts or results, and feel they could have done better. They work hard and suffer much from the faults they attach to themselves, even claiming responsibility for mistakes which are not theirs.

For Overconcern with the Welfare of Others

Chicory for those who are over concerned for the needs of others, friends, relatives or children, continually correcting them and wanting them to conform with their ideas. They are possessive, demanding and can be self-pitying.

Vine for strong, capable people, who are self-confident and powerful, certain they are right. They can be dictatorial and overbearing, dominating and directing others with their conviction, even during illness.

Vervain for those with strong ideas, fixed opinions, those who are always right and wish to teach and convert those around them. They can be over-enthusiastic and over-powering but, during illness, their determination helps them to struggle more than others.

Beech for perfectionists, who need to see more good in all around them and who are easily critical and intolerant. They tend to overlook the positive aspects of other people, over-reacting to minor details and lacking understanding of individual idiosyncrasies.

Rock Water for strictness and self-denial. They shun many of the pleasures of life for fear they will interfere with their work; they drive themselves hard and feel the need to live their lives as an example to others. They want to be strong and fit and will do whatever they believe is necessary to keep themselves so.

Directions

Take two drops of the chosen remedies and place them in a small bottle filled with water and a little brandy if you want to keep it for some time. Take four drops of this in a little water, or any convenient way, four times daily or when necessary.

Rescue Remedy

This is the remedy of emergency, for calming emotions during a crisis or trauma. Add four drops of Rescue Remedy to a quarter of a glass of liquid and sip every few minutes or as often as necessary. Hold in the mouth a while before swallowing. Alternatively, place four drops under the tongue or in a spoonful of water, or rub it on the lips, behind the ears or on the wrists.

13   *Herbs for Beauty*

For thousands of years women have prepared cosmetics and perfumes from the natural resources available to them, to care for their skin, hair, eyes and lips and to enhance their natural beauty. The ancient Egyptians are known to have used herbs and oils; the beauty box of the Queen Thuthu (1400BC), which was found in her tomb at Thebes, contains pumice stone for removing rough skin, eye pencils of wood and ivory used for applying kohl and antimony to the eyes, a bronze dish for mixing ingredients such as lapis lazuli powder for eye shadow, as well as three cosmetic pots she probably used for henna, scented oils and creams.

The ancient Greeks were also well versed in the use of herbs and oils for making beauty preparations; they made a study of the connection between health and beauty. Hippocrates, the famous Greek physician, developed the science of dermatology and advised exercise, healthy diet, massages and baths to improve and maintain health and beauty. The Romans dyed their hair with myrtle and walnut husks, darkened their eyes with kohl, bathed their heads with extracts of myrtle and juniper berries to prevent their hair from thinning and rubbed alkanet root on their cheeks to make them rosy.

The first cold cream ever recorded was made by Galen, a famous Roman doctor of the 2nd century. It included oils, wax and water, the basic recipe of cold creams ever since. Then, as now, women used myriad combinations of herbs, oils, powders and other natural ingredients to keep the skin soft and supple, to sweeten the breath, make the hair shine, brighten the eyes and perfume the body. They were concerned to delay wrinkles, prevent thinning or greying of the hair, to keep the skin free of blemishes and acne and protect the skin from wind and sun.

Natural ingredients such as honey, oils and fats, herbs and spices, grains and meals, fruits and vegetables, milk and vinegar, which were used in the ancient world, provide an alternative way to care for your appearance today. Modern aids to beauty involve the use of hormones, detergents, artificial colouring and synthetic perfumes as well as chemicals which can cause allergic reactions and may have been tested on animals. You can make beauty products using natural ingredients fairly simply at home, giving you complete control over what you put on your skin. They can be made up in small, trial amounts and making them is both satisfy-

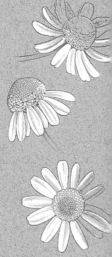

Chamomile
Matricaria chamomilla

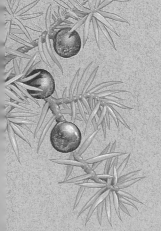

Juniper
Juniperus communis

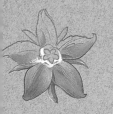

ing and enjoyable. Fruits and vegetables from your own garden or local grower are perfectly suitable; fragrant herbs such as rosemary and chamomile are easy to grow in pots and ingredients such as elderflowers may be harvested from hedgerows.

Beauty and health

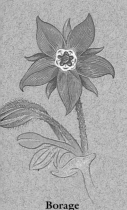

Borage
Borago officinalis

Our outward appearance is really only a manifestation of our inner state of health, of both body and mind. Beauty exists as much in the mind, or the heart, or even the soul, as it does in the physical body. Our inner thoughts and emotions are expressed through the light in the eyes, the movements of the face muscles, and the way we hold each part of our body. If we feel angry, worried, resentful, fearful, jealous or sad this will show clearly in our faces and body language, undermining not only the health of our inner selves, but also marring our outer beauty.

If you are aware of inner tensions and strains in your life, it is important to look at them and attempt to resolve them. Make sure you set aside time in your day to relax and let go, to do things purely for your pleasure. If you see stress and tension showing up in the face, causing taut muscles, wrinkles, tense lines and loss of skin tone, massage away the tensions in your face and body with dilute essential oils of either lavender, geranium, melissa or ylang ylang, or add a few drops to a warm bath and luxuriate in it for a few minutes. Herbal teas of chamomile, lavender, lemon balm, skullcap, vervain, borage or linden blossom can be drunk freely to soothe tensions and lift spirits, as well as to relax taut muscles throughout the body.

A healthy diet and lifestyle are vital to health and a beautiful complexion, to the shine in the eyes and hair. Plenty of fresh air, exercise, rest and relaxation, adequate sleep and a nutritious diet will help protect against the effects of aging and the accumulation of toxins in the system, which congest the tissues causing acne and blemishes. Plenty of polyunsaturated fats are essential, and will not increase oiliness of the skin. They are found in nuts and seeds, whole grains, cold-pressed nut and vegetable oils, fatty fish, beans and pulses. Vitamin C is vital to beautiful skin; it builds collagen and elastin, which are structural substances giving tone and elasticity to the skin keeping it free from wrinkles. Eat plenty of fresh fruit and vegetables, especially blackcurrants, watercress, parsley, citrus fruits and greens, all high in vitamin C. Vitamin A keeps the skin healthy, supple, free from acne and ensures rapid healing. It is found in watercress, carrots, parsley, dandelion leaves and fatty fish. B vitamins help balance the function of the skin; a dry and flaky skin, or cracked or peeled lips could indicate a deficiency.

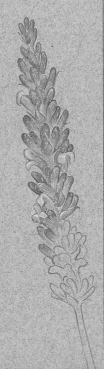

Lavender
Lavendula officinalis

The skin

Our skin is wonderfully suited to fulfil a variety of functions. It is our first line of defence against damage from infection, chemical pollution, extremes of temperature and light, and physical injury. It secretes antiseptic substances to ward off invading micro-organisms, and is home to beneficial bacteria which discourage the proliferation of less favourable ones. It has an acid mantle which is vital to the health of such defence systems, and for this reason it is important that the pH of the skin is not disturbed by over cleaning, heavy creams, perfumes, deodorants and the like.

When the weather is very cold, blood vessels in the skin contract and help keep heat inside the body. When it is very hot the blood vessels dilate and the blood suffuses to the surface of the body, losing heat into the atmosphere and keeping the body cool.

The skin is also a major organ of excretion, with several million sweat glands through which the average adult excretes about one pint (600 ml) of liquid every day. During vigorous exercise or in hot weather this can increase by ten times or more. Sweat contains water, mineral salts, nitrogenous wastes and other toxins – in fact it is similar in content to urine. Diaphoretic herbs such as chamomile, yarrow, linden blossom and catmint can be taken as hot teas to increase perspiration, and thereby clear toxins from the system, as well as bring down a fever. Sweat contributes to the function of the protective acid mantle covering the body, helping to ward off harmful bacteria, and maintains the balance of electrolytes and mineral salts in the blood. If you do not take sufficient vigorous exercise to produce a sweat on a regular basis, a greater burden rests on the other organs of elimination – the lungs, bowels and kidneys.

The skin is also an organ of sense: it is richly supplied with sensitive nerve endings which relay messages to the brain about sensations from the outside world: heat or cold, pleasure or pain. It is the point of contact between our inner and outer worlds, so it is hardly surprising that many skin problems arise not only through physical abuse of the skin but also through emotional disharmony. The skin reflects our inner state on both physical and emotional levels.

Skin care

The surface of your skin needs to be kept moist as well as clean, to protect it from the harmful effects of drying wind, burning sun and environmental pollution. All preparations used either to cleanse, tone, moisturize or nourish the skin should be used in moderation. Always remember that your skin is alive, breathing and eliminating, and that its delicate balance of pH, moisture and immunity can easily be damaged by too much cleansing, toning, and moisturizing which can clog the pores.

The preparations you use on your skin will vary according to your skin type, the time of year, your general health and the atmosphere you live in. Beware of using the same product for too long, as your skin can become sensitive to it. When applying anything to your skin, always be gentle; do not drag the skin or rub it too vigorously. Avoid extremes of temperature such as facial saunas or cold water splashes to wake you up in the morning. Make-up is best avoided as far as possible as it tends to clog up the pores; it dries and ages the skin as well as making it look dull and lifeless.

Cleansing

Removing dirt and make-up is best done once a day at night, unless your skin is very oily, in which case it may be necessary to cleanse in the morning as well. Cleansing creams and lotions are preferable to water and most soaps, which can over-dry the skin and damage its pH, especially if your skin is dry and sensitive. However, unperfumed natural soaps and rainwater are suitable for many people for face washing.

Toning

Regular toning after cleansing, a bath or facial steaming, is important to keep the skin firm and fine in texture. It counteracts any tendency to large pores, and sagging of the skin, and will help eliminate excessive oiliness and any residue left from the cleanser. Skin tonics are generally prepared with astringent fruits or herbs which have a refreshing and stimulating effect on the skin.

Moisturizing

Light oil, creams or lotions can be applied to the skin regularly to protect the skin from the effects of winds, sun, central heating, and environmental pollution. Avoid using heavy oils or creams as they do not allow the skin to breathe properly. It is best only to moisturize in the morning and leave the skin to breathe freely at night.

Skin types

It is important to ascertain what kind of skin you have so that you can tailor your beauty preparations to your own individual needs.

Normal skin

Normal skin is smooth, soft and supple and has a healthy shine and a fine texture. It generally is free of problems and requires only the simplest care to keep it looking good. Even normal skins, however, tend to become more dry and sensitive with age.

Dry skin

Dry skin tends to be more delicate than normal skin, and has less glow. It is thin, flaky and prone to fine lines. It can feel taut across the face especially after cleansing or toning, and requires careful moisturizing. It needs gentle care, only mild cleansing, and light oils or lotions for moisturizing.

Dry skin is often caused by overuse of soap on the skin, or frequent exposure to the harsh winds or the drying effect of air conditioning or central heating without the protection of moisturizers. It can also be related to stress, tiredness or poor diet.

On dry skin you need to use soothing and hydrating herbs such as comfrey, rose and chamomile to soften and lubricate the skin.

Oily skin

Oily skin tends to be shiny, sallow and coarser in texture than normal skin, often with enlarged, open pores prone to blackheads and acne. It tends to wrinkle less than other types of skin, staying supple longer, and is less vulnerable to the drying effects of the wind and sun.

Oily skin is caused by excess sebum secreted by overactive sebaceous glands, and may be related to hormonal imbalance, poor diet or stress. To improve an oily skin, you need both internal and external treatments.

Avoid rich, greasy and fried foods, junk foods, and sugar; eat plenty of fresh fruit and vegetables. Cleansing teas of herbs such as dandelion, cleavers, and borage are also helpful. On the skin you should use in your preparation astringent herbs which reduce oiliness, tighten the skin, help close the pores and heal blemishes. Such herbs are calendula, witch hazel, yarrow, horsetail, sage and elderflower.

Oily skin requires more thorough cleansing than other types of skin as grease attracts dirt and is a breeding ground for acne and infection. However, cleansing that is too vigorous can over-stimulate the sebaceous glands, causing them to produce even more oil, so cleansing must always be gentle.

Combination skin

Some parts of the face may have normal to dry skin, while others, particularly around the nose, mouth and chin where there are more sebaceous glands, tend to be oily. If you have this type of skin you will need certain beauty preparations for the dry to normal areas, and others for the oily ones. Alternatively you can use those herbs which are suited to all skin types, including chamomile, comfrey, elderflower, fennel and rose. Cucumber is also useful for combination skin.

Sensitive skin

Sensitive skin tends to be on the dry side, finely textured and prone to rashes or allergic reactions. There may be broken capillaries in the skin and red, inflamed patches. Gentle care is required when looking after such skin; use light lotions for cleansing and moisturizing and mild toners which are soothing and healing. Suitable herbs are chamomile, coltsfoot, rose, fennel, comfrey, elderflower, and borage. Cucumber is also soothing and healing and helps restore the acid mantle of the skin, important for its protection.

Mature skin

As the skin ages so it tends to lose its tone and elasticity and its ability to hold moisture, and so it becomes more dry. This process is accelerated by poor diet, stress, unhealthy lifestyle, pollution, central heating, grimacing and lack of adequate moisture in the skin. It is important to include plenty of protein in your diet as well as vitamins A, B, C, and E to provide the building blocks for skin cells to ensure skin regeneration.

Mature skin can be cleansed, toned, softened and nourished to maintain a healthy glow. Useful herbs include comfrey, marshmallow, rose, fennel, elderflower and chamomile. Cucumber and vitamin E in wheatgerm oil are very beneficial. Dilute cider vinegar and lemon juice, as well as cucumber, should be used regularly on the skin.

Brewer's yeast taken daily will help prevent premature aging of the skin. Antioxidants such as vitamins C and E also help prevent premature aging, so be sure to include plenty in your diet.

Recipes for skin preparations

Once you have chosen a recipe, make it up in small amounts to try out on your skin, as everybody's skin reacts differently. Larger amounts need to be stored in the refrigerator where some will keep for several weeks, or even months, depending on the ingredients. You should always use distilled water when making recipes.

Should you need to warm your ingredients while making up recipes, place the bowl or jar containing your mixture in a pan of hot water and place on a low heat if necessary. Both fresh and dried herbs can be used in beauty preparations though twice the quantity of fresh herbs are required to make-up for their extra moisture. Make sure to label and date your preparations as soon as you have made them and make a note of each recipe and how well it suited you.

To prevent bacterial contamination, ensure that your hands are clean while making up recipes and also when dipping your fingers into creams and lotions.

Cleansers

Apply lotions with clean fingers or cotton wool and massage gently into the skin to loosen dirt and remove make-up. Avoid dragging the skin and use light, stroking movements upwards across the face. Wipe off with soft tissues or cotton wool, or use tepid herbal infusions to rinse off.

For oily skin

For simple cleansers you can use tepid infusions of either elderflowers, yarrow, sage, lady's mantle, calendula or chamomile to rinse the face. Rose water is also useful. Cucumber is an ideal cleanser for oily skin. Mix a little cucumber pureé with half a pint of milk and keep it in the refrigerator for up to three days. Shake well before use. Alternatively if you grate half a cucumber and boil it in half a pint of milk gently for three minutes, cool, sieve, and bottle it, it will keep for a week.

Fennel helps to remove dirt and impurities from oily skin. Bran, oatmeal, or cornmeal can be used daily as facial scrubs to help absorb excess oil on the skin. Take a small handful of fine oatmeal and mix a little water, milk or buttermilk with it to make a paste, and wash the face gently with it. This will help prevent blackheads.

Almond milk cleanser

2 teaspoons ground almonds
¼ pint of rose water

Blend for 2 minutes, strain and bottle.

Buttermilk and fennel cleanser

½ cup (125 ml) buttermilk
2 teaspoons fennel seed

Heat the milk and crushed fennel seed slowly for 30 minutes in a double boiler. Leave to cool and infuse for 2 hours. Strain and bottle; this keeps in a refrigerator for up to a week.

For dry to normal skin

Sweet almond oil is cleansing and nourishing and is excellent for removing dirt and make-up. Remove excess oil with elderflower or chamomile in tepid infusion.

Orange flower cleansing cream

1 oz (25 ml) soya oil
1 oz (25 ml) almond oil
1 oz (25 ml) orange flower water
1 oz (25 g) cocoa butter
1 tablespoon (15 g) beeswax
5 drops essential oil of neroli

Mix and warm the oils. Melt the cocoa butter separately, then stir into the oils. Melt the beeswax and stir it into the oil mixture. Add the orange flower water, leave to thicken and cool. Stir in the essential oil as the mixture thickens; spoon into jars. Neroli stimulates the formation of new skin cells.

Glycerine and rose water cleansing cream

4 tablespoons (60 ml) lanolin
2 oz (50 ml) almond oil
1 tablespoon (15 ml) glycerine
3 tablespoons (45 ml) rose water
6 drops essential oil of rose

Melt the lanolin in one pan and heat the glycerine and almond oil to the same heat in another. Mix the two together, slowly stirring all the time. Add the rose water gradually, leave to cool and stir in the rose oil.

For dry skin

Apricot oil is nourishing and moisturizing and makes a good cleanser. Wash off any excess oil

Rose

Rosa species

Note Avoid during pregnancy.

PARTS USED: Hips, leaves, flowers

CONTAINS: Vitamins C, B, E, K, tannins, pectin, carotene, fruit acids, fatty oil, nicotinamide

KEY USES: Relaxant, nutrient, mild laxative and diuretic, astringent, refrigerant, detoxifying, decongestant, nervine

The beautiful perfumed rose has many medicinal uses. The leaves and petals have a cooling effect and can be used in tea to bring down fevers and clear toxins and heat from the body when they produce rashes and inflammatory problems. Rose also enhances immunity, helping to restrain the development of infections through their cleansing action. An infusion of rose petals can relieve cold and flu symptoms, sore throat, runny nose and blocked bronchial tubes. An infusion or syrup of the petals or hips strengthens the lungs in their fight against infection and is particularly useful for those prone to chest problems. Roses also help fight infection in the digestive tract and help re-establish the normal bacterial population of the intestines. Rose petals and seeds have a diuretic action, relieving fluid retention and hastening elimination of wastes via the kidneys.

Rose petals have a decongestant action in the female reproductive system. They can be used to relieve uterine congestion causing pain and heavy periods, as well as for irregular periods, infertility and to enhance sexual desire.

An infusion makes a useful astringent remedy for diarrhea, enteritis and dysentery. Interestingly, rose petal tea has also been used as a laxative, as well as a liver remedy, promoting bile flow, stimulating and cleansing the liver and gallbladder, and relieving problems associated with a sluggish liver, such as headaches and constipation.

Rose hips and petals have an uplifting, restoring effect on the nervous system, and can relieve insomnia, lift depression, dispel fatigue and soothe irritability.

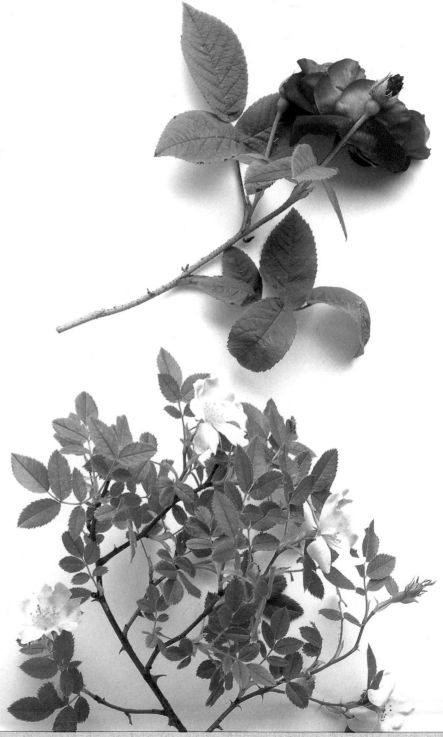

with a tepid infusion of chamomile or elderflower. Lemons will help restore the acid pH of the skin.

Chamomile cleansing milk

½ *cup (125 ml) full fat milk*
2 *tablespoons (30 ml) chamomile flowers*

Heat together very gently in a double boiler for half an hour, but do not allow to boil. Leave to cool for 2 hours, strain, refrigerate and use within a week.

Lemon cleansing milk

½ *small pot of natural yoghurt*
½ *tablespoon (7.5 ml) lemon juice*
1 *tablespoon (15 ml) safflower or almond oil*

Blend the ingredients together and use within 3 days.

For any skin type

Buttermilk makes an excellent cleanser and can be mixed with juice or purée of lemons, strawberries, tomatoes, honey or beaten egg white.

Olive oil cleanser

2 *teaspoons olive oil*
1 *teaspoon honey*

Mix together and apply; rinse off with a tepid infusion of chamomile or elderflower.

Sage cleansing lotion

1 *teaspoon olive oil*
1 *teaspoon honey*
2 *drops cider vinegar*
2 *teaspoons sage infusion*

Combine the oil and honey, and warm. Add warm sage infusion and the vinegar; stir well.

Toners and fresheners

Rose water, elderflower water and lavender water all make useful toning lotions. All are available from the pharmacist or from natural beauty products suppliers.

Cucumber juice

Wash a cucumber (organically grown for preference) and put it through a juice extractor (or in a blender, then strain off the juice). Wipe the juice over your face and leave it to dry.

Horsetail toner

1 *tablespoon oatmeal*
2 *tablespoons (30 ml) horsetail infusion*

Simmer oats in a cup of water for 5 minutes. Strain and use the water as gruel. Combine one teaspoonful with horsetail infusion and bottle. Keep in a cool place for 2-4 days. Apply it to the face and neck and leave for 10-15 minutes. Rinse with tepid water or rose water, pat dry.

Rose water and witch hazel toning lotion

4 *tablespoons (60 ml) lemon juice*
4 *tablespoons (60 ml) witch hazel*
4 *tablespoons (60 ml) rose water*
3 *drops essential oil of lavender*

Mix all the ingredients together and bottle. Shake well before using. This lotion will help to restore the acid skin mantle, close the pores, tighten and freshen the skin.

Several herbs can be used in tepid infusions as skin fresheners; these include chamomile, yarrow, sage, mint, lady's mantle, elderflowers and fennel. Add one or two drops of tincture of benzoin, to help preserve the lotion a little longer, per cup of infusion.

Face masks

If you have normal to dry skin and keep it cleansed and toned regularly, you need only occasionally use face masks for deeper cleansing and conditioning. If your skin is particularly oily you could use a face mask about once a week to tone the skin, particularly after steaming the face.

When you have chosen and made your recipe, spread the mask mixture evenly over clean skin, avoiding the delicate areas around the eyes and lips. Lie down and relax, leaving it on for about ten minutes or until it sets. Rinse off thoroughly with tepid water and apply toners or fresheners to enhance the tonic effect. Herbal infusions to suit your skin type can be mixed with fuller's earth to make "mud" packs.

For any skin type

Egg yolk and lemon face mask

½ *lemon*
1 *egg yolk*

Hollow out a space in the cut lemon just big enough to hold the egg yolk. Put the unbroken egg yolk in and leave overnight. Cover your face and neck with the egg yolk which will have absorbed some of the oils from the lemon. Leave for about 10-15 minutes. Rinse. This combination will cleanse, nourish and tone the complexion.

Comfrey face mask

4 *tablespoons (60 ml) comfrey leaf infusion*
½ *teaspoon arrowroot*
2 *teaspoons (10 ml) apricot oil*

Stir the arrowroot into the warm comfrey infusion; heat in a bowl or jar in hot water until it thickens slightly. Remove from the heat, add the oil and shake well; cool. Apply to face and neck.

For sensitive skin

Chamomile and honey face mask

2 tablespoons unprocessed bran
3 tablespoons (45 ml) chamomile
   infusion
1 teaspoon (5 ml) runny honey

Mix ingredients together and apply. After 10 minutes rinse off with chamomile infusion.

Marshmallow face mask

2 tablespoons (30 ml) strong decoction of marshmallow root
2 tablespoons natural yoghurt
fine oatmeal

Mix the infusion and yoghurt together. Stir in enough oatmeal to make a paste. Apply to the face.

For oily skin

Egg white and lemon face mask

1 egg white
½ teaspoon honey
1 teaspoon lemon juice

Beat the egg white stiff, and add a few drops of lemon juice and the honey.

*Brewer's yeast and witch
hazel face mask*

4 oz (120 g) brewer's yeast
1 tablespoon (15 ml) witch hazel
2-3 drops peppermint oil

Mix together into a paste and apply.

Strawberry face mask

4 oz (120 g) mashed fresh strawberries
2 tablespoons (30 ml) powdered milk
1 tablespoon (15 ml) lemon juice

Mix together and apply. Rinse off with a little lemon juice or cider vinegar in warm water.

For dry skin

*Brewer's yeast and comfrey
face mask*

3 teaspoons (15 ml) strong comfrey
   leaf infusion
1 teaspoon runny honey
1 teaspoon brewer's yeast
1 teaspoon natural yoghurt
1 teaspoon avocado or olive oil

Blend together the honey and yeast. Then add the yoghurt and comfrey, stirring until it makes a paste. Pat your face with the oil then apply the paste.

Egg yolk and olive oil face mask

1 egg yolk
1 teaspoon olive oil

Beat the two ingredients togeth-er, and apply.

Peaches and cream face mask

1-2 ripe peaches
whipped cream

Mash the peaches with enough cream to make a paste.

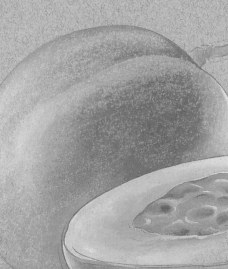

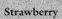

Strawberry

Peach

Moisturizers

Simple moisturizers can be made using the oils of avocado, wheatgerm, almond, safflower, apricot, sunflower and olive which are all moisturizing and penetrating. Apply the oil lightly to the skin, leave to soak in for a few minutes and then wipe off any excess. Egg yolk, cream, melon juice, brewer's yeast, buttermilk, honey, oatmeal, almond meal and peach juice are also moisturizing.

For dry to normal skin

Rose moisturizer

1 teaspoon beeswax
1 teaspoon lanolin
1 tablespoon (15 ml) almond oil
½ teaspoon (2.5 ml) wheatgerm oil
3 tablespoons (45 ml) rose water
6 drops essential oil of rose or rose geranium

Melt the beeswax and lanolin together while stirring. Warm the oils and gradually mix into the wax mixture. Slowly add the warm rose water while stirring. As the mixture cools and thickens, stir in the oil of rose. Spoon into jars.

Elderflower and buttermilk lotion

4 tablespoons (60 ml) buttermilk
2 teaspoons elderflower infusion
1 teaspoon apricot oil
2 teaspoons almond oil

Combine in a glass jar. Screw lid on and shake well.

Avocado moisturizer

1 ripe avocado
1 teaspoon honey
½ teaspoon lemon juice
natural yoghurt

Put the stoned avocado in the blender, add the honey and lemon juice and enough yoghurt

to make it into a stiff cream. Cool for half an hour, massage into the face and neck, leave on for a few hours, then rinse.

For any skin type

Buttermilk and calendula lotion

2 teaspoons (10 ml) buttermilk
2 teaspoons apricot oil
½ teaspoon (2.5 ml) almond oil
1 teaspoon calendula infusion (steep until cold)

Put the ingredients in a jar, screw the lid on and shake well.

Witch hazel and rose lotion

1 teaspoon (5 ml) almond oil
1 teaspoon rose water
1 ½ teaspoons (7.5 ml) witch hazel
1 teaspoon honey

Warm the ingredients and combine them in a glass jar, screw on the lid and shake well.

Elderflower and cucumber lotion

2 tablespoons (30 ml) almond milk
1 teaspoon (5 ml) almond oil
1 teaspoon cucumber juice
1 drop tincture of benzoin

Combine ingredients in a jar, screw on the lid and shake well.

For oily skin

Avocado and nettle moisturizer

1 teaspoon beeswax
2 teaspoons emulsifying wax
4 teaspoons (20 ml) avocado oil
2 tablespoons (30 ml) strong nettle infusion
4 drops essential oil of cedarwood

Melt the waxes together, warm the oils and stir in to the waxes. Mix in the infusion. Allow to cool and mix in the essential oil.

Witch hazel and buttermilk moisturizer

4 tablespoons (60 ml) buttermilk
2 teaspoons (10 ml) witch hazel
1 teaspoon (5 ml) apricot oil
2 teaspoons almond oil

Put the ingredients in the jar, screw on the lid and shake well.

Preparations for acne and blemishes

You can help to keep your skin clear by using an oatmeal scrub to wash your face, or oatmeal mixed with buttermilk as a cleanser. By maintaining the right acid balance of the skin you will help keep acne at bay. Rinse your skin regularly by using a lotion of 1 teaspoon cider vinegar diluted with 2 tablespoons of distilled water.

Compresses

Dip cotton wool into a warm herbal infusion of any of the herbs recommended for oily skin, (see p.251) or else chamomile, burdock or comfrey. Hold the cotton wool against the face for up to 15 minutes.

Both castor oil and honey will help bring spots to a head. Dab spots with either, night and morning. You can add a little wheatgerm to warm honey to aid its drawing properties, and spread it over the face. Leave it on for 15 minutes or so while you relax, then rinse with tepid water. Lemon juice with equal parts of rose water or elderflower water can be used to cleanse the face. It is antiseptic and astringent and helps prevent blackheads and acne. Egg white and lemon juice will also help control blackheads and tone oily skin. Juice half a lemon and whip up an egg white, heat the two together in a basin until they thicken; keep the mixture in the refrigerator.

Elderflowers

Sambucus nigra

ALSO KNOWN AS: Black elder, bore tree

PART USED: Flowers

CONTAINS: Essential oil (including palmitic, linoleic and linolenic acids), triterpenes, flavonoids (including rutin), pectin, mucilage, sugar

KEY USES: Diaphoretic, astringent, decongestant, antispasmodic, detoxifying, diuretic, relaxant

Elderflowers taken in hot infusion make a wonderful remedy for the onset of upper respiratory infections – colds, tonsilitis, laryngitis and flu. With the first signs of malaise, aching, sore throat, chills, restlessness and fever, elderflowers will stimulate the circulation and cause sweating, cleansing the system by elimination of toxins through the pores of the skin and in this way they resolve fever and infection. They are also recommended at the onset of eruptive diseases such as measles and chickenpox, to bring out the rash and speed recovery. They also have a decongestant action, reducing and moving phlegm, and can be taken in hot infusion (combined with yarrow and peppermint) for an ideal remedy for colds, catarrh, sinusitis, hay fever and bronchial congestion in chest infections and asthma. The relaxant effect of elderflowers is a bonus where asthma is concerned, relieving bronchospasm and catarrh.

Elderflowers enhance the action of the kidneys and so act further as a decongestant, relieving fluid retention in the body and eliminating toxins and clearing heat from the system via the urinary system. They have been used in rheumatism, gout and arthritis.

Elderflowers have a long history of use as a relaxant, soothing nerves, allaying anxiety and lifting depression. A hot infusion at night time will help induce a restful sleep and is particularly useful for restless or irritable children at the onset of infections.

Elderflowers in infusion or ointment are used externally on cuts and wounds, chilblains, skin eruptions, sunburn, and irritable skin.

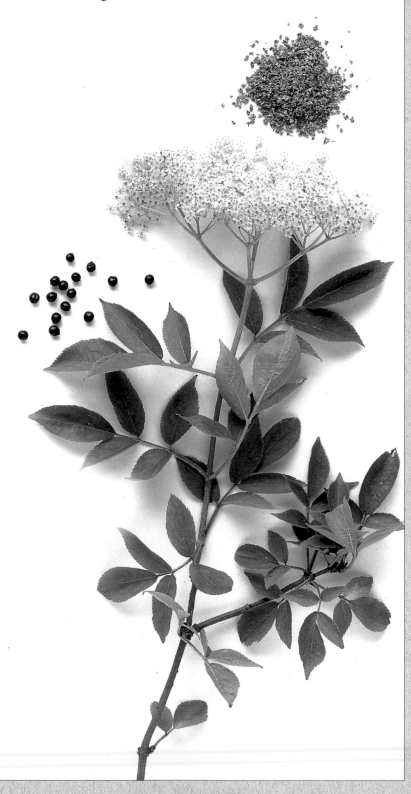

Hair care

The condition of your hair is a good indication of your general health and nutrition. Hair loses its shine when you are tired and run down, unwell or unhappy. Hormonal changes, sun, chlorine, wind and chemical hair treatment can also affect the condition of your hair. A healthy diet is essential to beautiful hair so make sure yours includes plenty of vitamins A and B, minerals such as calcium, iron, iodine, zinc, and silica, as well as protein and essential fatty acids.

The kind of shampoo you use is also important. Many commercial shampoos are largely made up of alkaline detergents which strip the natural oils from the hair and scalp. Avoid washing your hair frequently as this can overstimulate the scalp and increase oiliness of the hair. Choose a natural bristle brush as nylon brushes damage the hair and cause split ends.

Rosemary
Rosmarinus officinalis

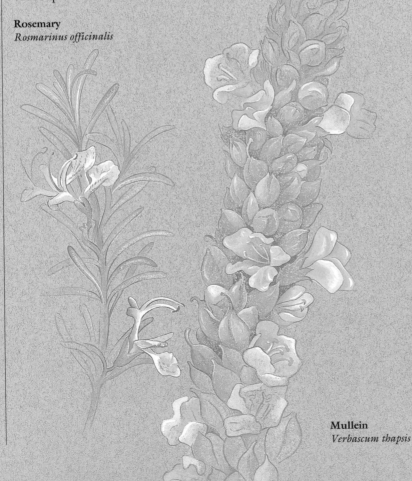

Mullein
Verbascum thapsis

Shampoos

Castile soap shampoo

2 dessertspoons herb
juice of half a lemon
150 g castile soap
1 litre boiling water

Infuse the herbs in the boiling water and leave to cool. Strain, and add the lemon juice. Grate the soap and dissolve it in the infusion. Gently bring it to the boil, stirring from time to time until the water is clear. Remove from heat and beat until the mixture is fluffy. This is a very gentle shampoo suitable even for babies.

Soapwort shampoo

1 oz dried soapwort root
1 pint boiling water
1 oz dried herb

Pour the boiling water over the soapwort, cover and steep for 12 hours. Bring to the boil and simmer for 15 minutes. Remove from heat and stir in the required herbs, cover and leave to cool. Strain into a jug for use. Soapwort shampoo will keep in the refrigerator for 3-4 days.

Herbs for use for shampoos and rinses for all hair types:

nettles	linden blossom
calendula	rosemary
southernwood	yarrow
burdock	horsetail

For dry hair

Comfrey leaf or root and marshmallow contain plenty of mucilage which softens and conditions brittle hair; it soothes and heals sensitive or irritated scalps. Burdock, nettle and sage are also helpful when your hair tends to be dry. Apply rosemary hair oil regularly before washing to restore shine to dark hair.

Rosemary hair oil

2 tablespoons (30 ml) strong
   rosemary infusion
6 tablespoons (90 ml) almond oil
30 drops of lavender oil

For oily hair

Excess oil in your hair is caused
by overactive sebaceous glands in
the scalp. Watch your diet and
cut down on fatty, greasy foods
and animal fats. Hormone imbalance, poor thyroid function,
stress and tiredness may also be
problems. Take a supplement of
brewer's yeast and kelp to
improve the condition of your
hair. Infusions of lemon balm,
yarrow, calendula, horsetail,
lavender, mint, rosemary and
witch hazel can be added to your
shampoo recipe; they can also be
used as hair rinses, as can lemon
juice. Add 1 teaspoon of sea salt
to every 50 grams of shampoo
that you use to reduce oiliness.

Hair rinses

Use herbal infusions to pour over
the hair as the last few rinses after
shampooing. You can also comb
them through the hair each
morning or night when you are
not washing your hair.

To give shine to the hair

rosemary   nettles
calendula   horsetail
sage   parsley

*To bring out blonde highlights and
give sheen*

chamomile   calendula
yarrow   mullein flowers

*To bring out shine and highlights
in dark hair*

rosemary   sage
nettles   rasberry leaves
black tea   elderberries

To disguise grey hairs in dark hair

rosemary   black tea

Treatment for thinning and dropping hair

Stimulate the circulation and
nerve supply to the scalp by
brushing and massaging it regularly. You can use olive oil with
essential oil of rosemary for regular massage (2 drops of essential
oil to each teaspoon of olive oil).

*The following herbs can be used as
hair lotions to massage in to the
scalp:*

nettles   ginger
parsley   thyme
cloves

Check your diet and make sure
you have adequate exercise, rest
and relaxation. If you are unwell,
this may be the cause of hair loss.
B complex, particularly
pantothenic acid, helps to stimulate hair growth. Consult the
Diet chart on p.70–73. Allergic
conditions of the skin can give
rise to hair loss. If you suffer
from a skin problem it is important to seek treatment for it.

Treatment of dry, brittle hair

Give your hair a treat in the form
of either almond oil, coconut oil,
olive oil or castor oil rubbed well
into the hair and scalp; leave it on
overnight or for at least a couple
of hours before washing it. After
shampooing, rinse the hair with a
little lemon juice or cider vinegar
in the water to restore the natural
pH balance of the hair.
   Brushing your hair very thoroughly from the back of your
head to the forehead will stimulate blood circulation in the scalp
and relieve tension there. To
increase the B vitamins and

iodine in your diet take
supplements of brewer's yeast
and kelp.

Dandruff

A few white flakes of dead hair
cells in the hair is normal; only
when it becomes excessive is it a
problem. Dandruff may be related to an upset in the pH balance
of the scalp, or associated with
oily hair and acne in adolescents.
It is related to hormone
imbalance, fatty diet, stress and
toxins in the system.
Brush the hair vigorously each
day to condition the scalp and
only use shampoos with a castile
soap or herbal base, as detergents
in commercial shampoos can further irritate the scalp and upset
the pH balance. Never use hair
spray.

*Use shampoos and hair rinses with
any of these herbs which will help to
heal and soothe any irritation of
the scalp:*

rosemary   cleavers
thyme   nettle
burdock   elderflowers
horsetail   chamomile
comfrey

Add cider vinegar to the final
rinse to restore the pH of the hair
and scalp. Use castor oil, olive oil
or linseed oil on the hair once a
week for a few hours before
washing.

14 Housekeeping Herbs

One of the great pleasures of living with herbs is having them in the house and the garden, smelling their delicious scents on your clothes and in your toilet preparations. The variety of scents and the delicacy of their colours can enrich our homes, whether we plant them in the garden or enjoy them indoors as houseplants.

Growing plants in the house or garden is a reminder of how close is our relationship with the plant world, and discovering this relationship is both beneficial and enriching in our lives. So much of the modern environment contains chemicals which, it appears, can be harmful to the health of many people. Some are sensitive to the chemical ingredients of air fresheners, skin cleansers, fly killers, or household cleansing products of many kinds. The natural ingredients of herbs, in contrast, are well adapted to the systems of the human body and mind, and have a gentle, balanced action. While equally effective, they avoid the harsh, irritant components of some modern products. They also tend to be more quickly biodegradable, and can be made at home and stored in re-used containers, therby avoiding excessive, wasteful packaging.

Many of the herbs used in house are delightfully scented and aromatic. They include many favourite plants of the cottage gardens of our ancestors: lemon balm, rosemary, and the various species of fragrant rose. The appreciation of cottage garden plants is growing rapidly, and many people now want to grow these attractive plants, whether in a typical country garden or on the balcony in a busy modern city.

There is a range of herbal home-care products that you can make at home, without fears about toxicity and at little cost. They include pot-pourris, cleansers and polishes, and all are very effective, pleasant and safe to use. They are not meant to be tasted, however, so remember to keep them out of the reach of children.

Perhaps the most pleasing of all the ways we can enjoy herbs is simply being among them, growing them in the garden or walking among them in the countryside. Those fortunate enough to have a garden can enjoy the sweet fragrance of lavender, lemon balm, roses, thyme or rosemary on a warm spring or summer day. The sheer enjoyment as you breathe in their delicate scents can bring a unique kind of healing to different aspects of your being.

A herb garden in spring is very productive and itself a healing place to be.

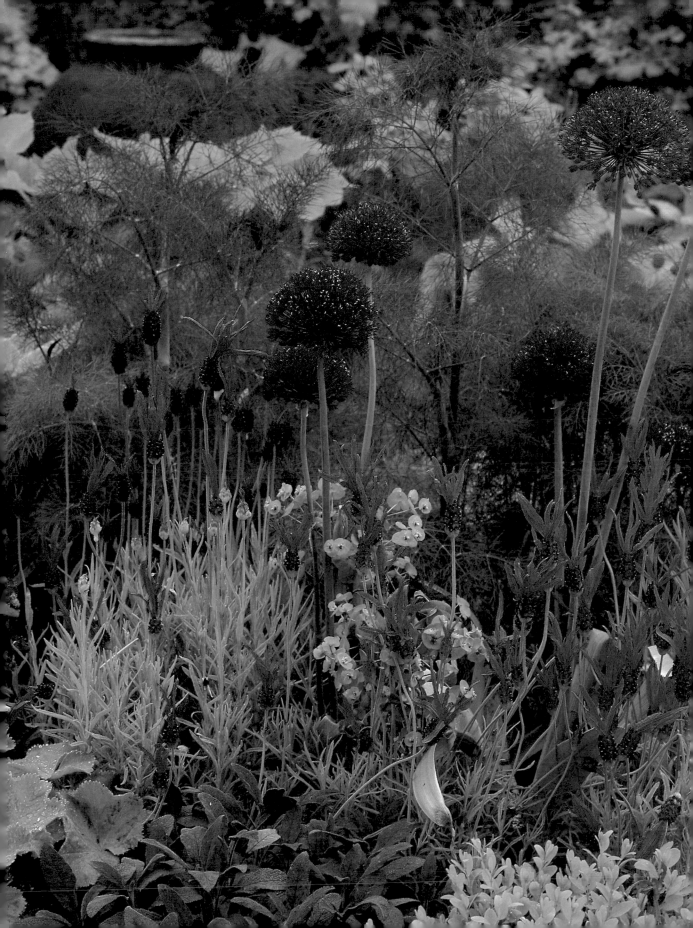

Herbs to grow

Growing your own herbs is very satisfying; you will have fresh herbs to provide an instant medicine chest from spring to autumn, while others can be dried or frozen to provide remedies through the winter months.

When you are planning where to plant your herbs, bear in mind that most of them like a sunny position, ideally facing south and sheltered to the north and east from the cold, particularly from the frost and wind. Choose a spot where the ground slopes down slightly towards the south, so that the herbs requiring a sunnier position can be planted at the top and those that prefer less sun and damper soil can go at the bottom. If you decide to plant your herbs either among your flower borders or in your vegetable garden, make sure that they are not shaded by taller plants.

Most herbs will grow well in almost any soil and any garden, but they generally thrive in a light, well-drained soil.

Even within the confines of small gardens there are many different forms your herb garden can take. If space is very tight, herbs can be grown successfully on a patio, in spaces between paving slabs, or in all manner of containers, so long as they are watered freely during dry spells.

If your have enough space, time and energy, you can follow the traditional pattern of monastery or physic gardens. The best known design for a formal herb garden, which was popular in England during Elizabethan times, is the knot garden. Choose low-growing herbs, with contrasting leaf colours, textures and flower shapes, and plant them in rows that interlace with each other like a knotted rope.

A semi-formal herb bed makes a neat and tidy herb garden. Paths can be used between beds to make the herbs easily accessible and the garden very attractive. It is wise in any such garden to restrict the growth of invasive roots, such as those of tarragon or mint, by putting pieces of slate or tile vertically in the ground around the plant.

Herbs planted between vegetables or flowers are both very attractive and beneficial to the other plants. Some will deter insects such as blackfly and aphids; others will encourage bees which are essential pollinators of many fruit crops.

Sowing and propagating herbs

Some herbs, such as coriander, basil, dill, calendula, borage, and parsley, can be treated as annuals. Sow seeds each year, usually towards the end of spring or in early summer. Sow the seeds close together in the bed, thin out the seedlings when they appear, but leave the plants close enough so that they can support each other as they grow.

The phases of the moon were taken into consideration when sowing seeds and transplanting seedlings in the past. Today many people are paying attention to such matters again, and it seems that both sowing and transplanting are best done when the moon is waxing rather than waning.

Herbs that are not annuals can be easily propagated by cuttings taken during the summer.

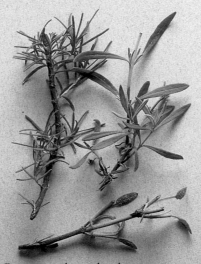

Rosemary, lavender, hyssop, sage, and thyme fall into this category. Take a cutting 3-4 inches (7.5-10 cm) long from the previous year's growth, and trim it just beneath a node (the point at which leaves grow from the stem). Dip it in hormone rooting powder if you wish, and put it into a pot of potting compost or equal parts of sand and a growing medium. Spray your cuttings with water in the evenings until the roots have formed. Once the cuttings have rooted, you can plant them out where you want them in your herb garden or pot them on for transplanting in the following spring. Hardwood cuttings can be put straight into open ground in the summer; water them well and frequently until the roots are established and protect them from excessive sun and wind. You can also take cuttings in late autumn and keep them over winter in a greenhouse or cold frame, ready for planting out in the spring.

Some herbs can be propagated by root division. Mint, lemon balm, chives, tarragon and marjoram fall into this category. Divide these plants and replant them either in the spring or autumn.

Harvesting herbs from your garden

When harvesting herbs, choose plants that look as healthy and vibrant as possible. Select those that are free from disease and infestation, and preferably those that are growing as far away as possible from busy roads or sprayed fields.

The time to harvest your herbs and the method of collection will depend on which part of the plant you need. The leaves and flowers of herbs should be gathered just as the plant is bursting into bloom, on a dry day once the dew has dried. A flat basket is

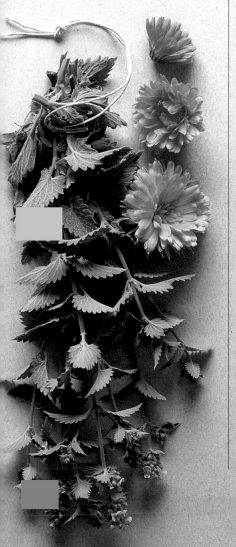

the best container to collect a substantial amount of herbs for making medicines or storing, as its shape makes it easier to avoid bruising or crushing the leaves or flowers.

During the growing season leaves and flowers can be gathered and used fresh straight from the garden. Harvest extra amounts for drying or freezing to last you through the winter months.

Seeds are collected once they have "set" and the flower is past its best. Cut off the whole flower head when harvesting, tie it up in a paper bag and hang it upside-down in a dry, well-ventilated place. The seeds will drop into the bag as the flower head dries.

Roots and rhizon. (the root-like stems of some species) are normally collected in autumn once the aerial parts of the plants have died down, or in spring before they shoot up and while the plant's energies are under the ground.

Drying herbs

The aim of the drying process is to reduce the moisture in the plant before it starts to die, so that it can be stored for a few months without deteriorating and retain its therapeutic properties, its aroma and taste.

The best places for drying herbs are shaded, well-ventilated rooms that are free from moisture or condensation. For this reason avoid using the kitchen, bathroom, utility room, damp sheds or garages. The drying room should have a steady temperature of about 90°F (32°C) so an airing cupboard is ideal, or you could use a shaded greenhouse where the temperature does not fall below 72°F (22°C). If the atmosphere is too cold, the plants will absorb moisture from the air and take too long to dry.

Dry the herbs as soon as possible after you have harvested them. Spread out the leaves and flowers on a tray leaving plenty of space between them, and cover them with muslin or fine wire netting. Alternatively, place them in a shallow box without a lid. Turn them frequently – once or twice on the first day and once daily thereafter.

Some herbs can be hung upside-down in small bunches from hooks or beams. Tie the bunches loosely with string so that air can circulate between the stalks. If the bunches are tightly fastened the stalks may go mouldy or rot. Rosemary, marjoram, mint, lavender and sage can all be hung to dry.

Barks, roots and rhizomes should be washed thoroughly, patted dry and chopped up before being spread out to dry.

Storing herbs

Crumble the leafy herbs between your hands, remove the stalks and twigs, and store them in wooden or cardboard boxes, jars with airtight lids or paper bags. Roots, rhizomes and barks should be broken up into small pieces and stored similarly. Carefully label all herbs before they are dry.

Freezing herbs

Herbs, particularly those with soft leaves, are ideal for freezing.

You can successfully freeze:

marjoram	*borage*
comfrey	*coriander*
mint	*fennel*
basil	*dill*
lemon balm	*parsley*

Pick the leaves or flowers, wash them, chop them or leave them whole, and place them to freeze in small plastic bags.

Culinary herbs

The herbs most commonly used in cooking are basil, bay, chives, marjoram, mint, parsley, rosemary, sage, tarragon and thyme. These ten herbs should provide for most of your culinary needs and are all relatively easy to grow. Parsley needs to be sown twice – once in Spring and then again in Summer – to ensure you have enough to pick regularly. Basil, an annual, should be sown indoors or under glass and transferred to the garden once the danger of frost has passed. Parsley, chives (and also dill) can be grown indoors or in a greenhouse to ensure a fresh supply in winter.

There are many lesser known but equally delicious herbs which will enhance your cooking.

For cooked dishes:

chervil	lemon balm
lovage	coriander
sweet cecily	

Herbs for summer drinks, cake decorations and jam making:

angelica	borage
calendula	mint
peppermint	nasturtium
rose geranium	

Aromatic and pleasant tasting herbs excellent for making herbal teas:

angelica	chamomile
fennel seed	lemon balm
lemon verbena	peppermint
lovage	meadowsweet
rosemary	sage
thyme	catmint
hyssop	

Herbs for soup:

basil	bay
chervil	chives
coriander	dill
lovage	marjoram
parsley	nettles
sage	tarragon
thyme	sorrel
garlic	

Herbs for bread:

basil	coriander
dill	fennel
marjoram	parsley
thyme	aniseed
garlic	

Herbs for salads:

lovage	dandelion leaves
chickweed	sorrel
coriander	mint
parsley	basil
calendula flowers	borage
garlic	salad burnet
nasturtium leaves and flowers	

Herbs for cooking with fish:

dill	basil
bay	lemon balm
lovage	thyme
tarragon	sorrel
rosemary	sage
garlic	

Herbs for cooking with poultry:

basil	bay
dill	lovage
marjoram	parsley
rosemary	garlic
sage	tarragon
thyme	

Herbs for cooking with lamb:

basil	bay
thyme	rosemary
marjoram	mint
sage	tarragon

Herbs for cooking with pork:

basil	coriander
dill	fennel
marjoram	rosemary
sage	tarragon
thyme	

Herbs for cooking with beef:

basil	sage
dill	garlic
chervil	marjoram
parsley	rosemary
tarragon	thyme

Herbs for cooking with eggs:

basil	chervil
chives	dill
coriander	garlic
marjoram	parsley
rosemary	

Herbs for cheese dishes:

chives	garlic
chervil	dill
coriander	mint
sage	tarragon
thyme	rosemary
basil	marjoram

Herbs for vegetable dishes:

parsley	chives
marjoram	garlic
thyme	basil
coriander	dill
lovage	mint
rosemary	sage
sweet cecily	tarragon
thyme	ginger

Herbs for desserts:

sweet cecily	mint
ginger	calendula
lemon balm	lovage

Dill

Anethum graveolens

PART USED: Seeds

CONTAINS: 4% volatile oil which includes carvone and limonene

KEY USES: Carminative, antispasmodic, digestive, relaxant, galactagogue

The name dill is said to derive from a Saxon word *dilla* meaning to lull. Dill water is an old and still famous remedy, made from a distillation of the seeds, to soothe colic, flatulence and abdominal pain in small babies. The volatile oil in the seeds has an antispasmodic action, relieving spasm in muscles in the digestive tract, and it also enhances digestion. Dill can be used for indigestion, wind, and colic in adults as well as in babies and children. It will also relieve nausea, hiccoughs, constipation and an upset stomach. When chewed, the seeds will reduce bad breath.

Dill also has tranquilizing properties and has a reputation for inducing sleep in babies and children – another reason for every mother to be well acquainted with dill water. It also increases milk supply in breastfeeding mothers. In the East it is given to women prior to childbirth to ease the birth. In menstruating women it relieves painful periods, and brings on delayed or suppressed periods.

Dill can be used externally in warming liniments to increase circulation in the limbs, and to soothe muscular tension and joint pain.

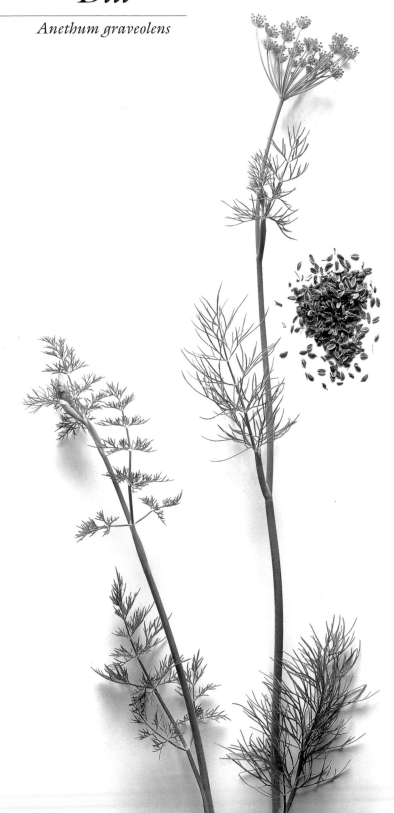

Herbs in the house

In addition to the well-known traditional uses of herbs for culinary and medicinal purposes, herbs have been invaluable through the ages in many forgotten domestic roles. They have been employed to enhance natural beauty, to freshen and perfume the air, to repel insects in wardrobes and cupboards, to clean cooking utensils, and to strew on floors to keep away unpleasant smells and infectious diseases.

Herbs for cleaning

Very often the common name of a plant gives a good indication of its traditional use. Horsetail, for instance, was called scouring rush or pewterwort. It would be bound in bunches and used for scouring pans, because it contains silica and is excellent for cleaning and polishing pots and utensils. It is also used to clean and polish pewter, and to scour saucepans and baking pans.

Recipe for metal polish

Make a strong infusion of horse-tail using 1 ounce of herb to 1 pint of boiling water. Leave it to infuse for 2-3 hours, bring to the boil and simmer for 15 minutes, then strain. Pour over the metal or pewter articles to be cleaned and allow to soak for 5 minutes. Let them dry and then polish the surfaces gently with a soft cloth.

Acidic plants such as rhubarb (*Rheum palmatum*) and sorrel (*Rumex acetosa*), when boiled in water, will clean stained pans and leave them with a high polish. Be careful not to leave a strong rhubarb solution in an aluminium pan or cook rhubarb to eat in one, as it will dissolve the metal which could ruin your pan and certainly pollute your dessert.
    Herbs can also be used for cleaning and polishing furniture

and floors. For removing the white spots which appear on varnished furniture, rub the surface with a few drops of linseed oil mixed with an equal amount of turpentine. To clean and polish furniture, including leather upholstery, use enough beeswax dissolved in turpentine to give a polish with a creamy consistency. Add a few drops of essential oil of lavender, pine or rosemary to the polish so that a delightful fragrance will permeate the room.

Thyme furniture wax

4 oz (110 g) beeswax
1 pint (570 ml) turpentine
12 oz (350 ml) strong thyme
    infusion
½ oz (15 g) olive oil based soap
a few drops essential oil of thyme

Grate the beeswax into the turpentine and let it dissolve over the next few days. Alternatively, warm the beeswax and turpentine carefully over a flameless heat in a bain marie, or in a jar standing in a pan of water on the stove, until the wax melts. Never use turpentine near flames as it can easily catch fire. In a separate pan heat the infusion until it's nearly boiling, add the grated soap and stir until it has melted. Allow the mixture to cool and then stir it gently to a creamy consistency. Stir in the oil of thyme, and pour it into a labelled jar.

Soapwort (*Saponaria officinalis*), also known as latherwort, contains saponins, substances which when mixed with water produce a soapy solution. This provides a gentle base for shampoos and also soap for washing fabrics. It has been used to clean upholstery and to restore valuable old tapestries and brocades, as it can restore old vegetable dyes to their former brightness.

Soapwort cleaner

½ oz (15 g) dried soapwort root
1 ½ pints (0.75 l) water

Soak the soapwort root in the water overnight, bring to the boil in an enamel pan and simmer for 20 minutes. Allow to cool, then strain. For upholstery or tapestry, apply with a sponge, and then rinse. Use the infusion cool to wash delicate fabrics, and rinse out afterwards in cool water.

It is easy to make natural disinfectants at home for general use about the house; they are much kinder to the environment and your hands than chemical cleaners.

Lavender disinfectant

20 drops essential oil of lavender*
1 teaspoon (5 ml) isopropyl alcohol
4 pints (2 l) tepid water

*or thyme, eucalyptus, clove, rosemary, or lemon

Various herbs can be used for washing hands and removing stains from the hands. Try lemon juice rubbed gently into the skin.
    Elderflower water helps bleach the skin, while fine oatmeal with a little water added to it makes an excellent substitute for soap – rub the hands with it until they are clean. Coconut oil rubbed into the hands and then rinsed off leaves the skin soft and supple.

Herbs to sweeten the air

In past times, rooms for human habitation would have their floors strewn with herbs such as lavender, juniper, rosemary, wormwood and tansy. These traditional strewing herbs were used to impart their fragrance to an otherwise unpleasant smelling atmosphere in the home. They helped to repel insects as well as disinfect the atmosphere by giving off antiseptic aromas, and were used to counteract infection.

Antiseptic and sweet-smelling herbs, such as cloves, were traditionally made into pomanders; other herbs were held in the hand, tied around the neck, or hung on belts while walking through fetid streets to prevent contamination. Some herbs were dried and burnt in pots or barrels to fumigate the atmosphere in hospitals or homes of the sick. Eucalyptus, rosemary leaves and juniper berries were used in this way.

Herbs are still used today in herb bags placed among linen and clothing to impart their delightful fragrance and to repel insects. Another well-perpetuated custom is to place bowls of certain herbs around the house. The welcome practice of bringing fresh flowers into the sickroom may have originated with the use of aromatic medicinal herbs in flower to repel infection and freshen the atmosphere, and not simply as today, to please the senses. Herbs such as lavender, rosemary, linden blossom, wormwood and mint were scattered in cupboards to sweeten the air, dispel mustiness and repel insects and moths.

Pomanders

Many will be familiar with orange pomanders studded with cloves, which children are sometimes taught to make today. These and many other kinds of pomander originated in the Middle Ages in France, where they were carried as protection against plague. They were made from lemons, limes, apples and oranges and often worn around the neck, or on a belt, and lifted to the nose to disguise unpleasant odours when necessary. They were also believed to ward off bad luck.

Orange pomander

Seville oranges are best for this, but any thin-skinned orange can be used. Take two lengths of narrow tape or ribbon and tie them around the orange so that they divide it into 4 equal segments.

Dry the orange for a couple of days above a stove and then push cloves into the surface. First, follow the edges of the tape so that you get an even pattern. If you find it hard to push the cloves in, make a little hole first with a needle. Cover the whole surface with cloves, placing them close together so that the heads almost touch. Then mix a powder consisting of equal parts of cinnamon powder and orris root powder, roll the orange in the mixture and wrap it up in a paper bag. Leave it for 2 weeks in a dry place such as an airing cupboard. After this time, remove the paper, shake off the powder, replace the ribbon or tape if you like with a clean, pretty ribbon, making a loop from which it can be hung. You can hang your pomander in a cupboard, wardrobe, cloakroom or anywhere else you will enjoy its scent.

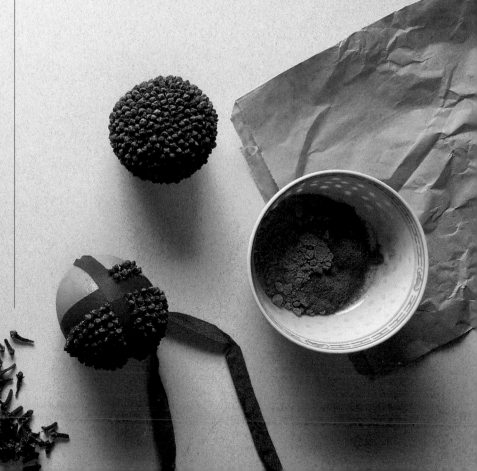

Pot-pourri

Pot-pourri is a mixture of sweet-smelling flowers and leaves with aromatic spices, used to sweeten the atmosphere. Traditionally pot-pourri is placed in large ceramic bowls or kept in jars or pomanders. Rose petals have usually been the main ingredient, but you can choose any kind of scented leaves, flowers or spices to make pot-pourri. Once you have dried and blended them, you will need to add a fixative to retain the aroma of the mixture. The most common fixatives are common salt, orris root powder or gum benzoin.

To make a normal, dry pot-pourri, the leaves and petals must be thoroughly dry and retain much of their colour or scent, or both. Spices, peel and wood chips have a stronger aroma than most leaves and flowers, so use them in moderation – about 1 tablespoonful (15 ml) to 4 cups (1 l) of flowers and leaves. Whole spices need to be ground or grated to release their aroma.

When making up the pot-pourri, combine the leaves and flowers, then add the fixative to the spices and blend it all together with your hands. Use 1 tablespoon (15 ml) of orris root powder to every cup (225 ml) of flowers and leaves, or half an ounce (15 g) of gum benzoin to 4-6 cups (1-1.5 l) of flowers and leaves. Then sprinkle on a few drops of essential oils of your choice. Lavender, rose, sandalwood, pine, lemon, ylang ylang, jasmine, frankincense, geranium, lemon grass, cedarwood, ginger, bergamot and cypress are the favourites. Store the mixture in tightly-closed jars in a warm, dry, dark place for six weeks.

To make a "moist" pot-pourri, which will retain its aroma and colour for longer than dry pot-pourri, use partially dried leaves and flowers of a limp and leathery character. Put a layer of petals, leaves, or both, in the base of a jar, then a half-inch layer of fixative made from a mixture of orris root and sea salt. Then put another layer of petals and leaves and repeat the process until the jar is full. Put a weight on top of the mixture, screw the lid on, and store in a warm, dark place to "fix". Open it up and stir it every day. After six to eight weeks, take it out and add dried flowers, spices and essential oils of your choice, seal it up again and leave for another two weeks. After that time, put the pot-pourri in a transparent glass container with a lid. Keep the lid on except when you want to smell the fragrance, and it should keep for years. You can refresh it by adding a few drops of essential oil.

Choose your ingredients from the following:

flowers	leaves	seeds, spices, peel
roses	wormwood	cinnamon
carnations	rosemary	coriander
honeysuckle	sage	ginger
jasmine	bergamot	nutmeg
lavender	coriander	fennel
lily of the	bay	cardamon
valley	thyme	vanilla pods
pinks	choisya	allspice
stocks	scented	vetiver root
wallflowers	geranium	citrus peel
sweet peas	marjoram	sandalwood
thyme	curry plant	shredded cedar wood
linden blossom	hyssop	
sweet cicely	woodruff	
calendula	basil	
clary sage	lemon verbena	
borage	lemon balm	
hyssop		
mock orange		

Traditional herb pot-pourri

8 oz (250 g) thyme
4 oz (125 g) rosemary
2 oz (50 g) lavender
4 oz (125 g) mint
1 oz (25 g) lemon balm
½ oz (15 g) orris root powder

Olde English pot-pourri

1 lb (500 g) damask rose petals
4 oz (125 g) common salt
4 oz (125 g) coarse salt
4 oz (125 g) brown sugar
½ oz (15 g) storax
½ oz (15 g) benzoin
½ oz (15 g) orris root powder
½ oz (15 g) ground cinnamon
½ oz (15 g) cloves
1 oz (25 g) lemon verbena

Woody pot-pourri

1 lb (500 g) cedar wood or sandal-
*   wood shavings*
2 oz (50 g) crushed coriander seeds
2 oz (50 g) ground cinnamon
2 oz (50 g) rose petals
2 oz (50 g) lavender

Soothing pot-pourri

2 cups (450 ml) lemon verbena
2 cups (450 ml) rose petals
1 cup (225 ml) lavender flowers
1 cup (225 ml) calendula petals
1 cup (225 ml) linden blossom
1 cup (225 ml) chamomile flowers
1 oz (25 g) angelica root, finely
*   chopped or powdered*
4 tablespoonfuls (60 ml) orris root
*   powder*

Keep the pot-pourri you have made in jars or open bowls; alternatively you could fill a porcelain pomander to hang in a cupboard or wardrobe.

Linen sachets

Fabric sachets filled with fine herbs, small petals or powdered mixtures, or scraps left from making pot-pourri, can be made for placing in drawers and amongst linen. A good linen sachet mixture is made from equal parts of mint, lavender and lemon verbena, or from a mixture of one part each of rose petals and carnations with half a part of powdered cloves.

Bouquet sachet

2 oz (50 g) damask rose petals
2 oz (50 g) lavender flowers
2 oz (50 g) philadelphus (mock
*   orange) blossoms*
1 oz (25 g) orris root powder
2 tsp (10 g) powdered cloves
2 tsp (10 g) cinnamon powder
2 tsp (10 g) powdered allspice
2 tsp (10 g) powdered coriander

Spicy sachet

1 oz (25 g) powdered cloves
1 oz (25 g) grated nutmeg
1 oz (25 g) powdered cinnamon
1 oz (25 g) powdered caraway seeds
6 oz (170 g) orris root powder

Rose sachet

2 oz (50 g) lavender flowers
2 oz (50 g) rose petals
2 oz (50 g) orris root powder
5 drops essential oil of rose

Sachets can also be filled simply with dried lavender flowers, famous for repelling insects and moths in drawers and wardrobes and for keeping your clothes smelling sweet.

Herb pillows

Mattresses in past times were sometimes stuffed with aromatic herbs to bring the owner a restful sleep and to repel disease-carrying organisms. Herb pillows can easily be made today from aromatic herbs which will sweetly fragrance the bedclothes and encourage a relaxing sleep. Herb pillows, or cushions, are usually smaller than normal bed pillows, and can be tucked under or by the side of a standard pillow.

Take a plain cotton pillowslip to stuff with your chosen herbs, and make another cover in the same size in attractive material that can be easily washed.

Choose mixtures of relaxing herbs from:

rosemary	thyme
rose petals	lavender
lemon verbena	lemon balm
chamomile	catmint
linden blossom	hops

Enhance the scent of your chosen herbs with spices, ground citrus peel, and a few drops of essential oils such as geranium, lavender, neroli, ylang ylang or melissa. Add a couple of teaspoons of orris root powder to your mixture as a fixative.

Herbal sleep pillow

1 cup lavender flowers
1 cup rose petals
1 cup hops
1 cup linden blossom
1 cup lemon balm
2 teaspoons orris root powder
3 drops oil of bergamot

Mix together enough herbs in these proportions to fill the size of pillow size you have chosen.

Herbs for repelling pests and insects

The homes that we find warm and comfortable are equally pleasant places for many insects and other creatures. Herbs have always been used to deter unwanted insects such as ants and moths, and larger creatures too. Traditional herbal preparations are preferable in many ways to modern insect repellents; chemical sprays are generally toxic and not recommended for use in the kitchen, or where children play. Among the many herbs that can help deter flies are lavender, mint, bay, mugwort, cloves, wormwood, rue, eucalyptus and elder. You can add them to potpourri, sew them into sachets or hang them in bunches from beams and hooks.

Sweet and sticky elecampane root makes a useful alternative to fly paper.

To prevent moth grubs from eating your cloths, use lavender, rosemary, wormwood, southernwood, woodruff and cloves. Fill sachets with the herbs or sprinkle them into the bottom of drawers, covered with a layer of muslin or cloth. Cedar wood shavings and ground sassafras root will also repel moths.

Moth bags

1 cup rosemary
1 cup ground vetiver root
1 cup cedar shavings or
  southernwood
5 bruised bay leaves

Mix these together and tie into bags.

Another good mixture to repel moths is made from equal quantities of dried lavender, tansy and rosemary.

To repel all sorts of insects, including moths, use sweet smelling woodruff, vetiver root, crushed bay leaves, tansy, cloves and sweet flag root – a piece of this root can be placed in your drawers of clothes. Dried pyrethrum or feverfew flower heads act as a contact poison for all insects, and yet are perfectly safe for children and domestic animals. Use the powder in sachets or sprinkle it in cupboards.

If your kitchen is prone to invasion from ants, sprinkle some crushed catmint along the ant trails and the ants will keep away as they dislike the smell. It is a different matter with cats, of course! Ants also hate pennyroyal, rue and tansy.

To keep mosquitoes and gnats away when you are out of doors, you can apply oil of lavender or citronella to the skin. Dilute the oil with a little ethyl alcohol (one part alcohol to two parts oil). Pennyroyal and elderflower infusion can also be used as a mosquito-repellent wash for the skin. You can also rub fresh leaves of lemon balm, pennyroyal or basil on the skin to keep away insects, and if you are bitten the same leaves can be rubbed on to relieve itching and swelling. Other remedies for insect bites and stings include lavender oil, plantain, yarrow, hyssop and rosemary.

For fleas, either on your pets or in your house, you can hang herbs from beams or hooks, fill sachets or herb pillows to place in a dog basket – use pennyroyal, rue, southernwood, chamomile, eucalyptus or cedar shavings. You can also try the traditional remedy of burning herbs on an open fire over low embers to repel fleas – use fleabane, mugwort or wormwood. Burning hemp agrimony (*Eupatorium cannabinum*) will keep away wasps.

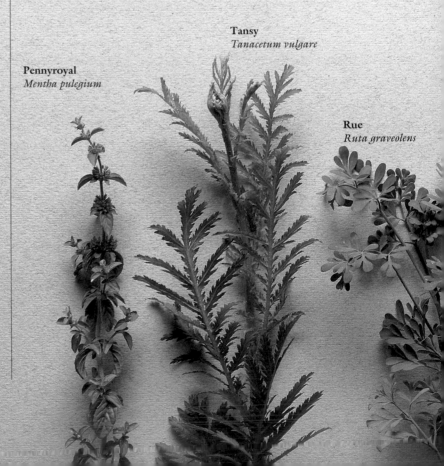

Tansy
Tanacetum vulgare

Pennyroyal
Mentha pulegium

Rue
Ruta graveolens

Mint and tansy strewed or hung in your food cupboard will help keep away mice. Peppermint oil is also useful and was used in the past to drive out rats. A few bay leaves in flour and rice, and also beans and pulses, will prevent infestation by weevils.

Fragrant preparations for the bathroom

Sweet-smelling herbs can be incorporated into natural deodorants, body lotions, bath fragrances and hand creams.

Natural deodorants do not inhibit perspiration, which is a vital pathway for the body's elimination of poisons and wastes.

Herbs can be used, however, to prevent perspiration from developing unpleasant odours by inhibiting the growth of microorganisms that act on perspiration when it is stale.

Herbal deodorant stick

1 ½ tablespoons beeswax
½ tablespoon cocoa butter
1 tablespoon coconut oil
½ teaspoon thyme oil
½ teaspoon rosemary oil
½ teaspoon lavender oil
½ teaspoon peppermint oil
3 drops castor oil

Melt the beeswax in a glass jar standing in hot water. Add cocoa butter and let it melt, then stir in the oils. Pour the mixture into an empty deodorant stick plastic case and leave it to cool and set.

Vinegar is mildly antiseptic and can be mixed with herbal infusions and essential oils to help maintain the acid balance of the skin. Use herbs such as peppermint, eau de cologne mint, thyme, rosemary, marjoram, lavender, sage, clove or cinnamon to make body lotion. Infuse the herb or herbs in cider vinegar and

leave them to macerate for seven to ten days on a sunny windowsill, then drain off the oil. Dilute one part of the infusion with two parts of water and use in a spray-top bottle. Add a few drops of essential oil of your choice to the vinegar mixture to increase the fragrance if you wish.

Aromatic body lotion

25 drops lavender oil
25 drops rosemary oil
15 drops clove oil
50 ml ethyl alcohol
110 ml rose water
2 tablespoons mint leaves

Dissolve the essential oils in the alcohol. Add the rose water and mint leaves and leave to macerate for 1-2 weeks, then strain into a bottle with spray top.

Herbal baths

Aromatic herbs can enhance the relaxing and tonic effects of a warm bath at the end of a long day. Not only do they help to cleanse the body as it soaks, but also certain herbs can ease tense muscles, uplift the spirit, dispel lethargy and improve the function of the skin. Many a legendary beauty in history was reputed to have kept her skin lovely and youthful by bathing in herb-scented waters. One such famous French beauty gave the following recipe as her secret.

Beautifying bath mixture

a handful each of:
rosemary   mint
comfrey root   thyme
dried lavender

Mix the herbs together loosely in a muslin bag, cover with boiling water and leave for 10 minutes. Add to the bath water and relax in it for 15 minutes daily.

If you want to relax tense muscles, add to the bath a few drops of essential oils of either lavender, rose, ylang ylang, geranium, melissa, rosemary or jasmine.

On the other hand, if you feel tired and lethargic and are planning to go out for the evening, add more stimulating oils such as clove, cinnamon, thyme or ginger. These will help to increase the circulation if you feel particularly cold.

To soften the skin, strong infusions of soothing herbs such as comfrey, marshmallow, chamomile or elderflower can be added to bath water. Milk infusions also help to keep the skin soft and supple. You can make milk and herb sachets which hang over the hot tap so the water runs through. Add three tablespoons of full fat powdered milk to a muslin bag with 2 oz dried (4 oz fresh) herb, either elderflower, chamomile, rose petals, sage or lemon balm.

Vinegar baths help soften the skin, and they also soothe itching skin and relieve aching muscles. Bring one pint of cider vinegar and two handfuls of fresh herbs to the boil. Remove from the heat and infuse overnight, strain and bottle. Add one cupful to the bath.

Herbal oils can also be added to the bath, but create slightly more work as they leave a residue on the sides of the bath. To make herbal bath oils, infuse herbs of your choice in almond oil for two weeks on a sunny windowsill. After that time, press out the oil and bottle it.

St. John's wort oil is excellent in baths because it soothes nerves, relieves any nerve pain, and soothes irritation of the skin. Although the hypericum flowers used to make the oil are bright yellow, after two weeks the oil turns bright red and has been called "heart of Jesus oil".

The Herbs and Ailments

The bullet points on this chart tell you which herbs are indicated for the ailments described in this book. The ailments are listed according to the chapter in which they occur and in the order they are described.

Chapter	Ailment	ARNICA	ASHWAGANDHA	BETH ROOT	BLACK COHOSH	BLACK HAW	BLESSED THISTLE	BLUE COHOSH	BORAGE	BURDOCK	CALENDULA	CATMINT	CAYENNE PEPPER	CHAMOMILE	CHASTE TREE	CINNAMON	CLEAVERS	COMFREY	CORN SILK	CRAMP BARK	DANDELION	DANG GUI	DILL	ECHINACEA	ELDERFLOWERS	FALSE UNICORN ROOT
The Well Woman	STRESS				•		•		•			•								•						
Puberty	ACNE									•	•			•	•		•	•	•		•			•	•	•
The Menstrual Cycle	PREMENSTRUAL SYNDROME				•	•				•	•			•	•	•		•		•	•					•
	PAINFUL PERIODS				•	•		•		•	•			•	•	•				•		•				•
	HEAVY BLEEDING			•							•			•						•						
	AMENORRHEA						•							•	•	•						•				
	MENSTRUAL HEADACHES				•					•		•	•	•						•						
	SPOTTING										•			•												
Preconception and Fertility	INFERTILITY		•												•	•						•			•	•
	THREATENED MISCARRIAGE					•	•							•								•				
Pregnancy and Childbirth	ANEMIA									•											•					
	CONSTIPATION									•				•							•					
	CRAMP																			•						
	NAUSEA													•	•	•										•
	VARICOSE VEINS									•	•						•	•							•	
	HEMORRHOIDS					•					•	•		•			•	•		•						
	INSOMNIA											•		•												
	THRUSH										•			•			•						•			
	STRETCH MARKS										•															
	BLADDER/KIDNEY PROBLEMS							•			•			•					•	•			•			
	HEARTBURN													•		•										
	EDEMA																•		•		•					•
	HIGH BLOOD PRESSURE																		•	•						
	BIRTH CONTRACTIONS				•	•		•			•									•						
	TENSION AND ANXIETY													•						•						•
	PAIN IN CHILDBIRTH													•												
	RIGID CERVIX				•			•																		
	RETAINED PLACENTA				•	•	•																			
Postnatal Care and Motherhood	PAIN AFTER CHILDBIRTH				•																					
	TORN PERINEUM	•									•							•								
	POST-PARTUM HEMORRHAGE			•		•																•		•		
	UTERINE INFECTION			•															•					•		
	AFTER PAINS																									
	POSTNATAL DEPRESSION								•						•											•
	BLADDER PROBLEMS			•																						
	STRESS								•					•												
Breastfeeding and Infant Care	POOR MILK SUPPLY						•		•			•		•	•								•			•
	SORE, CRACKED NIPPLES																									
	ENGORGED BREASTS										•						•				•					
	INFLAMED BREASTS/MASTITIS				•						•			•			•	•			•			•	•	
	DIAPER RASH										•			•					•							
	CRADLE CAP								•																	
	COLIC											•		•		•							•			
	VOMITING											•		•		•								•	•	•
	DIARRHEA													•		•										
	CONSTIPATION											•		•		•					•					
	ALLERGIES													•												
	SLEEPING PROBLEMS																									
	TEETHING											•		•												
	FEVER								•			•		•											•	

FEVERFEW	GARLIC	GINGER	GINKGO	GINSENG	GOAT'S RUE	GOLDEN SEAL	HAWTHORN	HOPS	HORSETAIL	HUANG QI	LADY'S MANTLE	LAVENDER	LEMON BALM	LICORICE	LINDEN BLOSSOM	MEADOWSWEET	MOTHERWORT	MYRRH	NETTLE	OAK BARK	PARTRIDGE BERRY	PASSIONFLOWER	PEPPERMINT	PLANTAIN	POKE ROOT	PULSATILLA	RASPBERRY LEAVES	ROSE	ROSEMARY	SAGE	SAW PALMETTO	SHATAVARI	SKULLCAP	SLIPPERY ELM	ST. JOHN'S WORT	THYME	VERVAIN	WILD OATS	WILD YAM	WITCH HAZEL	WOOD BETONY	WORMWOOD	YARROW	YELLOW DOCK
				•				•				•	•		•		•					•				•			•				•		•		•	•			•			
												•					•	•	•					•	•				•	•			•			•	•		•	•			•	•
		•						•					•	•			•					•	•		•	•			•	•			•		•		•	•	•		•	•		•
		•				•					•	•	•				•				•					•	•		•			•	•				•		•					•
						•					•		•							•	•						•		•				•				•							•
		•										•					•												•	•		•	•				•	•				•	•	•
		•						•			•	•	•		•	•						•	•						•				•			•	•				•	•		•
																	•				•						•																
		•		•							•		•	•							•						•		•		•	•	•				•	•	•					•
											•										•						•					•											
								•											•								•						•				•							•
		•																					•				•						•										•
									•							•			•																			•						
		•						•				•	•			•							•				•		•				•	•		•			•					
							•								•					•			•	•					•						•									
									•		•			•					•	•															•					•				•
													•		•							•											•				•							
																													•							•								
									•			•	•			•						•		•			•		•				•			•	•							
		•											•	•		•							•											•										
									•							•								•			•																	
							•						•		•				•			•					•						•					•					•	
•						•																				•			•			•						•			•		
												•	•		•		•				•	•					•						•		•		•		•					
												•			•		•				•								•	•														
																	•				•	•											•		•									
																					•						•																	
												•														•							•						•					
																																			•					•				
						•																																•					
						•												•																		•						•		
													•													•			•				•		•		•	•						
														•								•							•				•					•			•			
	•				•								•		•				•								•				•						•							
											•													•										•								•	
	•	•				•					•	•												•		•							•		•								
												•															•								•								
								•					•		•																												
		•										•	•		•	•													•							•								
		•											•			•								•			•							•										
		•										•	•		•	•								•					•					•										
																																					•					•	
												•	•		•																											•	
													•		•																				•							•	

The bullet points on this chart tell you which herbs are indicated for the ailments described in this book. The ailments are listed according to the chapter in which they occur and in the order they are described.

		ARNICA	ASHWAGANDHA	BETH ROOT	BLACK COHOSH	BLACK HAW	BLESSED THISTLE	BLUE COHOSH	BORAGE	BURDOCK	CALENDULA	CATMINT	CAYENNE PEPPER	CHAMOMILE	CHASTE TREE	CINNAMON	CLEAVERS	COMFREY	CORN SILK	CRAMP BARK	DANDELION	DANG GUI	DILL	ECHINACEA	ELDERFLOWERS	FALSE UNICORN ROOT
Adult Life and Menopause	STRESS				●																					
	LOW ESTROGEN							●							●							●				●
	HOT FLASHES/NIGHT SWEATS				●																					
	DEPRESSION/MOOD SWINGS						●		●																	
	VAGINAL DRYNESS										●							●								●
	LOSS OF LIBIDO												●			●										
	OSTEOPOROSIS								●												●					●
Later Years	POOR CIRCULATION												●													
	STRESS																									
	LOW IMMUNITY																									
First Aid	ABRASIONS										●							●							●	
	BITES/STINGS										●										●					
	BOILS									●											●					
	BRUISES/SPRAINS	●									●							●								
	BURNS																	●				●			●	
	CHILBLAINS												●													
	COLD SORES									●	●					●				●				●		
	FAINTING/SHOCK	●											●												●	
	HAY FEVER												●											●	●	
	HEADACHE												●													
	HEAT RASH																									
	NOSEBLEED										●															
	SPLINTERS										●								●							
	SUNBURN										●			●												
	TOOTHACHE																							●		
	TRAVEL SICKNESS																									
	WOUNDS																	●								
Healing Yourself	BENIGN MAMMARY DYSPLASIA			●						●	●				●						●					●
	BREAST ABSCESS			●						●	●					●					●			●		
	ENDOMETRIOSIS				●			●			●			●	●					●	●					●
	CYSTITIS													●					●							
	KIDNEY INFECTION													●										●		
	PROLAPSE			●						●																
	VAGINAL/VULVAL INFECTIONS			●						●	●			●		●	●		●	●		●		●		
	THRUSH									●	●			●		●	●				●					
	GENITAL HERPES									●	●					●					●			●		
	GENITAL WARTS										●					●					●			●		
	PELVIC INFLAMMATORY DISEASE							●			●													●		●
	BACTERIAL INFECTIONS																									
	FIBROIDS			●				●			●				●	●				●	●	●				●
	OVARIAN CYSTS				●			●							●						●					●
	CANCER					●								●	●	●								●		●
	BREAST CANCER										●						●				●					
	UTERINE CANCER									●	●															
	CERVICAL CANCER									●	●															
	LOW IMMUNITY																									
	NAUSEA AND VOMITING																									
	LIVER DAMAGE																									
	HIV/AIDS									●	●			●		●	●		●		●	●		●		

FEVERFEW	GARLIC	GINGER	GINKGO	GINSENG	GOAT'S RUE	GOLDEN SEAL	HAWTHORN	HOPS	HORSETAIL	HUANG QI	LADY'S MANTLE	LAVENDER	LEMON BALM	LICORICE	LINDEN BLOSSOM	MEADOWSWEET	MOTHERWORT	MYRRH	NETTLE	OAK BARK	PARTRIDGE BERRY	PASSIONFLOWER	PEPPERMINT	PLANTAIN	POKE ROOT	PULSATILLA	RASPBERRY LEAVES	ROSE	ROSEMARY	SAGE	SAW PALMETTO	SHATAVARI	SKULLCAP	SLIPPERY ELM	ST. JOHN'S WORT	THYME	VERVAIN	WILD OATS	WILD YAM	WITCH HAZEL	WOOD BETONY	WORMWOOD	YARROW	YELLOW DOCK

Glossary

acne vulgaris inflammation or infection of the sebaceous glands

adaptogenic helping to restore balance within the body

aerobic exercise exercise which raises the heart rate

after-pains pains occurring after childbirth due to contraction of the uterus

afterbirth the placenta and membranes expelled from the uterus after childbirth

allergen a substance which provokes an allergic response

alterative producing beneficial effects through detoxification and improving nutrition

amenorrhea lack of periods

amino acid one of the building blocks of protein

analgesic pain relieving

anodyne pain relieving

anorexia chronic failure to eat

antacid a substance which reduces stomach acid

anthelmintic destroying worms

anti-inflammatory reducing inflammation

antibacterial destroying the growth of bacteria

antibiotic destroying bacteria

antibody protein produced by the body to fight antigens

antifungal treating fungal infections

antigen a toxic substance stimulating production of antibodies

antihistamine neutralizing the effects of histamine in an allergic response

antilithic dissolving stones or gravel in the kidneys

antimicrobial destroying or stopping the growth or micro-organisms

antineoplastic having anti-cancer properties

antioxidant substance which reduces the damage done by free radicals

antipyretic reducing fever

antiseptic preventing putrefaction

antispasmodic preventing or relieving spasms or cramps

areola the dark ring around the nipple

astringent contracting tissue, reducing secretions or discharges

autonomic independent and spontaneous

benign harmless

bioflavonoid plant constituent aiding absorption of vitamin C

bitter increasing appetite and promoting digestion

Braxton-Hicks contraction a painless uterine contraction occurring after about 20 weeks of pregnancy

Caesarean section delivery of a baby through an incision in the abdomen and uterus

carcinogen a cancer-producing substance

cardiovascular relating to the heart and blood vessels

carminative easing cramping pains and expelling wind

Caucasian belonging to one of the light-skinned races

chemotherapy treatment of disease by chemicals directed against invading organisms or abnormal cells, especially cancer

chiropractor a therapist who manipulates the body, especially the spinal column

cholagogue increasing flow of bile into the intestines

colostrum a clear fluid, rich in antibodies, produced in the breasts before the milk

congenital existing from birth

constipation difficulty in passing stools

corpus luteum body developing in the ovary after the ovum is released, becoming glandular only if the ovum is fertilized

decoction a liquid made from woody parts of plants, and water

defecation the expulsion of solid waste from the bowels

demulcent soothing irritated tissues, especially mucous membranes

dermoid a cyst containing hair, skin or teeth, usually occurring in the ovary

diaphoretic promoting perspiration

dilation and curettage (D and C) an operation where the cervix is widened and the contents of the uterus scraped out

diuretic promoting the flow of urine

Doderlein's bacilli micro-organisms living in the vagina which maintain its acidity

douche to introduce liquid into the vagina by means of a sponge or tampon (never used in pregnancy)

ectopic pregnancy the implantation of an embryo outside the uterus, usually in the fallopian tubes, causing severe pain and miscarriage

emetic causing vomiting

emollient soothing and healing the skin

emmonagogue promoting menstrual flow (and to be avoided in pregnancy)

endometrium the lining of the uterus

endorphin a protein made in the pituitary gland and having pain-relieving properties

episiotomy incision of the perineum during childbirth

estrogenic resembling the actions of estrogen

expectorant promoting expulsion of mucus from the respiratory tract

febrifuge reducing fever

fecal matter waste expelled from the bowels

fetus the term used to describe a baby in the womb once the organs start to develop (before which it is an embryo)

free radicals shortlived unattached molecules which can damage body cells

galactagogue increasing milk flow

gestation the period from fertilization to childbirth

hemoglobin the red pigment in blood which carries oxygen

hemophilia a condition in which the blood fails to clot properly

HIV human immunodeficiency virus, the virus which causes AIDS

holistic an approach to therapy which considers the body, mind and spirit of the patient

homeopath a practitioner who treats illness with very tiny amounts of substances which would cause that illness in a healthy body, thus stimulating the patient's body to fight the illness itself

hypertension chronic high blood pressure often caused by stress

hypnotherapy a therapy which involves putting the patient into a mild trance state

hypoglycemia a condition where the blood sugar level falls too low

hysterectomy the removal of the uterus, or the uterus and ovaries

incontinence lack of control of urine flow

incubation period the time between initial infection with an invading organism and the display of symptoms

infusion herbal tea

iu international unit for drug measurement

IUD inter-uterine device; a contraceptive method where a small object is placed in the uterus to prevent implantation of a fertilized egg

laparoscopy an inspection of internal organs by means of a fine tube inserted through the wall of the abdomen

laxative promoting evacuation of the bowels

let-down reflex the stimulation of milk release by the hormone oxytocin, itself stimulated by a baby crying, sucking, or simply being near

libido drive or energy for pleasure, especially sexual pleasure

ligament fibrous tissue connecting bones or cartilages

lochia discharge from the vagina in the first two weeks after childbirth

lubricant a substance which reduces friction

luteinizing hormone (LH) a pituitary hormone stimulating the growth of the corpus luteum in the ovary

malignant potentially harmful

menarche the first menstrual period, and the time it occurs

menopause the last menstrual period, and the time it occurs

metabolism the chemical changes which take place in the body's cells, especially the release of energy

miscarriage loss of a fetus between the 12th and 28th week of pregnancy

nervine calming the nerves

organic describes food that has been produced to exacting standards without the use of artificial pesticides or fertilizers

osteopathy a therapy in which abnormalities in the human framework (bones, muscles, ligaments) are treated by skilled manual adjustment

ovulation the release of an ovum from the ovary

oxytocin pituitary hormone stimulating uterine contraction and the production of milk

palpitations abnormal heartbeat caused by exertion, agitation, or disease

pap smear test, cervical smear an examination of cells at the neck of the womb; they are removed painlessly by scraping with a spatula

parturient facilitating childbirth

partus preparator preparing for childbirth

perinatal relating to the time immediately before or after childbirth

perineum the tissue between the anus and vulva

pH a value indicating acidity (below pH 7) or alkalinity (above pH 7)

placenta the tissue connecting the fetus with the uterus

posseting regurgitation of undigested milk in babies

post-partum hemorrhage bleeding after childbirth

postnatal relating to the period after childbirth

poultice a soft, wet mass applied to the site of pain or injury

premenstrual relating to the days before a menstrual period

purgative producing vigorous emptying of the bowels

putrefactive causing to decay and rot

radiotherapy treatment of disease, usually cancer, with radiation

rubefacient gently irritant, producing redness of the skin

salicylates antiseptic and pain-relieving chemicals

sebaceous gland skin gland which produces oily sebum

sedative reducing nervousness and anxiety, inducing sleep

sitz-bath a hip-bath, in which one sits up to the waist in water

stillbirth the delivery of a dead fetus or baby

stomachic stimulating, strengthening or toning the stomach

stool the feces evacuated from the bowel

stypic stemming bleeding

tincture herbal extract preserved in alcohol

tonic invigorating, toning the body and promoting wellbeing

toxin poison

trace element mineral required by the body in very small amounts

vasodilator widening blood vessels, lowering blood pressure

venous blood blood in the veins, having had oxygen removed

vulnerary promoting wound healing

Where to Find Help

The American Herbalist Guild
PO Box 1683, Soquel, CA 95073

American Aromatherapy
Association
*Box 606, San Rafael
CA 94915*

American Herb Association
*Box 353, Rescue
California 96672*

American Herb Product
Association
*7353 El Tomaso Way
Buena Park, California 90620*

Herb Research Foundation
*1007 Pearl Street
Suite 200, Boulder, CO 80302*
303 449 2265

International Herb Growers and
Marketers Association
*Box 281, Silver Springs
PA 17575*

Northeast Herbal Association
*Box 146, Marshfield
VT 05658-0146*

Rocky Mountain Herbalist
Coalition
*Salsina Star Route, Boulder
CO 80302*

South-West Herbalist
Association
Box 74, Ojo Caliente NM 87549

Educational Programs

California Institute of Integral
Studies
Herbal Studies Program
*765 Ashbury, San Francisco
CA 94117*
Director: David Hoffmann

California School of Herbal
Studies
*P.O. Box 39, Forestville
CA 95476*

New Mexico Herbal Center
*122 Tulane SE, Albuquerque
NM 87106*
Director: Tieraona Klar

Rocky Mountain Center for
Botanical Studies
*1705 14th St. #287, Boulder CO
80302*
Director: Feather Jones

Southwest School of Botanical
Medicine
*122 Tulane SE, Albuquerque NM
87106*
Director: Michael Moore

Where to Find the Herbs

Frontier Cooperative Herbs *Box 299, Norway IA 52318*

Herb Pharm
347 East Fork Road, Williams, OR 97544
503 846 7178

Herbalist & Alchemist Inc.
PO Box 553, Broadway NJ 08808
908 689 9020

Herbs ETC
1340 Rufina Circle, Santa Fe NM 87501

McZand Herbal
PO Box 5312, Santa Monica CA 90405

Nature's Apothecary
997 Dixon Road, Boulder CO 80302
303 440 7422

Nature's Sunshine Products Inc.
PO Box 1000, Spanish Fork UT 84660

Nature's Way Products Inc.
10 Mountain Springs Parkway PO Box 2233, Springville UT 84663

Naturpharma, Inc. (Nature's Herbs)
1113N, Industrial Park Drive PO Box 336, Orem UT 84059

Planetary Formulas
PO Box 533, Soquel CA 95073

Rainbow Light Nutritional Systems
207 McPherson Street Santa Cruz, CA 95060

Starwest Botanicals Inc.
11253 Trade Center Drive Ranco Cordova CA 95742

Sunrider International
3111 Lomita Boulevard Torrance, CA 90505

Traditional Medicinals
4515 Ross Road, Sebastopol CA 95472

The Hay Diet

or food combining

This is a system of eating devised at the turn of the century by an American doctor, Dr. Hay. It is based on the premise that different kinds of foods require different mediums for their proper digestion, and so should not be mixed together in the same meal.

Starches should not be combined with either proteins or acid foods, and meals containing starches should be eaten at least four hours from meals with proteins or acid foods.

The Hay diet has been used successfully in the treatment of problems such as overweight, high blood pressure, digestive ailments, allergies, candida, chronic catarrh, and joint problems.

It is expounded very well in the book Food Combining for Health by Doris Grant and Jean Joice (Thorsons).

Further Reading

Conrow & Hecksel
HERBAL PATHFINDERS: VOICES OF
THE HERB RENAISSANCE
WOODBRIDGE PRESS, 1983

Duke, James A
HANDBOOK OF MEDICINAL HERBS
Boca Raton, FL:CRC Press, 1985

Foster, Steven
ECHINACEA, NATURE'S IMMUNE
ENHANCER
Healing Arts Press, Rochester,
1991

Fulder & Blackwood
GARLIC - NATURE'S ORIGINAL
REMEDY
Inner Traditions, Rochester, 1991

Gardner, Joy
HEALING YOURSELF DURING
PREGNANCY
Crossing Press, 1989

Graham, Judy
EVENING PRIMROSE OIL
Inner Traditions, Rochester, 1984

Grieve, M
A MODERN HERBAL, VOLUMES 1
AND 2
Dover Publications, New York,
1971

Hobbs, Christopher
FOUNDATIONS OF HEALTH: THE
LIVER AND DIGESTION HERBAL
Botanica Press, Capitola, 1992

Hoffmann, David
AN ELDER'S HERBAL
Inner Traditions, Rochester, 1992

Hoffmann, David
SUCCESSFUL STRESS CONTROL
Healing Arts Press, Rochester,
1986

Hoffmann, David
THE ELEMENTS OF HERBALISM
Element Books, Shaftesbury,
1990

Hoffmann, David
THE HERBAL HANDBOOK
Inner Traditions, Rochester, 1988

Hoffmann, David
THE NEW HOLISTIC HERBAL
Element Books, Shaftesbury,
1983

Hudson, Tori
GYNECOLOGY AND NATUROPATHIC
MEDICINE
TK Publications, Beaverton, 1992

Mabey, Richard
THE NEW AGE HERBALIST
Macmillan, New York, 1988

McIntyre, Anne
HERBS FOR MOTHER AND CHILD
Sheldon Press, London, 1988

McIntyre, Anne
THE HERBAL FOR PREGNANCY AND
CHILDBIRTH
Element Books, Shaftesbury,
1992

McIntyre, Michael
HERBAL MEDICINE FOR EVERYONE
Penguin, 1989

Mills, Simon
OUT OF THE EARTH: THE
ESSENTIAL BOOK OF HERBAL
MEDICINE
Viking, New York, 1992

Moore, Michael
MEDICINAL PLANTS OF THE
DESERT AND CANYON WEST
Museum of New Mexico Press,
1989

Moore, Michael
MEDICINAL PLANTS OF THE
MOUNTAIN WEST
Museum of New Mexico Press,
1979

Murray, Michael
THE HEALING POWER OF HERBS
Prima, Rocklin, 1991

Parvati, Jeannine
HYGIEIA, A WOMAN'S HERBAL
Freestone, Monroe, 1978

Potts, Billie
WITCHES HEAL
Du Reve, Ann Arbor, 1988

Riggs, Maribeth
NATURAL CHILD CARE
Harmony Books, New York,
1989

Theiss, Peter and Barbara
THE FAMILY HERBAL
Inner Traditions, Rochester, 1989

Tierra, Lesley
THE HERBS OF LIFE
Crossing Press, Freedom, 1992

Tierra, Michael
PLANETARY HERBALOGY
Lotus Press, 1988

Weed, Susun
HEALING WISE
Ash Tree Publishing

Weed, Susun
WISE WOMAN WAYS FOR THE
MENOPAUSAL YEARS
Ash Tree Publishing, 1992

Weed, Susun
WISE WOMAN HERBAL FOR THE
CHILDBEARING YEARS
Ash Tree Publishing, 1986

Index

Bold figures indicate herb profiles

Acknowledgements

Photographers
Cover and all other photographs by Philip Dowell, except for: p.15 Clive Boursnell, Garden Picture Library; pp.45, 49, 115, 153, 166 Camilla Jessel; p.101 Francis Leroy, Science Photo Library; p.2 Marie Read, Bruce Coleman Ltd; p.263 Ron Sutherland, Garden Picture Library (designed by Nula Haycock and Matthew Bell).

Artists
Richard Bonson pages 22-41 inclusive, and pages 56, 82, 105, 107, 108, 109, 125, 149, 150, 155, 173, 191, 201, 207, 213, 229, 242. **Sally Launder** pages 55, 57, 59, 60, 63, 64, 67. **Tony Lodge** pages 120, 121, 122, 133, 137, 141, 145, 192, 248/9, 255, 258, 260. **Bridget Morley** pages 81, 87, 93, 94, 117, 134, 161, 164/5.

The author wishes to thank Virginia Sandbach for typing the manuscript and giving moral support; Maureen Carter and Niky McIntyre whose help made writing the book possible; and Michael, Zaira and Zoe for their tolerance of her long working hours.

The publishers would like to thank Dr David Hoffmann and Dr. Helen Dziemidka for their helpful commentson the text, Mary Warren for the index, Gill Smith for photo research, Juliet Bailey and Charlie Ryrie for illustration research, and the members of the family who kindly allowed us to photograph them. And for their help, we would like to thank Focus Foods, Halesworth, Suffolk; Hawthorn Herbs and Wild Flowers; Salley Gardens, West Bridgford, Nottingham; Maggie and Alannah Lythgoe.

Note: The extract on p.200 is from *Everywoman's Book*, Paavo Airola, Health Plus Publishers, Phoenix, Arizona, 1979

*"This book's a treasure chest."**

Nutrition For Women: The Complete Guide

by Elizabeth Somer, M.A., R.D.

HOW EATING RIGHT CAN HELP YOU LOOK AND FEEL YOUR BEST

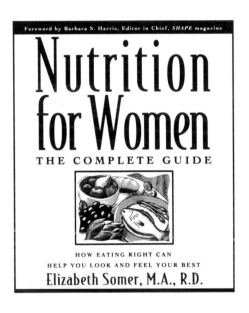

Includes:
- The "Healthy Woman's Diet"
- Nutrition and women's health issues
- Nutrition and specific life events
- Glossary of over 200 health, medical, and nutritional terms
- Over 100 tables, charts, and worksheets

isbn 0-8050-3563-X•$14.95•pb•496pp.
Available at all bookstores

*from the foreward by Barbara S. Harris,
Editor in Chief of *SHAPE* magazine

A Henry Holt Reference Book
Henry Holt and Company, Inc.
115 West 18th Street
New York, NY 10011